"As a Certified Natural Health Professional for more than eight years, I would be delighted if everyone would recognize these basic principles of the damage we do daily to our scalp and hair quality, and approach all other health concerns and "dis-ease" with the same principles of understanding.

The general public has little idea about how our lifestyles and environment damages our overall health and vitality, including what we put in ourselves, what we put on ourselves, and what air we breathe. "Our LONG HAIRitage" is a highly recommended gift of knowledge for anyone wanting to improve their quality and abundance of hair."

Char Revell Thompson, CHNP, Herbalist, Reiki Master

Our LONG HAIRitage

Bringing Peace and Health to Your Head

Roger Sigler

WestBow
PRESS
A DIVISION OF THOMAS NELSON

WestBow Press books may be ordered through booksellers or by contacting:

WestBow Press
A Division of Thomas Nelson
1663 Liberty Drive
Bloomington, IN 47403
www.westbowpress.com
1-(866) 928-1240

Because of the dynamic nature of the Internet, any web addresses or links contained in this book may have changed since publication and may no longer be valid. The views expressed in this work are solely those of the author and do not necessarily reflect the views of the publisher, and the publisher hereby disclaims any responsibility for them.

Any people depicted in stock imagery provided by Thinkstock are models, and such images are being used for illustrative purposes only.

Certain stock imagery © Thinkstock.

ISBN: 978-1-4497-1482-6 (sc)
ISBN: 978-1-4497-1483-3 (dj)
ISBN: 978-1-4497-1481-9 (e)

Library of Congress Control Number: 2011928525

Printed in the United States of America

WestBow Press rev. date: 5/26/2011

Table of Contents

Preface

||

Back in the Summer of 2003 I was ignorant about hair loss, thinking it to be a genetic issue like everyone else. But after seven years of research and writing, it is a relief to understand that most causes are manmade. I learned quickly how our scalps are abused by the pressures and products of modern society. The result is a book backed by hundreds of references. I cite from many sources, including science, holistic health, medical research, chiropractic care, preventative health, psychology, historical writings, Holy Scripture, biblical references, and other ancient texts. I wanted to be thorough. The benefit to the reader is a high-quality self-help book with plenty of information to make positive changes in their lives, the lives of others, and in this world. You will learn the secrets how to have a full head of hair for life. Baldness is not inevitable.

I express my deepest thanks to all those who helped me on this project. First, I thank my endorsers in various alternative/preventative care fields: Char Thompson, Dr. Mick Mahan, and Dr. John Parks Trowbridge. I appreciate their time reading and commenting on the manuscript. Preliminary versions of the book were reviewed by Scott Lowery, Peggi Merkey, Robert Piazza, and Ed Sherrill. Their comments and suggestions were particularly beneficial. Thanks to all those who gave permissions to use their photographs: Dr. John Bezzant, Dr. Jeffrey Melton, and Dr. Christoph Lehman for the cancer images; Mick Box of Uriah Heep (my favorite rock star); and my friends Amanda King, Cohl Brazil, Delisle Doherty, and Yohance Hunter. A variety of images included in this book are found in "The Secret Museum of Mankind" (Salt Lake City: Gibbs Smith Publisher, 1999). According to author David Stiffler, all images are in the public domain, and they are being used as such. Other public domain images were found in "The Bible and Its Story" (New York: Francis

R. Niglutsch, 1908) and elsewhere as indicated. Special thanks to them for their permission to use these vital images.

Finally, a special thank you is due to my family, my wife Selene, Katlin, and Zach. I appreciate their patience and endurance as I became quite zealous about this project.

Chapter 1: Hair We Go

ıllılıllıllıllıllıllıllıllıllıllıllıllıllıllıllıllıllıllıllıllıllıllıllıllıllıllıllıllıllıllıllıllıllıllıllıllıllıllıllıllıllıllıllıllıllıllıllıllıllıllıll

There is a way which seemeth right unto a man, but the end thereof are the ways of death (Proverbs 14:12).

I f you really want to prevent hair loss, heal the scalp, and even possibly re-grow lost hair, then you must read this book. You will learn many incredible things about the design, significance, symbolism, and purpose of human hair. Once you understand these purposes, and how hair is made, then you will learn how to properly care for the hair. Even more importantly, you will learn what you must do to prevent hair loss naturally, right now and in the future. The greatest myth ever is that baldness is inevitable.

My research on this subject began in the summer of 2003 when my wife, a hair stylist for twenty-five years, said, "There must be manmade causes of hair loss." At the time she uttered those words, she had no idea how right she was. Along with millions of others, I was led to believe that baldness was nothing more than a genetic issue. But this is just not true. I was already becoming quite aware of natural alternative health methods for many manmade ailments. With this knowledge and my background in science, I began my journey researching hair loss. I was surprised by what I found, because after months of study, I discovered that my wife's words are absolutely correct. In fact, I would now say that most causes of thinning hair and baldness are preventable and can be addressed when you know how. This book gives you the knowledge to take action and deal with the manmade causes of hair loss.

Trichology is the study of hair. When one considers the statistics, hair loss appears to be much more prevalent since the advent of the twentieth century than in times past. *The London Centre of Trichology* puts it this way: "The statistics with younger men losing their hair, and at a much quicker rate are high." They state that three out of ten men thirty years of age already are becoming quite bald.[1] Some poor souls even begin balding as teenagers or young men in their early twenties. Generally, by age fifty, about 50 percent of modern men are mostly bald. In the United States alone, this means that somewhere from 40 million to 50 million men between the ages of twenty and sixty-four will have balding problems. One in five, or 20 million to 25 million, females will also have thinning hair problems. In 1998, Dr. Morton Walker found that balding women believe they "look freakish." He also related "contrary to popular myth," more than half of all balding men are also affected psychologically.[2]

Trichologists are hair and scalp specialists who approach hair loss in a holistic way. Dr. David Kingsley, a trichologist in New York, was himself affected psychologically by hair loss. Much of his research studied this very fact. He states that several men and women said "they had seen other hair-loss specialists who showed no empathy for their condition."[3] The truth is about 25 percent of bald men would trade five years of life for a full head of hair![4] What about the appearance of bald men? Have we become so accustomed to seeing male pattern baldness (MPB) that we think it to be normal?

With an unprecedented amount of global baldness, Rachel Bergsman, author of "The Disaster of Hair Loss: Take It Easy," clearly recognizes this truth: the "problem is that the more we care about our hair, the less hairs we appear to have on our head."[5] She is correct. Many of the problems associated with hair loss are generated by the hair-care industry, such as dyes, relaxers, other chemicals, and excessive cutting. In America's cities, there is quite literally a hair salon or barber on just about every block and around every corner. Does this not seem to be a little too much care? Bear in mind too that commercial advertisers and marketers do not care about you. They need to sell products to earn money. Ask yourself, do I really need all those products to look good?

But should we just blame the hair care industry for our demise? Hair care is big business, but it certainly is not the only problem in modern

1 "Male Hair Loss Prevention Diagnosis, Women's Hair Loss Treatment—Trichology Consultants." Accessed April 15, 2006, http://www.london-centre-trichology.co.uk/male-hair-loss.asp.

2 Morton Walker, Bald No More (New York: Kensington Publishing Corporation, 1998), 44–45.

3 David H. Kingsley, The Hair-Loss Cure, A Self-Help Guide, (Bloomington, IN: iUniverse, 2009), xii.

4 Walker, Bald No More, 42.

5 Rachel Bergsman, "The Disaster Of Hair Loss: Take It Easy," accessed June 19, 2010, http://www.articlesphere.com/Article/The-Disaster-Of-Hair-Loss--Take-It-Easy/27570.

culture contributing to baldness. The social pressures of super-short hair on men in modern society are particularly disastrous to the scalp.

The history of hair and hair loss is a very amazing, illustrative, and instructive part of this book. Indeed, there is a correlation with baldness in history when super-short hair was worn. The origins of excessive cutting are presented as proof. Currently, the American military, private schools, some public schools, the Christian education system, and certain corporations have all promoted unnaturally short hair. By their example, this leadership has not only led us to baldness, but they have also caused other skin diseases, including the most harmful and mutilating of all, cancer, including deadly melanoma. When it comes to hair, most men follow each other like sheep and thereby have become addicted to scissors and razors, as if hair serves no purpose. Many even in the medical and hair-loss industry treat their own hair as if it is a waste product, by evidence of their close-cropped heads. This is why these so-called professionals show no compassion for your hair - they do not even care about their own. The few courageous souls who ward off this modern abusive society are often called unprofessional, rebels, or sinners. Personally, I think it is better to be a so-called rebel than have a weathered head prone to warts and cancers.

Despite what these people and organizations teach by example, hair is not a waste product, and long hair is no crime. The real Creator is for long hair. In fact, God-given, long, majestic, beautiful hair is exactly what the scalp is designed to produce, and for good reasons. The great irony is that longer hair is much healthier, physically and spiritually. Even most trichologists have not been trained to recognize this essential fact.

Our ancestors realized it, though; they had healthy heads of long hair as the Creator intended. It is written in Scripture and in the genetic code. The long hair ways of Jesus and the Nazarites, and the ancient Hebrews, Assyrians, Babylonians, Spartans, Native Americans, the founding fathers of the United States, and a host of others all demonstrate this fact. Paintings, sculptures, and photographs of men prior to the twentieth century show that when they wore long hair (or at least shoulder-length hair) when young, they retained a full head of hair when old with little to no receding hairline. The fight against hair loss will never be won until society recognizes the dismal results of close-cropped hair and the importance of long hair to strengthen the scalp and protect the head. Longer hair prevents hair loss and other disease. If you want to prevent hair loss and skin cancer or have always liked long hair and need support or have been persecuted for long hair, then this book is for you.

Besides haircut madness, other twentieth-century ideas never experienced in prior times entered the scene. Enormously large, stress-ridden cities arose; most people live in these polluted areas. Stress causes hair loss. Chemical-laden shampoos and other hair care products were invented and hit the market. The development of artificial foods and spraying of natural crops with poisons occurs on a regular basis. And what should we think about fast food? All these things were introduced in the twentieth century as well, and they all contribute to hair loss. This book addresses the nutritional and other internal aspects of hair loss as well as the external acts upon the skin's surface.

With all this hair loss, sadly, not even one out of five balding men and women seek help. Apparently, they believe that little can be done or it must be too expensive. In other words, they believe the great myth: that baldness is nothing but a genetic issue. More often than not, those who do seek help tend to seek the heavily advertised expensive choices: drugs, surgery, wigs, or toupees. People have been systematically taught that these are their only choices even though all these methods are unnatural. So first we are taught to constantly cut the hair and use chemicals on our heads, which eventually withers hair follicles, leading to hair loss. Then we are told the only way to fix the problem is with more unnatural methods. Thus, the modern hair-care industry makes money, coming and going, at your expense. The simple truth is that your scalp is damaged and must be healed.

What about drugs, surgery, wigs, or toupees? Is this what you really want to do? Why spend hundreds or even thousands of dollars for these things if you do not have to? Before going to these extremes, get the facts and do the things suggested in this book. Surgery should always be the last resort. Prevention of hair loss is a key theme because prevention is far better and easier than re-growing hair. But there is hope. Based on powerful testimonies, if you have been thinning or balding for fifteen years or less, then it is possible to heal the scalp and grow your own hair back within two years. Backed by either clinical research or testimonials, high-quality products to help rejuvenate your scalp are discussed. The main requirement is patience while you heal the scalp over this time period.

The book is somewhat detailed but written in easy-to-understand terms. It is advisable to read it thoroughly from the beginning to the end. In this way, you can absorb all the facts. There are important things you need to understand about this remarkable creation called hair. During research, related issues were uncovered. Chief among them is the issue of skin cancer of the head, ears, and neck, and how to prevent this naturally. Like a forest, long hair provides cover and shade. Learn how sunscreens are no substitute for hair, for it turns out that certain dangerous chemicals within them actually increase skin cancer risk. Read on and be enlightened. Then take simple steps now to stop your hair loss, heal your scalp, prevent skin cancer, and even re-grow your hair.

Chapter 2: Physical Characteristics of Hair

||||||||||||||||||||||||||||||||||||||||||||||||||||||||||||||||||||||||||||||||||||||||||||||||||||||||||||||||||||||||||||||||||||||||||||||||||||||

And God saw every thing that he had made, and behold, it was
very good (Genesis 1:31, KJV)

Many modern men treat their head hair as an insignificant waste
product. This is evidenced by excessive cutting and shaving. The
implied statement is that hair serves little to no purpose. This means that
male hair is not "very good," in spite of the Creator saying "everything"
He made is indeed "very good." In fact, what good is it to say that the
human body is the temple of God (1 Corinthians 3:16-17; 6:19) if the hair
is to be destroyed?

Today, most people simply conform to the styles of the times without
any regard to the consequences to the scalp. While males are taught to just
cut it off, females are taught that they need several hair products to make
their hair look good. But these acts of continual interference are primary
causes of thinning hair. Sadly, a great majority of health care professionals
of all backgrounds are clueless. Even most of those who preach preventative
health are just as unaware. This is because the focus has been on inner
health only, such as inspiration, nutrition, exercise, stress management, and
peace with God. Yes, all these things are vital for ultimate health. However,
the skin is the only organ of the body directly affected from stresses placed
on it, not only from inside the body, but from the outside as well. It is the
skin where the hair is made. What happens or does not happen on and in
the skin of the scalp is vital for hair growth. As you will learn, a true body
by God includes scalp health.

The physical characteristics of hair, how it is made, its incredible
growth rates and lengths all show the Creator's handiwork. This
remarkable creation called hair is defined in a variety of ways. Physically
speaking, hair is a cylinder of cells comprising three major structures:

(1) the outside layer, the cuticle; (2) the middle layer, the cortex; and (3) the central medulla.[6] Hair is a specialized form of skin[7]. It is made in the hair follicle beneath the skin surface within a layer of the skin called the dermis (Figure 2-1).

The cuticle of the hair (outer visible layer) is covered by a multitude of fine, scale-like markings along the hair shaft. They represent the attachment of the root sheath during growth in the hair follicle. According to Walker, these markings are "highly characteristic of the individual," and are utilized in identification.[8] Hair is part of your natural identity. The forensic science laboratory of the Federal Bureau of Investigation (FBI) often analyzes hair under a microscope. In this manner they can identify individuals and animals by these unique markings on hair (Figures 2-2, 2-3). People are unique from each other, and human hair is different than animal hair.[9]

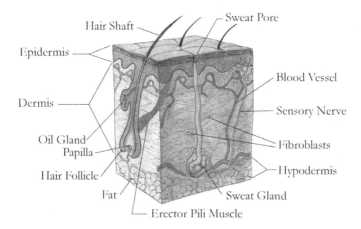

*Figure 2-1: Cross-Section of the Skin**. Modified Skin Cross-Section. Courtesy of National Institute of General Medical Sciences (NIGMS), National Institutes of Health, U.S. Department of Health and Human Services with modifications showing the *erector pili* (some spell *arrector pili*) muscle from the skin cross section by Patrice Hyde, M. D. @ http://kidshealth.org/kid/body/skin_noSW.html (September 11, 2005).

6   Morton Walker, Bald No More, (New York: Kensington Publishing Corporation, 1998), 66-67.
7   Loren Pickart, Reverse Skin Aging: Using Your Skin's Natural Power, (Bellevue, Washington: Cape San Juan Press, 2005), 112.
8   Walker, Bald No More, 66.
9   Douglas W. Deedrick and Sandra L. Koch, "Microscopy of Hair Part 1: A Practical Guide and Manual for Human Hairs," Forensic Science Communications, January 2004, vol. 6, no. 1, accessed May 8, 2009, http://www.fbi.gov/hq/lab/fsc/backissu/jan2004/research/2004_01_research01b.htm

In fact, hair is so different that Walker declares "human hair is not vestigial."[10] This means that human hair is not a purposeless, worthless leftover from some supposed animal ancestry. In fact, there is no evidence for the evolution of hair. However, belief in the origins of hair may determine a person's outlook on it.[11] Jerry Bergman explains that if a person believes he came from ape-like ancestors, then he may consider hair to be a worthless, useless evolutionary leftover. This abysmal negative attitude towards hair is most unfortunate. Indeed, human hair is unique as Bergman and others recognize, and it serves many purposes as you will soon learn. You are not an animal. Since the beginning of creation, mankind has always been mankind. Information within the body's DNA produces the right type of hair, which is extruded at the proper places on the human body. In reality, hair forms part of your identity and was created for special purposes discussed throughout this book. And since everything God made is very good, it must not be maltreated and wasted, a common practice of modern man by training.

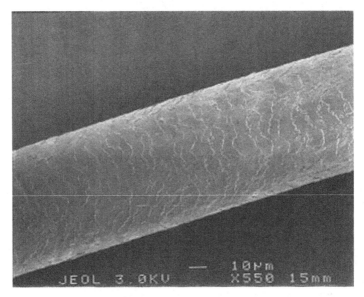

Figure 2-2: Normal Human Scalp Hair Magnified 550 Times. Note the scaly structure of the outermost layer of the hair shaft called the cuticle. Image from Deedrick and Koch, Forensic Science Communications, January 2004, vol. 6, no. 1 (FBI).

---

10   Walker, Bald No More, 57.
11   Jerry Bergman, "Why Mammal Body Hair is an Evolutionary Enigma," Creation Research Society Quarterly, v. 40, March 2004, 240-243.

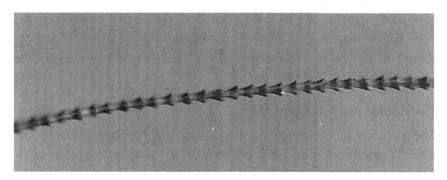

Figure 2-3: Bat Hair under the Microscope. Animal hair is different than human hair. This helps the Federal Bureau of Investigation (FBI) determine who was at a crime scene, including what types of animals. Image from Deedrick and Koch, Forensic Science Communications, January 2004, vol. 6, no. 1 (FBI).

Defining Hair

Standard definitions from the hair care industry are used herein. In his book "Human Hair," Vlado Valcović informs us that two basic types of hair occur in man: vellus hairs: the very tiny (almost invisible) hairs that help make skin feel silky and terminal hair, the obvious, visible hair.[12]

More specifically, vellus hairs are the short, very fine, silky and usually unpigmented hairs found on the seemingly hairless areas of the body, such as the forehead, nose, eyelids, and bald scalp. Terminal hairs are the thick, visible, pigmented hairs found on the scalp, beard, armpits, and pubic area.

Hair is also described when speaking about the portion above the skin surface and the place where the hair is made beneath the skin surface. The visible part of the hair seen above the skin surface is called the hair shaft, and the hair follicle is the place beneath the skin surface where the hair is manufactured, the root. Health and vitality of the hair follicles are extremely important with regards to the battle against hair loss.

Density of Hairs

The density of hair is defined as the number of hairs per unit area. Density is generally described as providing thick, medium, or thin coverage. When a person is described as having thick hair, this means there are many hairs per unit area, such that the scalp cannot be seen (remains adequately

---

12   Vlado Valković, Human Hair. Vol. 1: Fundamentals and Methods for Measurement of Elemental Composition (Boca Raton, Florida: CRC Press, Inc., 1988).

concealed) whether the hair is wet or dry. Thin hair represents sparse coverage so that the scalp can be seen through the hair. Generally, most people appear to have medium dense hair, which is neither thick nor thin, yet adequately covers the scalp.

Coarseness or Fineness of Hair

The diameter or circumference of the hair shaft is described as being coarse, medium, or fine. Coarse hair has the largest circumference and can feel heavy and rough. Fine hair has the smallest circumference and can feel very soft and silky, like feathers. It generally has a much thinner cortex than other hair textures and generally does not contain the inner medulla. Individuals with fine hair are more susceptible to hair loss. The most common type of texture is also called medium hair (not to be confused with density of follicles) and typically has lots of body and bounce.

Another interesting fact is that human body hairs differ among themselves and differ from head hair.[13] Head hair has a relatively small root and a tapered tip. Beard and moustache hair has an irregular structure, blunter tip, and larger root than head hair. Most body hairs are fine, but auxiliary hair (also called underarm or armpit hair) and pubic hair are coarse.

Every type of hair on the human body serves distinct purposes. Underarm hairs are usually (but not always) straighter than pubic hair. This straightness no doubt causes the hairs to roll as the arm swings. Apparently, one main purpose of underarm hair is to keep the skin itself from rubbing. Information in the genetic code tells the body what type of hair to produce at the proper location on your body. Hair growth rates and maximum hair length of each type of hair is predetermined genetically by the Creator's will.

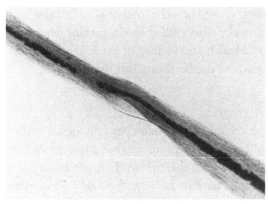

Figure 2-4: Microscopic View of Pubic Hair. Note the difference between this hair and scalp hair. Pubic hair is coarse, wiry, irregular, and asymmetrical in cross-section with many constrictions, twists and usually curved. Image from Deedrick and Koch, Forensic Science Communications, January 2004, vol. 6, no. 1 (FBI).

---

13   Valković.

Hair Length and Growth Rates

Obviously, terminal hairs are of utmost import to people, especially scalp hair, since this is the hair that can be seen. Hair growth rates and lengths of terminal hair depend upon hair type or location on the body (Table 2-1).

Table 2-1: Human Hair Length and Hair Growth Rates [14]

Hair Type or Location	Average Growth Rate	Average Length	Comments
Scalp	0.52 inches/ month (males); 0.53 inches/month (females)	Up to 1.5 m or 5 feet (normal range 4 inches to > 3 feet)	Scalp hair grows the fastest and longest of all human hair.
Beard and Moustache	0.32 inches/month (0.27 mm/day)	~2 to 8 inches (50 to 300 mm)	Beards grow slower and not as long as scalp hair.
Eyebrows	0.19 inches/month (0.16 mm/day)	7 to 16 mm (average is about 1 cm)	Full Growth in 30 days
Upper Eyelashes		8 to 12 mm	Full Growth in 30 days
Lower Eyelashes		6 to 8 mm	Full Growth in 30 days
Body Hair (chest; abdomen)	0.47 inches/month (0.40 mm/day)	0.12 to 2.36 inches (3 to 60 mm)	Body hair grows slower and is programmed to stay much shorter than scalp hair.
Limbs	~0.25 inches/month (0.20 mm/day)	0.12 to 2.36 inches (3 to 60 mm)	Programmed to stay much shorter than head hair.
Pubic Hair		0.4 to 2.36 inches (10 to 60 mm)	Programmed to stay much shorter than head hair. Usually curling.
Auxiliary (Armpit) Hair	0.35 inches/month (0.30 mm/day)	0.4 to 2.0 inches (10 to 50 mm)	These hairs are usually straighter than pubic hair and are programmed to stay short. Female's underarm hair is shorter than male's.

---

14 Based on data compiled (and edited) from Tables 1, 3, and 4 from Valković, Human Hair, 4-7.

Considerable variation of hair color, style, average growth rates, and average overall lengths are determined genetically per individual. To determine average growth rates, the number, size, and ethnicity of the study group is not known. For example, the scalp hair growth rate seems below the average reported by many hair stylists. Hair stylists generally believe the average growth rate of scalp hair is about 0.75 inches/month (0.64 mm/day), with no discernable difference between males and females. In fact, some males can grow hair longer and faster than some females. Interestingly, when a person is exposed to excessive heat in the summer or cold in the winter hair is "apt to grow more luxuriantly."[15] Hair grows faster during the summer than winter for both sexes.[16] This is evidence that one primary purpose of head hair is protection.

Although Valković's growth rates are slower, he does demonstrate that the scalp growth rate between males (0.52 inches/month) and females (0.53 inches/month) is practically none. If these growth rates are reasonably accurate, then after one year a woman's hair would be a mere 0.12 inches (1/8") longer than a man's. At these same rates and after four years (the average lifespan of a single hair - see below), the female's hair would be only one half inch longer than the male's, assuming that no cutting has taken place. According to Pickart[17], the average maximum length of head hair is 70 cm or about 2.3 feet if allowed to grow to maturity.

Valković also notes that beard and other body hairs do not attain full growth until middle age.[18] The original intent of this design was to be an important distinction between a young man and an older man. But his beard growth rate also appears on the slow side. For comparison sake, I measured my own hairs or hair growth. The results: beard growth rate is about 0.67 inches (5/8") per month; scalp hair exceeds 0.75 (3/4") inches per month; and some pubic hairs exceed lengths greater than three inches. The point here is that each and every person is unique; there are differences in physiology for each individual. Therefore, the growth rates and various hair lengths in Table 2-1 express only generalized truths. Again, individual growth rates and overall length for each person is written in the genetic code.

---

15   Charles T. Jackson and Charles Wood McMurtry. A Treatise on Diseases of the Hair (London: Henry Kimpton, 1913), 48.
16   Maggie Hira, "Does Hair Grow Faster in the Summer?" accessed June 20, 2010, http://www.ehow.com/how-does_4570190_does-hair-grow-faster-summer.html.
17   Pickart, Reverse Skin Aging: Using Your Skin's Natural Power, 113.
18   Valković, 5.

The aforementioned facts make it difficult to define hair in terms of length. A certain length may be called *long* hair on one person, but this same length may be called *short* on another. So we must appeal to nature itself for an answer. The first and foremost rule of science is simple observation. In this manner, Valcović has shown that the average growth rate of females is only slightly faster than the average growth rate of males: 0.53 inches/month for females vs. 0.52 inches/month for males. At birth the average hair length of males is about 2.4 cm (just under one inch) and females about 2.6 cm (a little more than one inch).[19] The difference is very slight, about 8 percent longer for females, in general. Obviously, some males are known to have longer hair than some females at birth. Nevertheless, based on Valcović's data it can be surmised that females are designed to have a slightly faster growth rate and are able to obtain a slightly longer length. But it should be kept in mind that this is the "average" reported by Valcović's scientific measurements.

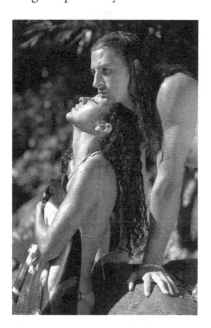

Figure 2-5: Couple with Similar Hair Length. This woman's hair is a little longer than the man's. If her hair was less curly, straighter like his hair, then it would extend a few more inches down her back. The observational evidence matches the scientific data showing that females are designed to grow hair just a little longer than males on average. However, there is little doubt that if this woman let hair her grow to maturity it would certainly reach down the full length of the back.

It is well known that females can grow hair to their mid-back or waistline, even lower in some cases. Simple observation illustrates that many males can also grow hair this long. Thus, hair to the mid-back or waistline is indeed in the realm of long hair. But what of the man who grows shoulder length hair? When compared to the man with waist-length

19   Valković, 6.

hair, hair to the shoulders would now be considered short or perhaps medium length at best. What is called long, medium and short hair for females seems to be practically the same for males. In terms of length, there is not much difference scientifically between the sexes (Figures 2-5; 2-6). The modern idea that a man's hair is *long* when worn over his ears or shirt collar is scientifically untenable. This erroneous idea may originate from modern western military standards.

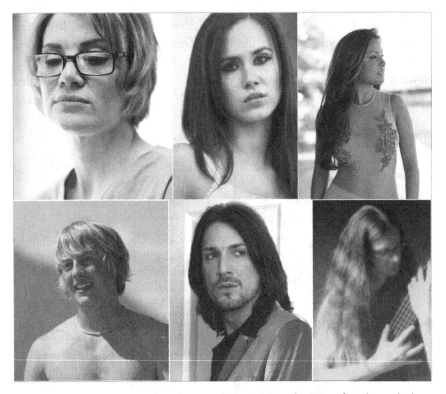

Figure 2-6: Comparison of Male/Female Hair Length. : Top: females with short hair (left), medium or shoulder-length hair (center), and long hair (right). Bottom: males with short hair (left), medium or shoulder-length hair (center), and long hair (right). This demonstrates that hair length has little to nothing to do with distinction between the sexes. The real distinctions are plain: shape or form of the body overall, facial hair (males), and softer, more rounded features for the female face.

Wig makers have helped define long hair. Sometimes people will donate their hair to charities such as Wigs for Kids and Locks of Love. Both organizations help children cope with their hair loss during cancer treatment. Locks of Love requires hair to be ten inches long (or greater) otherwise it is not long enough. Wigs for Kids prefers a minimum length of ten to twelve inches. Based on the work of these wig makers, long hair can be defined as lengths greater than ten inches.

This still seems on the short side, especially since the average maximum length hair can grow is about 28 inches (2.3 feet). A ten-inch hair compared to a three-inch hair would be considered long, but a ten-inch hair compared to a 28-inch hair would be short. So when it comes to head hair, length becomes a relative, arbitrary measure. If we truly wanted to define hair in terms of short, medium, and long then this must be done scientifically. The average maximum length of 28 inches can be divided into three equal parts. Based on scientific measurement, one could argue that head hair less than ten inches is short, from ten inches to less than 20 inches would be medium length, and 20 inches or greater would be long hair. Whoever thinks hair is long if worn over the ears or shirt collar is not basing this determination upon logic, reason, or scientific measurement. Why, hairs merely two to three inches in length can cover the ear and collar! These lengths of two to three inches are comparable to the length of armpit hair and pubic hair, which is genetically programmed to stay this short (Table 2-1). Must a man cut his head hair even shorter than his own body hair?

The Hair Cycle

On average, there are about 100,000 to 150,000 hair follicles on the head. Each of these hair follicles passes through a "hair cycle." The hair cycle can be divided into three phases: (1) growth (anagen); (2) rest (catagen); (3) shedding or hair loss (telogen). Each hair goes through a two to seven year growth phase: the average is four years of growth followed by an approximate three-month resting/hair loss phase prior to shedding.[20] About 90 percent are in growth phase and 10 percent in the resting phase at any given time. A person naturally sheds between 30 and 100 hairs per day, but this varies on an individual basis.[21]

In one experiment, one man and one woman started off with hair of the same length and went without a haircut for eighteen months (Figure 2-7).[22] Several things are evident in this experiment. The first thing we observe is very robust hair. It looks very healthy and full-bodied in both individuals.

---

20 Valković, 6, 9.
21 D.M. Podolsky, Skin: the human fabric. (The Human Body), (Tarrytown, New York: Torstar Books, Inc., 1984), 87.
22 A. Rook, and R. Dawber, Diseases of the Hair and Scalp, 2nd Ed., (Oxford: Blackwell Scientific Publications, 1991).

Secondly, in the case of these two people, her hair is longer than his. This means either her growth rate or growth phase (anagen period) is greater than his. Or perhaps his hair is designed to be shoulder length before it sheds. It would be helpful to see this experiment repeated over a four-year period, the average growth phase of hair. In this way we could have learned what the maximum hair length each could have achieved.

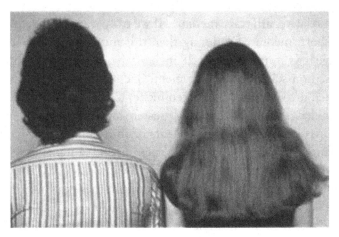

Figure 2-7: The 18-Month Hair Growth Experiment. Genetically, differences in hair length depend on growth rate, growth phase (the length of anagen), and maximum length by design.

Scalp hair is designed to grow long and grow fast (Table 2-1). Healthy scalp hair grows rapidly – about half an inch to more than one inch per month, or an average of about 0.75 of an inch per month. During the resting phase, the follicle stops making hair and the base moves upwards towards the skin surface to be shed. The old hair is removed as a new one begins to grow beneath. The new hair emerges from the same follicle and small tunnel-like opening, unless the skin and follicle become damaged.

The other interesting thing about hair is its fascinating design (Figure 2-1). The hair is made in the hair follicle. The hair grows and is then oiled (note the position of the oil gland). This oil called sebum covers the hair and scalp for its protection. The skin's design, aided by the oil glands, makes the skin nearly waterproof, "neither absorbing nor letting out moisture, except at the sweat pores."[23] Body oil protects the skin and hair from damage and infection. Thus, sebum is a form of anointing oil that God Himself made

---

23 Truman J. Moon, Biology for Beginners, (New York: Holt, Rinehart and Winston, Publishers, 1981), 405.

for your benefit. If long enough, the hair acts like a brush to anoint the neck, ears, forehead and cheeks. The oil spreads to cover the face. Overall, this system is designed to protect you from weathering and preserve your youthful appearance. Harsh detergents strip this oil away.

The Chemistry of Hair

Hair cells are called keratinized cells because the main constituent of hair is the protein keratin. It is the same protein that makes up feathers, claws, nails and hoofs. Hair is comprised of about 15 percent keratin. Like other proteins, keratin has very large molecules made up of smaller units called amino acids (arginine, histidine, and lysine) joined together in chains like beads on a string. This remarkable protein, keratin, is why hair is very resistant to wear and tear caused by the wind, sun, and other weathering effects.

Hair also contains fats, pigment (melanin), small amounts of vitamins, and traces of zinc and other metals. Hair also contains 10 to 13 percent water, which is extremely important for its physical and chemical properties. Water swells hair fiber considerably "as demonstrated by the thickening of the fiber diameter with increasing relative humidity."[24]

Scientifically, male hair is found to be different than female hair. In one study more than 2,000 hair samples were analyzed to determine the characteristics of male and female hair. "In general, hair level values of calcium, magnesium, manganese, potassium, copper, sodium, and zinc for female subjects, for all ages studied, tend to be higher than the corresponding values for male subjects ...."[25] Differences are very slight except female hair has two to four times more calcium and magnesium. The differences in composition may explain why female hair looks different than male hair, even when men wear longer hair. Apparently, men are designed with manly hair and females are designed with feminine hair.

The Strength of Hair

The strength of hair can be demonstrated in two ways: the strength of hair itself and its anchoring strength. The *anchoring strength* is the maximum amount of force, by pulling, that a single hair can take prior to plucking. The anchoring

---

24 Valković, 23.
25 D.J. Eatough, J.J. Christensen, R.M. Izatt, and C. Hartley, Level of Selected Trace Elements in Human Hair. The First Human Hair Symposium. Ed. Algie C. Brown. (New York: Medcom Press, 1974).

strength of chest hairs is a little more than 0.15 pounds per single hair.[26] This is the anchoring strength of chest hairs in the growing phase (anagen). This is probably close to the anchoring strength of scalp hairs. Thus, 100,000 hairs on your head, while still anchored, can hang an unbelievable amount of weight: 0.15 pounds/hair x 100,000 hairs = 15,000 pounds.

Hair is built to last. In some situations it is even better preserved than bones: "Structural features of hair can remain intact for thousands of years."[27] Wet hair can be stretched 1.33 times its original length.[28] This is a measure of its elasticity or tensile strength. According to the article *Hair Strength*, the hair shaft has approximately the same strength as copper wire of the same diameter.[29] Walker informs us that hair by itself is even slightly stronger than its anchoring strength. He says a single dry hair can support a weight of 100g or 0.2 pounds. Therefore, if the 100,000 hairs of the head are cut off and intertwined like a rope, they can collectively support 20,000 pounds, or ten tons, without breaking. This assumes of course that all hairs are in perfect, unweathered condition, which is never the case. To be conservative, even if just half of them are, this is still an incredible 10,000 pounds that can be hung by the hairs of the head. Was hair designed with such resilience, strength, and other weather resistant properties so that it could just be cut off continually and wasted?

Natural Hair

Natural hair is the hair that has been especially designed for you. In terms of head hair, this design includes color, straightness or curliness, coarseness, texture, density, and a mature length. Unaltered natural hair is sometimes called virgin hair by modern hairstylists. What is natural for one is not natural for another. Some have black tightly spiraled or coiled hair, while others have blonde straight hair, brown wavy hair, auburn straight hair, black curly hair, blonde curly hair, and many other combinations. In terms of length, this too is by design. Depending upon your own genetic code, some are able to grow longer hair than others. Longer hair is what the scalp is designed to produce. Again, length per person is determined genetically.

26 D.M. Chapman, "The anchoring strengths of various chest hair root types," Clin Exp Dermatol. 1992 Nov;17(6):421-3. PMID: 1486708, accessed August 31, 2005, http://www.ncbi.nlm.nih.gov/entrez/query.fcgi?CMD=Display&DB=pubmed.
27 Jerry Bergman, 241.
28 Morton Walker, How to Stop Baldness and Regrow Hair, (Stamford, CT: Freelance Communications, 1995), 21.
29 "Hair Strength," accessed October 26, 2004, http://www.keratin.com/aa/aa016.shtml.

Some, such as Sikhs, Rastafarians and Native Americans, would argue that uncut hair is natural. In this view, cutting the hair is not leaving the hair in its natural condition. On the other hand, trimming the hair does not cause pain, so can hair still be called natural if cut? This is a good question not so easily answered. For example, fingernails and toenails are also specialized outgrowths of the skin. What if these were never trimmed, if all cutting is unnatural? To answer this question we need to understand the similarities and differences between nails and hair. According to Loren Pickart, author of "Fingernail and Toenail Health for Stronger, Harder, Better-Looking Nails," the structure and growth of nails is similar to hair. But while nails are similar to hair, nails do not have a cycle of growth, non-growth, and shedding like hair does. In fact, "Nails grow continuously throughout your life," and never shed.[30] This is a big difference. Besides, nails and hair serve different purposes entirely. For example, the reason fingernails grow continuously is that they are the most basic natural hand tools. Like all tools, fingernails wear out with use. Thus they grow throughout life to fulfill basic needs. Thus, they must be kept trimmed and filed at a length needed to fulfill their job (e.g., peel fruit; pick a guitar; scratch; scrape). The situation with hair is arguably opposite.

As we have learned, each hair has a maximum length and time period that it will grow. After this, the hair falls out and new one emerges to grow in its place. For this reason, hair does not have to be trimmed in most cases. The possible exceptions to this might be those with locked hair (to be discussed shortly) and those with a missing growth factor in their genes.[31] The later apparently causes the individual to grow hair past the knees and to the floor or beyond. But for most people, the maximum length (usually between the shoulders and the coccyx) and shedding process of head hair is already in place via the DNA program of their body. Thus, for most, head hair does not need to be trimmed, naturally speaking of course. On the other hand, if split ends develop, then it may be better trim the ends just above the split before the situation worsens.

Visible differences in hair types of people are readily observable. Under the microscope the reasons why there are so many different types of natural hair become quite apparent. Most scientists classify hair into three broad categories: (1) Caucasoid, typical of those with fair skin; (2) Mongoloid, typical of Asians; and (3) Negroid, typical of those of African origins.

---

30 Loren Pickart, "Fingernail and Toenail Health for Stronger, Harder, Better-Looking Nails," accessed September 2, 2006, http://www.skinbiology.com/fingerandtoenails. html#Nail%20Biology.

31 Walker, Bald No More, 49.

Roger Sigler

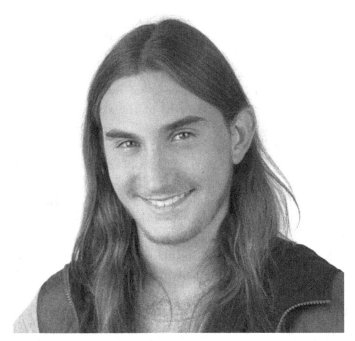

Figure 2-8: Young Man with Long, Straight, Natural Hair. His personal genetic code determines the straightness, coarseness, texture, maximum length, and color. Note also the small amount of facial hair typical for a young man. The beard does not attain its full length and thickness until middle age.

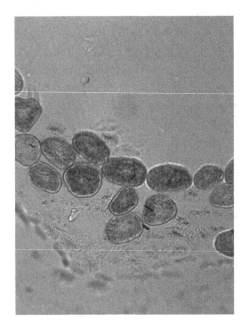

Figure 2-9: Microscopic Cross-Section of Caucasian Hair. Note the great variety of roundness. Some hairs are round, some are more elliptical. The rounder the hair shaft, the straighter the hair. Overall, this pattern will cause the hair to be slightly wavy rather than perfectly straight. Much oriental hair and Native American hair is rounder than this causing their hair to be very straight. Image from Deedrick and Koch, Forensic Science Communications, January 2004, vol. 6, no. 1 (FBI).

Caucasians have subrounded to elliptical hair follicles (Figure 2-9). The more rounded the follicle is, the straighter the hair will be (Figure 2-8). Asians and Native Americans generally have very round follicles in cross section. Therefore, they have very straight hair, straighter than Caucasians. It pleased the Creator to make a great variety of hair types. This is because from the standpoint of God's creativity, He does not want us all to look the same. It would be quite boring if we did. These should be obvious truths. The plea in the book "Dreads" is, "you don't have to have straight hair to be beautiful."[32] Ademole Mandella concurs and says quite correctly, "God made only good hair."[33] So why not wear your hair naturally, as God designed it especially for you? After all, your own natural hair, your crown, is part of you. If you have straight hair, wear it straight. If you have curly hair, wear it curly, and so forth. If you have blonde hair, keep it blonde. If brunette, keep it that way. This is the right thing to do as long as you can endure the pressures of those who falsify their hair.

Most blacks have coiled hair, which Nekhena Evans defines as a tight, spiral or coil formation.[34] She goes on to inform us that it should not be called kinky, woolly, peasy, knotty, or nappy. Evans feels that these words are negative cuts against blacks. That is why she prefers the term spiral. Some blacks have a tighter coil or spiral than others. A comb designed for relatively straight hair does not work on tightly coiled hair.

There are two ways most blacks can wear their hair naturally. The first is called an afro. A long-tooth pick is used to comb the hair in this fashion. The other is to allow the hair to intertwine together forming a lock. Hairlocking is a biological process that occurs when naturally coiled or spiraled hair is allowed to develop in its natural state, without combing, picking, or the use of chemicals.[35] In some people this is exactly what the hair is designed to do. People of all colors, including even some whites, from all around the world have hair that wants to naturally lock. Hairlocking is not a new phenomenon or fad. Locks can be traced to ancient times in many cultures of Africa, India, Asia, the Pacific Islands, Greece, and other places.[36]

---

32 Francesco Mastalia and Alfonse Pagano, Dreads, (New York: Artisan 1999), 61.
33 Ademole Mandella, Authentic Hair (New York: Cosmic Nubian Enterprises, 2002).
34 Nekhena Evans, Hairlocking, Everything You Need to Know (Brooklyn, NY: A&B Publishers Group).
35 Evans, 17.
36 Mastalia and Pagano.

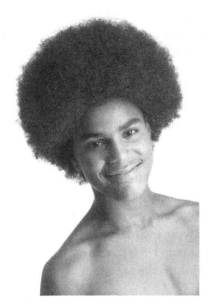 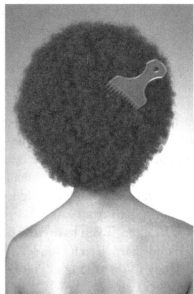

Figure 2-10: Young Teenage Male with Afro. A long-tooth pick is used to comb and dress the hair.

Most refer to locks as dreadlocks. The word dreadlock has different meanings to different people. On one hand, dreadful is the term the English used to describe the Africans' hair as they were captured and brought to U.S. shores.[37] According to Evans, many blacks prefer the term "Nubian locks" instead of dreadlocks to avoid this negative connotation. Others drop the 'a' out of the word, spelling it "dredlocks."[38] The modern worldwide popularity of dreadlocks can be traced back to Bob Marley, reggae and the Rastafarians, who adopted the hairstyle from the courageous Kikuyu soldiers in 1950s Kenya.[39] Locks and beards are a sign of the ancient covenant between God and man being part of "creation living."[40] Creation living to Bob Marley meant that hair is holy and taught people to respect their hair. His hair and beard was akin to a lion's mane, which invoked confidence, love, and commitment to Jah (a short form for Yahweh or God). God and His ancient Prophets would certainly agree.

---

37   Evans, 31-34.
38   Ayana D. Byrd and Lori L. Tharps, Hair Story, (New York: St. Martin's Griffin, 2001), 125.
39   Byrd and Tharps, 116-125.
40   Mastalia and Pagano, 8, 14, 55, 56.

No matter what locks are called the truth is that they are not dreadful. People with straighter hair do not seem to realize how difficult it is to comb out tightly coiled hair that wants to lock naturally. Besides, most people who wear locks or dreadlocks today have it professionally maintained at a salon. After years of freedom-fighting, thankfully, locks are now an acceptable and natural way to wear African hair in Jamaica. In the U.S., I give many thanks to those wiser corporations that allow naturally long hair, whether straight long hair or dredlocks. But much more work is needed in certain corporations and schools, who often expel those with long hair even though they claim to worship Jesus who had long hair as the Creator designed and allowed. Instead they seem to rejoice in baldness.

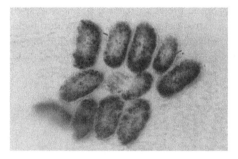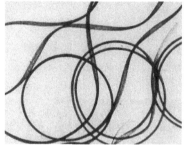

Figure 2-11: Microscopic Images of Tightly Spiraled Hair. This type of hair (called Negroid type by the FBI) is different than most of those with Caucasoid (whites) type hair and different from Mongoloid (Asian) type hair. Negroid hair is far less round in cross section than Caucasoid hair. This elongated portal flattened on the sides, causes the hair to form tight coils or spirals. Image from Deedrick and Koch, Forensic Science Communications, January 2004, vol. 6, no. 1 (FBI).

In the book "Dreads," Hilda Thompson said she had two choices: "Go bald or grow locks." This is after years of putting chemicals in her hair, when she decided to "go natural." This was a wise decision for her. Does anyone really want to go bald? A white woman, Kara Dodson, said "My hair locks naturally." Finally, after a tough time throughout life trying to force her hair to do things it was not designed to do, she let it lock. Like Bob Marley, many other men feel that long locks are like "the mane of a lion," and males and females alike feel free by wearing their hair in this manner.[41]

---

41 Mastalia and Pagano, 8-14, 48, 64, 87.

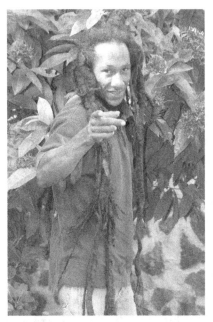

Figure 2-12: Man with Dreadlocks. Some prefer to remove the 'a' and spell it dredlocks. Dreadlocks grow into locks of various diameters. They should not be confused with Nubian or cultivated locks placed in strands of equal diameter.

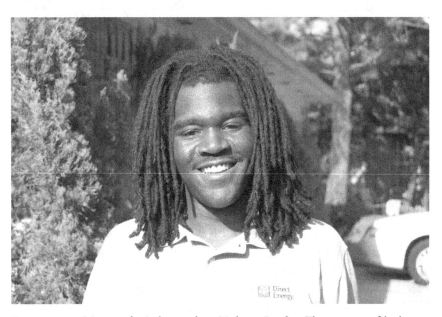

Figure 2-13: Man with Cultivated or Nubian Locks. These types of locks are usually called dreadlocks in America. However, cultivated locks are different than pure dreadlocks. Cultivated locks are placed in strands of roughly the same diameter and are professionally maintained at a salon by a loctician.

Nubian locks are named after Nubia, the homeland of Africa's earliest black culture. The Nubian's history can be traced from 3100 B.C. onward through their monuments and artifacts, as well as written records from Egypt and Rome. Nubia was located in the region of southern Egypt and northern Sudan. The modern inhabitants of this area still refer to themselves as Nubians. So this manner of hairstyling dates back to ancient times (Figure 2-14).

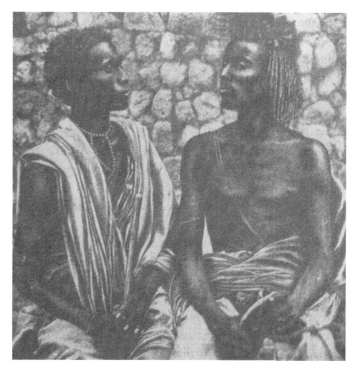

Figure 2-14: Descendants of a Famous Race of Antiquity: The Bisharin. This is a well-known nomadic tribe inhabiting the northeast part of the Sudan. The man on the right clearly wears locks or Nubian locks. Photograph from the late 19th century or early 20th century from "The Secret Museum of Mankind." Courtesy of David Stiffler.

As recorded in the "Guinness Book of World Records," the longest apparent dreadlocks on record are those of Swami Pandarasannadhi, the head of the Thiruvadu monastery in India.[42] In 1949 his hair measured 26 feet in length. However, this length needs to be qualified. His hair was

---

42 Guinness Book of World Records, Norris McWhirter (Ross McWhirter 1955-1975), ed., 1985 Edition: David A. Boehn et al, Eds. (New York: Sterling Publishing Co., Inc.).

locked, but it was "matted and crusted as a result of neglect." Recall that the life span of a single hair ranges from two to seven years. When hair is locked, all the old hairs that naturally fall out of the scalp *remain in the lock*. They do not fall to the ground like someone with straight, un-locked hair. This would give the impression of super-long hair when, in fact, no single hair of his head could achieve such a length. Thus, this person ended up with shorter hairs bound up within the same locked strand. Each individual hair in his locks would have been much shorter, probably no single hair longer than about three feet. A true world record must be based on hairs still anchored in the scalp, not those that have fallen out and are bound in the lock.

It should be stated that those in the Americas and Caribbean who wear cultivated locks or Nubian locks (sometimes still referred as dreadlocks) in the present time do not neglect them. They are maintained in a salon. Personally, I think locks should be kept trimmed at waist-length or higher. According to Ademole Mandella, locks start to weaken or atrophy in about seven to ten years anyway.[43] Master Loctician Ayanna Williams of Houston, Texas says this can happen sooner. And whenever it does, the ends are simply trimmed.[44] In this way the older hairs that have already fallen out of the scalp can be removed. Otherwise, the locks can get so long that they have to be carried over the shoulder.[45]

No matter your skin color or if you are male or female, long hair is natural hair even if the ends are trimmed periodically. The point is that all people should be allowed to wear their hair naturally. A brush and comb works well for people who have naturally straight hair, wavy hair, or hair with large curls. As already mentioned, a long-tooth pick is used to comb out tightly coiled hair in afro style. Besides the afro, some may wish to naturally grow their hair into locks. By perusing the thousands of photographs compiled by David Stiffler in "The Secret Museum of Mankind," quite a variety of hair styles and types can be observed.[46] Longer natural hair was worn by several of these cultures from around the world even as late as the late 19th and early 20th centuries. Those of African descent are shown with afros, while others wore locks.

---

43 Ademole Mandella, Authentic Hair (New York: Cosmic Nubian Enterprises, 2002), 191.

44 Ayanna Williams, personal interview with her at her salon "Knappi by Nature," Houston, Texas on June 21, 2005.

45 Mastalia and Pagano, 13.

46 David Stiffler, ed., The Secret Museum of Mankind, (Salt Lake City: Gibbs Smith Publisher, reprint edition 1999). Originally published (New York: Manhattan House, [1941?]).

Male Slovac farmers are shown with long, straight, blonde hair below the shoulders (Figure 2-15). Native tribes (erroneously called Indians) all over South America, Central America, and North America wore long natural hair. All over Asia it was the same. Based on design, it is okay to wear long hair. To avoid potential hair and scalp problems, there are two essential principles: (1) wear your hair in its natural state; and (2) longer hair is healthier.

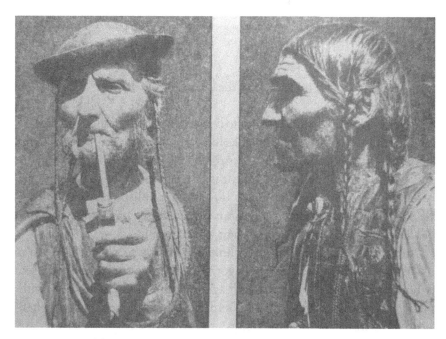

Figure 2-15: Old Slovac Men with Long Hair. Please note that these old men still have a full head of hair with no receding hair line. Photograph from the late 19th century or early 20th century from "The Secret Museum of Mankind." Courtesy of David Stiffler.

The foregoing begs for certain questions. Why is human head hair designed to grow long and grow fast? Why is it designed with such resilience, strength, and resistance to wear and tear? What are its purposes? What are the real causes of hair loss? Is baldness truly inevitable? These questions and many more are answered, but you must read on.

Chapter 3: The Root Causes of Common Baldness

... because it had no root, it withered away (Mark 4:6).

Some books about baldness claim to be the "complete guide" to hair loss.[47] They fall well short. In fact, books like these seem to simply regurgitate the same old rhetoric of drugs or surgery. Most of this information is readily available on the Internet. Little is offered about how to prevent hair loss in the first place, and not much is said about holistic methods to heal the scalp. So first you must understand what causes hair loss. Then you will learn the real ways to prevent hair loss naturally.

In the past, baldness has been linked primarily to old men due to a loss of virility. This loss of energy, vigor, and sex drive is apparently caused by hormone changes associated with aging. Baldness in conjunction with an increase in chest hair suggests a hormone driven process.[48] Other than the loss of virility, what other factors are involved? For example, why are there so many young men, even women and teenagers, losing their hair in modern times? This makes no natural sense at all. Could it be that an unhealthy lifestyle associated with modernism is the answer?

To understand the causes of baldness, you must acquire knowledge about the largest organ of the human body, your skin. Skin is designed to adapt admirably to its underlying contours as it forms a vast barrier between the person and his or her environment.[49] Skin is composed of three layers, the outermost epidermis, the dermis, and the subcutaneous fat layer, or hypodermis. Considering all three layers, Hori and colleagues indicate that

---

47 Antonio Avi Armani, How to Beat Hair Loss: The Complete Guide to Surgical, Medical, & Alternative Treatments for Hair Loss (Toronto: Redom Books, 1999).

48 Thomas Gutersohn, E. Paul Scheidegger, "Is Baldness Bad for the Heart?" Dermatology 2005; 211(1):72-74 (DOI:10.1159/000085583) S. Karger AG, Basil.

49 D.M. Podolsky, Skin: the human fabric. (The Human Body), (Tarrytown, New York: Torstar Books, Inc., 1984), 39.

normal scalp thickness in males is about 4.3 mm. That report also indicates that females have a thicker dermis and subcutaneous fat layer making the female scalp about 1.0 mm thicker than males.[50] Compared to most of the body, the scalp is the thinnest skin of all.[51] This thinness of the scalp compared to other places on the head obviously causes it to be a potentially very sensitive area. Thus proper treatment of your scalp, or better, your crown, is of utmost importance. The scalp must not be treated harshly. Otherwise, hair loss will ensue. A healthy scalp is vital for vibrant hair.

In his book, "Bald No More," Dr. Morton Walker considers common hair loss (androgenetic alopecia) a "disease."[52] Some may not think of hair loss as a disease because of its prevalence in men and because it is not life threatening. However, this belief is more emotional rather than scientific. According to "Webster's II New Riverside Dictionary," a disease is simply "a condition of an organism that impairs normal physiological functioning." Thus, the malfunction or dysfunction of any organ of the body can be called a disease. Just because we are dealing with a person's outward appearance does not mean that it is no less of a disease than the dysfunction of any other organ in the human body. Dr. Charles Brim even remarks that the ancient Hebrews considered baldness a "form of disease" thousands of years ago.[53] Although considered a disease, the good news is that common baldness is not contagious, a fact that was established more than 3,000 years ago (Leviticus 13:40-41).

Common baldness affects both men (male pattern baldness or MPB) and women (female pattern baldness or FPB). Internal and external processes can greatly affect this barrier organ we call skin. Oftentimes, the specialized outgrowths of the skin (i.e., hair and nails) are indicators of health. Brittle nails and brittle or dull hair sometimes indicates a lack of proper nutrition.[54,55] The skin organ, or outgrowths thereof, may also reveal much about the health of other organs of the body. Disease in the scalp may be related to disease in your internal organs. In any regard, thinning hair and baldness of the scalp are signs that the skin is not healthy.

---

50 Hiroyuki Hori, Giuseppe Morreti, Alfredo Rebora, and Franco Crovato, "The Thickness of Human Scalp: Normal and Bald." The Journal of Investigative Dermatology, Vol. 58, No. 6, 1972.

51 Lowell A. Goldsmith, ed., Physiology, Biochemistry, and Molecular Biology of the Skin, Vol.1. 2nd (New York: Oxford University Press, 1991), 5.

52 Morton Walker, Bald No More, (New York: Kensington Publishing Corporation, 1998), 50.

53 Charles J. Brim, Medicine in the Bible (New York: Froben Press, 1936), 159.

54 Phyllis A. Balch and James F. Balch, Prescription for Nutritional Healing (3rd ed. New York: Avery – a member of Penguin Putnam, 2000), 401-403.

55 Walker, Bald No More.

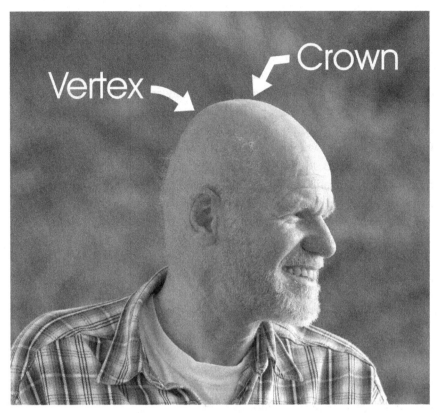

Figure 3-1: Position of the Vertex and Crown Area of the Head. The vertex is located where the whirl-shape or vortex of the hair is, if you still have hair. Vertex balding (i.e., the more or less rounded balding area on this backside/top position of the head) in young men may be a sign of health problems such as heart disease or prostate cancer.

The importance of head hair as an indicator of internal health is striking, especially in the vertex region of the scalp rather than the crown (see Figure 3-1). In "Is Baldness Bad for the Heart?" Thomas Gutersohn and E. Paul Scheidegger claim that there is a relationship between male pattern baldness and coronary disease.[56] In 1993, it was reported that the relative risk for a "coronary event," such as a heart attack, in balding men under 55 years of age is three times more likely than those not going bald.[57] By 2005 it was

---

56 Gutersohn and Scheidegger.
57 S.M. Lesko, L. Rosenberg, and S. Shapiro, "A case-control study of baldness in relation to myocardial infarction in men." JAMA. 1993 Feb 24;269(8):998-1003. PMID: 8429606, accessed October 18, 2005, http://www.ncbi.nlm.nih.gov/entrez/query. fcgi?CMD=Display&DB=pubmed.

confirmed that "a correlation between alopecia [loss of hair] and coronary disease exists."[58]

If there is a relationship between baldness and heart disease, then something must be wrong with processes inside the body of those individuals. Brian Simonis in his on-line book, "Immortal Hair," agrees. He says that men "who are balding in the crown area [he means the posterior portion of the top or vertex] are very likely to have some form of heart-related disease in their future. The root of the problem often stems from the types of fats that are consumed in the diet."[59] More than likely, poor nutrition and lack of vigorous exercise are involved. Of course, it should never be assumed that a balding man has a bad heart. Caution is warranted because there are other causes of thinning hair and baldness. Wendy Denmark-Wahnefried and colleagues also found a link between vertex balding and prostate cancer. Separate analyses, of two studies by this group, suggest an association between early onset vertex baldness (by age 30) and prostate cancer.[60]

DHT

Dr. Loren Pickart informs us that the causes of hair loss are more diverse than generally realized with most theories focusing on the metabolic actions of DHT (dihydrotestosterone).[61] The hormone testosterone is converted by 5-alpha reductase to DHT. Some call DHT: "testosterone times ten."[62] If you have ten times the needed testosterone, then this is obviously a hormonal imbalance. As this problem occurs, metabolism in the skin, hair follicles, and sebaceous glands are affected. According to Walker, these hormonal abnormalities occur especially with the body's metabolism of calcium and iron. This *too-much-testosterone,* or DHT, restricts blood flow to the papilla, the tiny organ that produces hair cells, at the base of the hair follicle (Figure 3-2). Thus, it is thought that testosterone overload is a

58   Gutersohn and Scheidegger, 72-74.
59   Brian Simonis, "Immortal Hair," accessed April 4, 2006 http://www.immortalhair. homestead.com/files/Entire_Hair_Loss_Book.htm.
60   W. Denmark-Wahnefried, J.M. Schildkraut, D. Thompson, S.M. Lesko, L. McIntyre, P. Schwingl, D.F. Paulson, C.N. Robertson, E.E. Anderson, and P.J. Walther,"Early Onset Baldness and Prostate Cancer Risk," Cancer Epidemiology, Biomarkers & Prevention. Vol. 9, 325-328, March 2000.
61   Loren Pickart, "Hair Biology, Hair Care, and Loss," accessed February 16, 2006 http:// www.skinbiology.com/hairbiology,care&loss.html.
62   Morton Walker, How to Stop Baldness and Regrow Hair (Stamford, CT: Freelance Communications, 1995), 17.

main cause of baldness for both sexes. Hormonal ravages certainly play a role with some people, for it is known that men castrated prior to puberty do not go bald.[63]

In contrast, a healthy papilla becomes engorged with blood and manufactures hair cells, which are forced up through the follicle.[64] Restricted blood flow has the opposite effect. Riquette Hofstein says it leads to "common thinning" or androgenetic alopecia, which accounts for about 95 percent of all hair loss cases. Common hair thinning affects both males and females. Estrogen obstructs the effects of DHT, so women do not suffer as much until menopause.[65] Also, the thicker subcutaneous fat layer, or hypodermis, in females probably helps them lose less hair than males. Dr. Loren Pickart's copper peptides, discussed later, increase subcutaneous fat.[66]

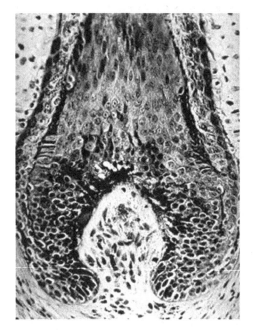

Figure 3-2: Micrograph of the Base of a Hair Follicle. A hair consists of cylindrical shaft and a root, which is contained in the flask-shaped chamber (i.e., hair follicle) in the corium and subcutaneous tissue of the skin. The base of the root is expanded into the hair bulb, which rests upon the papilla. The papilla (bottom-center) is the tiny organ that produces hair cells. Unrestricted healthy blood flow to the papilla is of utmost importance for the manufacture of hair in the follicle. Photograph courtesy of John L. Bezzant, M.D.

The popular idea that male pattern baldness is genetically determined, the so-called "baldness gene," is being dismissed:

---

63 Walker, Bald No More, 54.
64 Riquette Hofstein, Grow Hair Fast – 7 Steps to a New Head of Hair in 90 Days (Naperville, Illinois: Sourcebooks, Inc. 2004), 12.
65 Hofstein.
66 Loren Pickart, "Improving Hair Growth with Skin Remodeling Copper Peptides." Cosmetics and Medicine (Russia) (July 2004), accessed February 13, 2005 http://www.skinbiology.com/2004RussiaHairRemodeling.html.

But many men have high testosterone metabolite levels but never suffer hair loss. The ultimate factor in hair loss appears not to be DHT itself, but an already damaged hair follicle susceptible to the negative effects of DHT. A recent study of 3,000 individuals found no link between baldness and the genes (5-alpha reductase) controlling the production of testosterone metabolites.[67]

Hofstein agrees that the genetic code merely determines a tendency or sensitivity or predisposition for DHT problems and is not the main cause.[68] Now we are getting somewhere. It really depends upon how sensitive your skin organ is. The truth is that sensitive skin is a complex problem with genetic, individual, environmental, occupational, and ethnic implications.[69]

So DHT is not the main cause of hair loss and common balding, but can add its negative effects to an already existent problem. Most seem to agree on one thing, that the skin where the hair is made (follicle – see Figure 2-1) becomes inflamed, damaged, and unhealthy. Furthermore, as you age, the scalp becomes thinner and even more susceptible to skin damage.[70] The skin of a young person's scalp replaces itself naturally in fourteen days. The scalp of youth is thick and has rich blood supply. Nutrients are transported through the scalp much easier and wastes are readily eliminated when blood supply (circulation) is better. Likewise, a thicker-skinned scalp can take more abuse than an older person's thinner skin. In an average adult the skin replaces itself in about 28 days or longer depending on your age.[71] The normal range is thought to be 26 to 42 days.[72] So, two things are against a mature adult: (1) slower skin replacement (rejuvenation), and (2) thinner skin, especially the skin on the top of the scalp.

The importance of skin health cannot be overstated. Each individual hair is formed in the hair follicle beneath the skin surface. As long as the hair follicle functions properly, then the visible hair shaft will continue to be extruded. But, if your scalp is being damaged, its rejuvenation is

---

67 Pickart, "Improving Hair Growth with Skin Remodeling Copper Peptides."
68 Hofstein.
69 Ruth Winter, A Consumer's Dictionary of Cosmetic Ingredients (New York: Three Rivers Press, 2005).
70 Pickart.
71 David M. Homer, "Biolife Cleansing Guide: Understanding How Your Body Cleanses & Purifies Itself, Inner," accessed October 4, 2003 http://www.innerlifewellness.com/articles/internalcleansing1.html.
72 Lowell A. Goldsmith, ed., Physiology, Biochemistry, and Molecular Biology of the Skin, Vol.1. 2nd ed. (New York: Oxford University Press, 1991).

hindered. The health of the hair follicle below the skin surface is extremely important. Damaged, unhealthy hair follicles are the beginning of an unsuitable scalp for continued hair regeneration. You must treat your scalp properly, internally and externally. You must determine the causes of your hair loss. Your hair loss may not be related at all to another person's hair loss problem. Indeed, there is probably more than one cause. There could be two or three reasons, why you are losing your hair.[73]

Decreased Gene Expression?

People have been told that baldness is a genetic issue and nothing can be done other than taking drugs such as Rogaine and Propecia, or having surgery. It should be pointed out that this is the conventional sales pitch by those who sell either drugs or hair transplantation surgery. So the repetitive rhetoric by these firms is, no doubt, somewhat biased in their favor. The question we should be asking is why does the genetic code produce hair originally and then stop making hair at some point later in life? Would this not require a change in the genetic code of one's DNA (Deoxyribonucleic acid)? Midorikawa et al. found that there was indeed a "decreased gene expression" in 107 out of 1,185 genes apparently from the top of the scalp when compared to areas not affected by baldness.[74] The question is what causes a "decreased gene expression?" Is it strictly hereditary? Or could it be that certain other things cause the DNA's genetic code to become damaged leading to the "decreased gene expression"?

The truth is that processes inside the body cause hair loss and processes that act on the skin's surface cause hair loss. But whether the baldness is being caused by outside influences or internal processes, or both, the main point is that the bottom line may be an unhealthy modern lifestyle, which leads to the so-called "decreased gene expression." As already stated by researchers Hofstein, Pickart, and Morton Walker, the genetic code is definitely not the root cause of hair loss. So if all these things are not the real causes of hair loss, then what are?

---

73   David H. Kingsley, The Hair-Loss Cure, A Self-Help Guide (Bloomington, IN: iUniverse, 2009).

74   T. Midorikawa, T. Chikazawa, T. Yoshino, K. Takada, S. Arase, "Different gene expression profile observed in dermal papilla cells related to androgenic alopecia by DNA macroarray analysis," J Dermatol Sci. 2004 Oct;36(1):25-32. PMID: 15488702, accessed April 16, 2006 http://www.ncbi.nlm.nih.gov/entrez/query. fcgi?CMD=Display&DB=pubmed.

Internal Causes of Hair Loss

This section deals with processes inside the body that cause hair loss. The internal causes of hair loss include stress, poor nutrition, nutritional deficiencies, pesticides, herbicides, chemical poisoning, manmade chemical manipulations as found in street drugs, pharmaceutical drugs, over-the-counter drugs, too much alcohol, poor circulation, cancers of various organs such as the prostate, damage to the immune system, and spinal subluxations.[75][76][77][78] Men who take anabolic steroids to build muscle mass as in weight lifting are highly prone to hair loss.[79]

Again, DHT and a decreased gene expression are not the root causes of hair loss. They appear to be nothing more than symptoms of various other underlying problems. Valcović cites hormone problems such as too much testosterone or DHT, coupled with a "predisposing" hereditary pattern.[80] Sensitive skin is an inherited trait or someone with a predisposition for hair loss. Walker and Chinwah believe hair loss problems arise from dysfunctions of the endocrine system. Walker says too much androgen (a hormone produced from the endocrine system) causes hair loss in those with a predisposition (e.g., sensitive skin) to go bald.[81] The major glands of the endocrine system related to hair loss are the thyroid, thymus, and adrenals.[82] The two most important seem to be the thyroid and thymus glands.[83][84] The adrenal glands produce hormones to cope with stress.[85] Thus it may be surmised that the adrenals may play a role with stress related hair loss.

Hair loss results from dysfunctional processes inside the body and abusive acts on the skin's surface. In terms of those processes inside the body, two main systems must be maintained to reduce or stop hair loss.

---

75   Hezekiah U. Chinwah, "Baldness." Physicians Reference Notebook, ed. William A. McGarey (Virginia Beach: A.R.E. Press 1983), 60-63.

76   S. Mac-Mary, J.M. Sainthillier, P. Humbert, "Dry Skin and the Environment," Exogenous Dermatology 2004; 3:72-80 (DOI:10.1159/000086157) S. Karger AG, Basil.

77   Tobin, Desmond J. "Biochemistry of human skin – our brain on the outside." Chemical Society Reviews. 2006, 35, p. 52-67.

78   Walker, Bald No More.

79   Kingsley.

80   Valković, Human Hair. Vol. 1: Fundamentals and Methods for Measurement of Elemental Composition (Boca Raton, Florida: CRC Press, Inc., 1988), 25.

81   Walker, Bald No More.

82   Chinwah, 60-63.

83   Robert A. Leach, The Chiropractic Theories, A Synopsis of Scientific Research 2nd Ed. (Baltimore: Williams & Wilkins, 1986), 159.

84   Walker, Bald No More.

85   Alma E. Guinness, ed., ABC's of the Human Body (New York: The Readers Digest Association, 1987), 77.

These two systems are the central nervous system and the vascular (or blood circulatory) system. Dr. Hezekiah Chinwah believes that gland problems and spinal lesions called subluxations "are by far the most common causes of hair loss," and may be accompanied by other negative changes in the skin and nails. According to Chinwah, glands, such as the thyroid and thymus, malfunction due to poor diet, insufficient circulation, stress, infection, and toxic chemicals found in cosmetics and elsewhere. Chinwah cites the thyroid as an example. Apparently, a lack of certain elements, such as calcium, causes toxins to accumulate in the thyroid. This leads to "inflammation, congestion, and circulatory disturbances," which affects the scalp. The "outcome is hair loss."[86]

Maintenance of the central nervous system is of utmost importance for good health. It is the central nervous system that deals with basic disease process. Robert Leach says there is an overwhelming amount of evidence that links the nervous system to immunity by way of its control of endocrine function.[87] What happens is that your brain and your body talk to each other. The main way this is done is through the hypothalamus, a tiny cluster of cells in the brain. It coordinates activities in the nervous system with your vital organs of the endocrine system including the thyroid and thymus glands. "ABCs of the Human Body" informs us that the brain receives information through one set of nerves and sends out instructions for action through another set.[88] These nerves pass through the spinal column, exit through the vertebrae, and go out from there to all parts of your body, including the vertex portion of the scalp (Figure 3-1), thyroid and thymus. The nervous system controls all your activities. If this remarkable communication system (i.e., nervous system) is impaired (e.g., subluxations), then problems with your body and its functions result.

Thus, the proper curvature and alignment of the spine (your basic structural system, which impacts the nervous system) is of utmost importance. One of the early definitions of subluxation is "interference with the transmission of neural impulses," or simply put, "pressure on the nerves" caused by misaligned vertebrae (or a single vertebra) in the neck or back.[89] Dr. Chinwah remarks that spinal subluxations cause impaired circulation through the adrenals, thyroid, and thymus glands.[90] Furthermore, these glands secrete hormones (chemical messengers) directly

---

86 Chinwah, 60-63.
87 Leach, 182.
88 Guinness, 49-51.
89 Leach, 16.
90 Chinwah, 60-63.

into the bloodstream.[91] If there is a miscommunication between your brain and the glands at hand, then apparently an incorrect amount of hormones could be released into the bloodstream. Testosterone overload, which leads to hair loss, may very well be one of these incorrect amounts of hormones. Thus, a series of treatments "to correct spinal subluxation that may be causing circulatory, glandular and other organ dysfunction as well as hair loss" is encouraged by Chinwah.

According to Dr. Mick Mahan, corrective chiropractic care is the best strategy to ensure proper structure of the spine and the central nervous system.[92] After all, subluxations in the neck can not only affect your internal organs, but they can have a direct impact on the nerves that supply the follicles up the backside of the skull up to the vertex!

In summary, the remedy to internal causes of hair loss includes vigorous exercise, proper nutrition, and proper alignment of the spine. Outdoor exercise, with the benefit of fresh air, is encouraged. Chiropractic adjustments are the primary method used to correct subluxations of the spine. Also, it is important to get your blood moving by exercise. Think of sweat due to exercise as a good thing. Once you make these positive adjustments in your life, then you may be able to get off over-the-counter and pharmaceutical drugs, which also cause hair loss.

External Causes of Hair Loss

> Baldness is come upon Gaza ... how long wilt thou cut thyself?
> (Jeremiah 47:5)

This section deals with hair loss caused by things, which act upon the skin surface or directly on the scalp. Skin and follicle damage can occur in many ways. Valcović cites burns, scalds, trauma, fungal infection, and a host of inflammatory skin disorders that cause hair loss.[93] Stressful objects and substances such as noise, smoke, cosmetics, and visual display screens such as a computer monitor, cause a person's skin to age rapidly.[94] Obviously, aged skin means aged follicles and hair loss. In addition to this

---

91 Guinness, 76.
92 Mick Mahan, Discover Chiropractic, Houston, Texas. Verbal communication, 2006.
93 Valković.
94 S. Mac-Mary, J.M. Sainthillier and P. Humbert, P., "Dry Skin and the Environment." Exogenous Dermatology 2004; 3:72-80 (DOI:10.1159/000086157) S. Karger AG, Basil.

are hair dyes, cancers of the skin, moles, excessive traction by braiding,[95] many shampoos and other hair care products,[96][97] high heat, excessive hair cutting, short hair,[98][99] chlorine in the public water supply,[100] overexposure to the sun,[101][102] and chemical and mechanical "insults."[103] Does your scalp itch? If so, these things listed, and much more, all lead to hair loss via seborrheic dermatitis or a dysfunction of the sebaceous glands. Or, if the inflammation is within the hair follicle itself, then hair loss associated with this skin damage is called alopecia follicularis.

Earlier, the suggestion was made that the so-called decreased gene expression is actually caused by cell damage. It is now known that DNA in the cells becomes damaged by chemicals and overexposure to ultraviolet light, or too much sunshine. According to Sherwin Nuland, author of "The Wisdom of the Body," DNA altered by chemicals can lead to cancer.[104] As an example, tobacco smoke has been linked to skin diseases including premature gray hair and hair loss in mice. "Smoke-exposed mice had extensive atrophy of the epidermis, reduced thickness of the subcutaneous tissue, and scarcity of hair follicles." Cell death was especially severe "at the edge" of balding areas.[105] It should be pointed out that the typical receding hairline in men is also at the "edge" of baldness. Consider what might be the effects of other types of air pollution in urban environments. Who knows how these other micro-pollutants may act upon a person's scalp. Think about it when you see a dense yellow layer of smog lying over your city.

---

95 Walker, Bald No More.

96 Hofstein.

97 Arthur Rook and Rodney Dawber, eds., Diseases of the Hair and Scalp. 2nd Ed. (London: Blackwell Scientific Publications, 1991).

98 Pickart, "Improving Hair Growth with Skin Remodeling Copper Peptides."

99 Loren Pickart, Reverse Skin Aging: Using Your Skin's Natural Power (Bellevue, Washington: Cape San Juan Press, 2005), 113-119.

100 D.V. Riddle, "Evaluation of the Sprite RSF shower filter for chlorine removal characteristics," Kemysts Laboratory, June 1997.

101 D.I. Pattison and M.J. Davies, "Actions of ultraviolet light on cellular structures." EXS. 2006; (96):131-57. PMID 16383017, accessed April 16, 2006 http://www.ncbi.nlm.nih.gov/entrez/query.fcgi?CMD=Display&DB=pubmed.

102 Desmond J. Tobin, "Biochemistry of human skin – our brain on the outside," Chemical Society Reviews, 2006, 35, p. 52-67.

103 Tobin.

104 Sherwin Nuland, The Wisdom of the Body (New York: Alfred A. Knopf, 1997), 48.

105 F. D' Agostini, R. Balansky, C. Pesce, P. Fiallo, R.A. Lubet, G.J. Kelloff and S. De Flora, "Induction of alopecia in mice exposed to cigarette smoke." Toxicol Lett. 2000 Apr 3;114(1-3):117-23. PMID: 10713476, accessed April 16, 2006 http://www.ncbi.nlm.nih.gov/entrez/query.fcgi?CMD=Display&DB=pubmed.

Is ultraviolet radiation another contributor? Yes. There is much research that demonstrates conclusively that overexposure to the sun causes DNA damage in the skin, although a moderate amount of sunshine is greatly needed for good health.[106] Overexposure causes DNA damage, which can lead to mutations and skin cancer.[107] [108] D.I. Pattison and M.J. Davies, authors of "Actions of Ultraviolet Light on Cellular Structures," sum it up nicely in their research, saying, "Solar radiation is the primary source of human exposure to ultraviolet (UV) radiation."

They go on to tell us that "proteins and DNA" are the primary targets in cells. This is important because hair consists mostly of protein, and it is made in the hair follicle where muscles (also protein) are. Muscles are penetrated by nerves. Genetic damage caused by UV radiation "can trigger programmed cell death (or *apoptosis*) that is completed within hours of being injured."[109] Ironically, these damaged cells are called "sunburn cells." The genetic code of the DNA provides the instructions to make hair. Nerve supply from the brain controls the process. But if nerves, proteins, and DNA become damaged, then what do you think could happen? Presumably, this would indeed be a so-called "decreased gene expression" and your hair will fall out and not grow back. Thus, as you are beginning to see heredity plays a minor role, if any, in the case of baldness. For one thing, it should be pointed out that close-cropped short hair exposes the scalp to the powerful rays of the sun. Sunburn and other scalp trauma, including certain chemicals, can lead to permanent hair loss. Once the nerve endings are dead, is there any hope of regeneration? Only hair transplantation with undamaged hair follicle cells will probably work at this point.

Manmade Causes of Hair Loss

Have you noticed that nearly all causes of premature skin aging and hair loss are related to modernistic ideas, modern industry, and an unhealthy lifestyle? Chemicals including permanents and hair straighteners, hair dyes, hair sprays, shampoos, along with short hair, stress, subluxations due

---

106 Pickart, Reverse Skin Aging: Using Your Skin's Natural Power, 137.
107 D.I. Pattison and M.J. Davies, "Actions of ultraviolet light on cellular structures."
108 C. Nishigori, "Cellular aspects of photocarcinogenesis," Photochem Photobiol Sci., 2006 Feb; 5(2):208-214. Epub 2005 Dec 1. PMID: 16465307 [PubMed – in process] accessed April 16, 2006 http://www.ncbi.nlm.nih.gov/entrez/query.fcgi?CMD=Display&DB=pubmed.
109 Tobin, 56.

to stress, smoke, chlorine, poor nutrition, lack of exercise, and even some cancers, are actually manmade. Worse is the fact that these are either self-inflicted or caused by our fellow man. And the more you are associated with such things, the more prone you are to suffer.

But please keep in mind that these manmade causes of hair loss are dependent upon the sensitivity of one's own skin. This is really what an individual inherits genetically from his or her parents: skin and hair type. Obviously, some people have more sensitive skin than others, just as some have more sensitive hearts, kidneys, and lungs or any other organ. Those with sensitive skin need to take more care than those with less sensitive skin. Both, internal and external processes affect skin health.

Any one or any combination of these things contributes to hair loss. It is most interesting to note that there are as many manmade external causes as there are internal causes of hair loss. All these causes are real problems. Most, if not all, can be controlled to a large degree by you. You must be willing to change your habits and lifestyle to prevent and even reverse hair loss. Some items on the list of hair loss causes, for example poor nutrition and stress, are well known. But many items on the list are essentially unknown to most people. Who would have ever thought that spinal problems could lead to hair loss? And what about those innocent looking shampoos (that smell great) in those pretty bottles? Many of these causes will be dealt with in the pages that follow, but the issue regarding hair length is quite instructive and profound. Who would have ever guessed that hair length matters?

Short Hair and Scalp Atrophy

Atrophy – in general it is a "defect or failure of nutrition manifested as a wasting away or diminution in the size of cell, tissue, organ or part."[110]

It is commonly believed that cutting the hair has no effect on hair growth rate.[111] In the short term this is generally true. However, the long term effects of excessive hair cutting are another matter entirely. Biochemist Dr. Loren Pickart of *Skin Biology*, Bellevue, Washington is a skin tissue regeneration expert. In his "Improving Hair Growth with Skin Remodeling Copper Peptides," Pickart remarks that "excessive hair cutting" is a cause of hair loss.[112] Prior to his 2005 book being released, I spoke to him via telephone on two separate occasions. On both occasions

110 Dorland's Illustrated Medical Dictionary, 23rd Edition (Philadelphia and London: W.B. Saunders Co., 1957).
111 Valković.
112 Pickart, "Improving Hair Growth with Skin Remodeling Copper Peptides."

Dr. Pickart told me quite confidently that "longer hair is healthier," and short hair is a "primary cause of hair loss."[113]

The advent of the short hair problem in modern times began at the turn of the 20th century. According to Pickart, many years ago Russian physician Dr. George Michael came to the same conclusion: "longer hair is healthier." Some of the proof is in pictures, paintings, and sculptures prior to the 20th century that show elderly men and women, most with full-heads of hair. Women use to be proud of long locks of hair and grew it long, with beautiful, flowing locks cascading down the back, even to the waist line or base of the spinal column. Many men, whole nations throughout the ages, wore long hair too, or at least shoulder-length hair. When people wore their hair in this most natural way, balding was a much lesser problem, as the many photographs and ancient paintings in this book reveal.

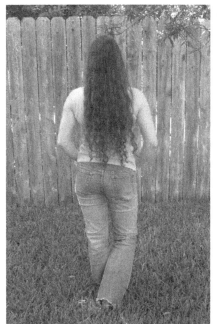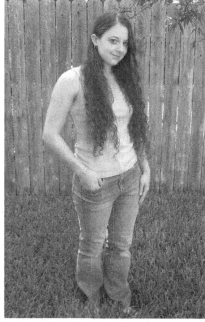

Figure 3-3: Young Woman with Truly Long, Naturally Wavy Hair. Her hair is natural because it is full length and unaltered by dyes, chemicals or heat, all of which damage hair.

---

113 Pickart, Loren. Two telephone conversations with him, the first on October 3, 2003 and the second about a year later on October 28, 2004. I spoke to him twice because I wanted to make certain I heard him correctly about the short hair problem, which is a great leading cause of hair loss. In thinking about the scalp, he said when muscles are inactive they tend to whither away.

There are muscles and nerves in the scalp. Longer hair is healthier for the scalp, and short hair invites injury. The scalp's incredible neuromuscular system (like all other muscular systems of the body) must be used - exercised for stimulation - to stay healthy. Besides the potential sun damage and cell death problem, short hair does not weigh enough to exercise the muscles of the scalp in order for it to function properly. The best way to strengthen scalp muscles is with the extra weight of heavier long hair. Morton Walker says hair loss can result from "disuse."[114] Pickart explains it thus: when muscles are "inactive" they tend to "whither away." Robert Leach informs us that the "most significant characteristic of muscle disease is weakness and atrophy of the involved muscles."[115]

By their very diminutive nature, weak muscles become susceptible to disease. In common language there is the adage of modern weightlifters, "either use it or lose it." By analogy, the same thing happens to the tiny muscles in the thin skin of the scalp, if they are not exercised. With longer hair the situation reverses. During those telephone interviews, Pickart said the extra weight of longer hair tugs on the follicle. Thus scalp muscles (e.g. *erector pili*) are exercised by the extra weight of longer hair just like arms and legs are exercised by weightlifters. Movement of hair seems to be of equal importance to the heavier weight of longer hair. Short hair leads to puny scalp muscles whereas long hair leads to larger, stronger scalp muscles. Long hair even stimulates the central nervous system.

Did you know that the nerves of the crown of the head originate directly in the brain? A new discovery in science informs us that hair is a neuro-transmitter. Believe it or not, skin is now being called our "brain on the outside."[116] Remarkably, Tobin informs us that skin and its appendages, especially hair, are both "a source and target of neuro-transmitters." This is especially important with regards to head hair. Nerves originating from the brain pass through openings or fissures through the skull and affect the scalp. Henry Gray's "Anatomy, Descriptive and Surgical" informs us that all the cranial nerves can be traced deeply into the substance of the brain, "their *deep* or *real origin*."[117] The 5th cranial nerve passes through the skull up the forehead and supplies the scalp, the crown. The condition of these nerves must be of great importance to follicular health. The signals of the nerves at each hair follicle end up in the brain. Thus, the extra weight of

114 Walker, Bald No More, 84.
115 Leach, 218.
116 Tobin.
117 Henry Gray, Anatomy, Descriptive and Surgical 1901 Edition, Pick and Robert Howden, eds., (Philadelphia: Running Press, 1974), 720, 728, 743.

long hair not only exercises the neuro-muscular system of the scalp alone, but may actually increase stimulation directly to the brain.

Incredibly, hair movement stimulates the central nervous system. In fact, "any movement of the hair sends an impulse to the brain."[118] This is because the nerve fibers that surround each hair follicle are mechanoreceptors. This means that these types of nerves respond to mechanical deformation or movement.[119] The extra weight of long hair combined with hair movement not only causes the scalp muscles and hair follicles to become larger and stronger, but even stimulates the brain. Just a little extra stimulation to the brain can go a long way. This is probably why long-haired musicians are a little more creative with their musicianship. In fact, the "Webster's II New Riverside Dictionary" tells us the meaning of the term longhair: an enthusiast of the arts and especially of classical music.

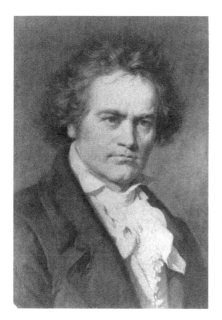

Figure 3-4: Ludwig van Beethoven, 1770-1827. He is one of the longhairs from which the term *longhair* is derived. Although much practice leads to perfection, musicians with long hair tend to be a hair more creative. U.S. Library of Congress, Prints and Photographs Division.

Along with the rise of the neo-Nazi skinheads, since the early 1990s there has been a tendency to crop the hair short, even exposing the skin of the scalp that can be burned by the sun, adding more stress to the brain rather than stimulation. As a general rule, this has led to choppy, less flowing, monotonous music. Young rock bands and musicians should

---

118 Podolsky, 82.
119 Richard S. Snell, Clinical Neuroanatomy for Medical Students, (3rd Ed. Boston: Little, Brown and Company 1992), 123-124; 417-419.

always be encouraged to wear long hair. In this way they will be a hair more creative than their uptight, short-haired competition. Young males in school and college should also be encouraged to wear long hair for that extra brain stimulation. The current situation is that females generally do better than males in school. Female enrollment at American universities has surpassed males for the first time in history. To remedy this situation, longer hair for males may bring about equal enrollment. If it is true that longer hair does stimulate the brain to a higher level, then who in their right mind would despise this? Only a menace would.

Obviously, brain stimulation is also the antithesis of stress. Therefore, long hair is a stress reducer. Since nerves are a two-way communication system, listening to or playing music, and other types of brain-stimulating activities (anti-stress) of the mind, should lead to better hair growth. But if short hair is kept short by excessive cutting, then extra weight is essentially never added to properly train these tiny scalp muscles and stimulation is reduced greatly. The scalp system could then become taxed or stressed. The result could be called scalp atrophy or a deadening condition of your natural crown. Unfortunately, many male scalps are trained to be weak from childhood by excessive hair-cutting. Eventually, death to the nerves means automatic death to the scalp, your crown.

In contrast, larger muscles in the scalp cause the hair follicles to become larger. A larger follicle means more space for blood flow to the papilla. As hair follicles become larger, the scalp flourishes by becoming thicker and thereby healthier. The skin is already stretched tight enough across the human scalp or crown. We do not need to cause it to become weaker and thinner by over-cutting. There is a big difference between the scalp and the sides and back of the head. The crown area feels thinner, tighter. But if you touch the sides and the back your head, you will notice that the skin is thicker and looser in these areas. It is vital to keep the crown of the head or scalp as loose and pliable as possible, similar to the sides and back of the skull.

Dr. Hori and his colleagues show just how drastic scalp atrophy of the crown is (Table 3-1).[120] In the initial stages of male pattern baldness (MPB), a 10 percent reduction in scalp thickness was found. At first glance, a 10 percent loss may not seem too bad. But if not corrected the situation gets progressively worse. Astonishingly, they found that those with advanced

---

120 Hiroyuki Hori, Giuseppe Moretti, Alfredo Rebora, and Franco Crovato, "The Thickness of Human Scalp: Normal and Bald," The Journal of Investigative Dermatology, Vol. 58, No. 6, 1972.

MPB have about a 35 percent reduction in scalp thickness. This reduced thickness occurs in every layer of the skin. The result is a thin, brittle scalp replete with cell death.

Table 3-1: Scalp Thickness in Male Pattern Baldness (MPB)

Skin Layers	Normal Scalp Millimeters (mm)	Initial Stages of MPB Millimeters (mm)	Advanced Stage of MPB Millimeters (mm)
Epidermis	0.072	0.065	0.053
Dermis	1.848	1.771	1.405
Subcutaneous Fat or Hypodermis	2.365	2.081	1.324
Total Skin Thickness	4.285	3.917	2.782

One reason human scalps are designed to grow long hair is to keep the scalp from becoming too thin, too brittle, too tight, and too weak. The combined weight of a full head of long hair not only stimulates the nerves and exercises the muscles but also, in a sense, pulls the scalp away from the skull. This makes the scalp thicker and the connective tissue more pliable, and thereby healthier. A thicker-skinned scalp means more blood circulation, thus, more nutrients find their way to the hair follicles.[121] When this happens, the scalp can now do what it was designed to do - grow the magnificent ornament of head hair, your crown. The scalp can now properly function. Atrophy of the scalp neuromuscular system is then lessened or eliminated. The neuromuscular system of the scalp becomes strong and healthy. Even normal daily hair loss occurs much less with longer hair (Table 3-2), as long as you have a healthy lifestyle overall.

Table 3-2: Longer Hair Reduces Shedding, Studies by Dr. George Michael (after Pickart, 2005)

Hair Length (Inches)	Number of Hairs Lost Per Day
4	87
12	26
Waist Length	16

---

121 Pickart, Reverse Skin Aging: Using Your Skin's Natural Power, 104-106.

According to Pickart, one of Dr. George Michael's remarks is "The longer the hair, the stronger the root."[122] Notice the incredible decrease in numbers of head hairs lost per day. Dr. Michael's research found that those with hair four inches in length lost an average of 87 hairs per day. But those with hair 12 inches in length lost only 26 hairs per day. What a disparity! This is remarkable proof that longer hair is healthier and reduces hair loss. In Rachel Bergsman's short essay she says that "hundreds of specialists" have been working on the problem of hair loss, but they "are not quite positive about the real root of the hair loss pandemic all over the world."[123] Well, it now appears that the "root" cause has indeed been discovered, and it is literally the root or follicle itself when in a weakened condition caused by excessively short hair. Consider this: a hair ten inches in length is ten times heavier than a hair one inch in length. Would a weightlifter's muscles become stronger and larger with a ten pound weight or something ten times heavier, a hundred pound weight? Obviously, the answer is the weight ten times heavier would produce larger stronger muscles. It is the same for each muscle attached to each hair follicle. Although scalp muscles are microscopic, the analogy still applies: a ten inch hair has ten times the weight of a one inch hair, and a five inch hair has five times the weight of a one inch hair, and so forth.

It becomes quite evident that longer hair strengthens the scalp's neuromuscular system. As a reminder, as long as the follicle is healthy, a new hair will replace the one that was lost regardless of length. However, longer hair makes a stronger root, a larger, healthier hair follicle, and apparently increases the growth phase (i.e., anagen period). A large, healthy follicle produces a new hair more readily than a weakened diminutive one. Thus, the evidence is clear that there is a better chance that each follicle will produce a new hair in longer-haired individuals during each repetitive hair growth cycle. Since most modern males, and even many females, wear very short hair, is it any wonder that many of them will eventually have hair-thinning problems and go bald? If you are a woman, and if you really want to have healthy, beautiful hair your whole life, then wear it twelve inches in length or longer. Obviously, if you are a man wear it as long as you think you can. Remember, head hair is designed to be longer than body hair. Longer hair is necessary for a healthy scalp. If you wear your hair four inches or shorter, this could lead to thinning hair in your future.

---

122 Pickart, Reverse Skin Aging: Using Your Skin's Natural Power, 117.
123 Rachel Bergsman, The Disaster Of Hair Loss: Take IT Easy, accessed June 19, 2010 http://www.articlesphere.com/Article/The-Disaster-Of-Hair-Loss--Take-It-Easy/27570.

Short hair is problematic in many ways. Short hair does not protect the scalp (skin) from the harsh chemicals in most shampoos, or the sun and other weathering and pollution affects. Because the hair is short, shampoo, overexposure to the sun, chemicals, and air-borne chemicals all have quick and easy access to the scalp, causing, as you will soon learn, inevitable skin damage or seborrhea. This inflammatory disease of the scalp is marked by the occurrence of an excessive discharge of sebum from the follicles forming white or yellowish, greasy scales or cheesy plugs within the follicles and on the scalp.

Understand that even the extraction of oil (called sebum) from the follicle is designed for longer hair. Consider this quote:

> The follicles of a man's head grow straight up; consequently, when oil is released from the scalp, it has no place to go. On a woman's head, it can slip down the hair shaft towards the end, on a man's head, it can only slide back to where it came from – the scalp.[124]

Well now, what is the real reason excess sebum builds up on a man's scalp? On a man's scalp *because the hair is cut too short*, the oil has no place to go except to buildup an excess amount on the scalp! The oil is designed to travel down the hair shaft of longer hair to protect the hair, scalp, and other parts of the head region. However, if the hair is too short, the oil builds-up on the scalp and in the follicle itself like wax, clogging the pores.[125] So after a hair is shed, the replacement hair cannot push through this waxy buildup within the follicle. If you think the answer is shampooing (especially with most store-bought products), think again and read *Scalp Trauma: Chemicals and Related Insults* chapter of this book, which explains how certain shampoos contribute to baldness. You will soon learn that short hair and over-shampooing are double jeopardy to a healthy scalp.

What is a man suppose to do? If your hair is short, the oil (sebum) can build up and cause hair loss. Short hair may also cause the hair to look oily since it has nowhere to go because the hair is not long enough for the

---

124 Accessed June 22, 2010 http://www.stophairloss.co.uk/ReasonsForHairLoss.htm This is from under the subheading: Causes of Hair Loss, where they list several reasons for hair loss. The reason for hair loss is a subject that no two doctors, scientist or clinics seem to be able to agree about, everyone seems to have their own opinion on the subject. See Explanation Two.

125 Riquette Hofstein, Grow Hair Fast – 7 Steps to a New Head of Hair in 90 Days (Naperville, Illinois: Sourcebooks, Inc. 2004), 21, 103.

amount of oil produced. Thus, you may be tempted to shampoo daily. But if you shampoo too much in an attempt to wash away the sebum, and with the wrong products, then this causes hair loss as well. Most shampoos add insult to injury. As you are beginning to see, the problems associated with short hair are great. Is it worth all these problems? In truth, the oil secreted by the sebaceous glands of the hair follicles is designed to anoint the hair and the skin of the head and neck to prevent damage.

If your scalp becomes unhealthy or damaged, then it cannot properly make hair. On the other hand, if your skin is healthy it will produce healthy hair. Do not despair. Even if your skin is damaged, there is hope. Once the skin is repaired, you have an excellent chance of re-growing your own hair. If you already have a healthy head of hair, future hair loss can be greatly reduced and even eliminated once you understand all the facts. To prevent hair loss you must follow the recommendations in this book: practice proper nutrition, exercise, use good shampoos (not store-bought products), grow longer hair, relax and reduce stress, and keep chemicals off your head.

Excessive hair cutting in modern times appears to be a revival of excessive hair cutting in ancient times. Several short-haired individuals of the past became bald. On the other hand, not everyone who wears short hair will go bald. It all depends on how healthy and pliable the connective tissue of a person's scalp remains over time. But for many, short hair can accelerate baldness, even those who begin life with a thick head of hair. A question that arises is why and when did men begin to cut their hair unnaturally short? This is an important question because of the unwarranted bias in much of the modern public against long hair.

Chapter 4: Shearing of the Sheep

||||||||||||||||||||||||||||||||||||||||||||||||||||||||||||||||||||||||||||||||||||||||||||||||||||||||||||||||||||||||||||||||||||||||||||||||||||||||||||||||||||||

Cut off thine hair, *O Jerusalem*, and cast it away, and take up a lamentation on high places; for the Lord hath rejected and forsaken the generation of his wrath (Jeremiah 7:29).

Mourning and Punishment

The origin of excessive hair cutting and shaving began in ancient times for the following reasons: (1) as a form of punishment; (2) as the mark of a slave; (3) in times of mourning; (4) as a religious ritual or idol worship; and (5) for military purposes. It seems to have begun in ancient Egypt.

In the Bible, baldness produced by shaving any portion of the head or face is forbidden. J.W. Kapp, author of "Baldness," says shaving "was practiced as a mark of mourning for the dead"[126] by certain peoples (e.g., Isaiah 15:2; 22:12); "as the result of any disaster" (Amos 8:10). Instead of shaving the head, some would actually pluck out the hair of their head and beard (Ezra 9:3). This would purposely cause an un-kept, disheveled, or even hideous appearance. "The custom [of hair removal] arose from the fact that the hair was regarded as a special ornament."[127] Thus, certain cultures thought it shameful for anyone to look "special" or "ornamented" in times of grief.

Even in modern times, reports circulated that some women who lost their husbands from the tragic World Trade Tower collapse in New York on September 11, 2001 cut off their hair. Renowned psychiatrist Dr. Karl

---

126 J.W. Kapp, "Baldness." The International Standard Bible Encyclopaedia, ed. James Orr, Vol. I. Hendrickson Publishers ed. 2nd Printing March 1996. 4 vols.

127 Kapp.

Menninger relates that cutting the hair to mourn the loss of a departed loved one is an act of "partial suicide."[128]

Baldness, or head shaving, was also instituted as a punishment against rogue nations and prisoners of war (Ezekiel 29:18). God's chosen people are strictly forbidden to practice head shaving and the hair was not to be cut in ways that mutilated the natural growth or its appearance (Leviticus 19:27; 21:5; Deuteronomy 14:1). Figuratively (e.g., see Jeremiah 47:5; Micah 1:16), baldness symbolizes the "barrenness" of a country.[129] Apparently, the physical barrenness of the head is somehow related to the spiritual emptiness of a country. Shaving and cutting the hair too short are processes of destruction. In fact, close-cropping the head is used symbolically or figuratively as the loss of something of great value (e.g., Micah 1:16).

Man Opposes Himself

> As the Lord liveth, there shall not one hair of thy son fall to the earth (2 Samuel 14:11; KJV).

During Old Testament time men and women both wore long hair and took great care in grooming their hair. It was not to be disheveled (Isaiah 3:24). On the practical side, because hair is strong, the Arunta tribesmen's hair was sometimes cut and made into string as stated in "The Secret Museum of Mankind."[130] At least this tribe considered hair a valuable commodity. But most hair-cutting seems to be a strange power struggle of man against man. In "The Histories" by Herodotus, he states that when the Argives were conquered, they:

> who before had worn their hair long by fixed custom, shaved their heads ever after and made a law, with a curse added to it, that no Argive grow his hair long ... until they recovered Thyreae; and the Lacedaemonians made a contrary law, that they wear their hair long ever after....[131]

---

128 Karl Menninger, Man Against Himself (New York: Harcourt, Brace & World, Inc., 1938) 244-245.
129 Kapp.
130 David Stiffler, ed., The Secret Museum of Mankind (Salt Lake City: Gibbs Smith Publisher, reprint edition 1999. New York: Manhattan House 1941?).
131 Herodotus, The Histories, Book 1, Chapter 82. A.D., ed. Godley, June 1, 2010 www.perceus.tufts.edu/hopper/ (Perceus Digital Library).

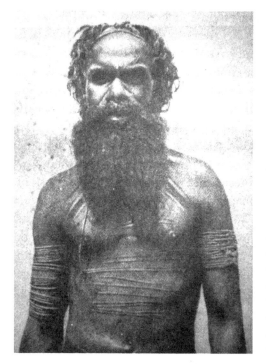

Figure 4-1: Arunta Tribesman. The hair of his head is shorter than his beard because he had to supply several fathers-in-law regularly with material for string-making. At least he is wise enough to leave a fair amount of hair on his head to avoid sunburn rather than crop it to the bone. Photograph from "The Secret Museum of Mankind," late 19th to early 20th century. Courtesy of David Stiffler.

In "Man Against Himself," Menninger acknowledges that cutting the hair is an act of "self-mutilation," and most people do it out of "deference to custom and convention."[132] Besides this, haircutting as a form of punishment, even self-punishment, is well established (Menninger; Rook and Dawber).[133][134] Rather than use hair for anything practical, not even to protect and shade the head, modernists simply cut it off and cast it away as a worthless thing. But head hair is valuable! When, where, and why did men begin to shave their faces and cut their hair terribly short?

Dr. Menninger goes on to say that the modern "widespread practice of shaving can be seen to be a deliberate cutting off of a part of the self."[135] So why cut a part of yourself away? Even back in 1913, Dr. Charles Jackson and Dr. Charles McMurtry determined that "physiologically, it is best not to shave, for if we do, we rob ourselves of a useful protection."[136] It gets

---

132 Menninger, 243.
133 Menninger, 245.
134 Arthur Rook and Rodney Dawber, eds., Diseases of the Hair and Scalp, 2nd Ed. (London: Blackwell Scientific Publications, 1991), 462.
135 Menninger, 244.
136 Charles T. Jackson and McMurtry, A. Treatise on Diseases of the Hair (London: Henry Kimpton, 1913), 56.

even worse. For "all hair removal methods" such as "tweezing" [plucking] and "shaving" "cause skin damage."[137] According to Dr. Pickart, these acts of hair removal allow viruses and bacteria to penetrate the skin. Warts then appear to have emerged from injured skin, such as the beard area of men. The shaving that was allowed was only on certain rare occasions, for instance at the end of a temporal Nazarite vow. The daily ritual of being so-called "clean shaven," as people do today, is foreign to design. The reasons God the designer of hair does not allow head shaving most of the time is for your health and a better outward appearance. This is because He is the Great Designer and Protector and knows full well that constant shaving and close-cutting can damage your face, neck and scalp (or crown). If you ever take the time to look at those who shave their beards or necks repeatedly, then you will see scars, pockmarks, warts and various other skin eruptions on the chin, cheeks, near the lips, or on the neck within the shaven areas of these men. Doing this daily means you can re-damage spots already damaged from the day before, even on a microscopic level. Is this truly what God wants?

Would you throw spears at your face? If you have tightly coiled hair, like those of African descent, or curly hair, you may be doing so. Razor-cut beard hairs act like sharp spear tips. When the spear-tips of razor-cut beard hairs curve back towards the skin, they perforate and damage your face.[138] The result is often permanent scarring. This nasty problem with beard removal is called barber's rash or pseudofolliculitis, which leaves unsightly scars. Is this what God had in mind? If you answered certainly not, you are correct. Bible scholar William Smith says it was a shame to lose the hair or beard, and to men of the East the beard is a badge of manhood and a mark of freedom.[139]

Those who force you to shave are violating and mutilating your appearance. Instead of the obvious solution of letting your beard come out from hiding, marketers invent all sorts of things to help you supposedly heal your damaged perforated skin, or help themselves through financial gain, depending on how you look at it. For example, Dinulos and Graham recommend shaving with an electric razor and applying "a depilatory

137 Loren Pickart, Reverse Skin Aging: Using Your Skin's Natural Power, (Bellevue, Washington: Cape San Juan Press, 2005), 122.

138 Rook and Dawber, 504.

139 William Smith, ed., A Concise Dictionary of the Bible, Comprising its Antiquities, Biography, Geography, and Natural History (Boston: Little, Brown, and Company, 1865).

chemical cream."[140] Halder's suggestion is intralesional injections of steroid and a topical chloramphenicol and steroid cream mixture. He also says scars or other severe lesions may require surgery.[141] So basically the experts' answers are chemicals, steroids and surgery! I would like to echo what television personality John Stossel often says: "give me a break"! How could the pagan custom of shaving have become so important? This is complete stupidity. Has America gone mad?

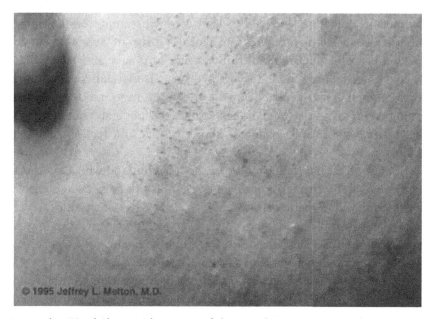

© 1995 Jeffrey L. Melton, M.D.

Figure 4-2: Toad Skin or Flat Warts of the Beard Region. Is toad skin attractive? According to Pickart, warts emerge from damaged skin areas caused by shaving. Men shave these warts repeatedly inflicting further damage. Young men also have the problem of shaving acne pimples along with whiskers - is this a good thing to do? Life would be easier for men if they let, or were allowed to let, their beard grow. Photograph courtesy of Jeffrey L. Melton, M.D. (drmelton.com).

The "Dermatologic Disease Database, the American Osteopathic College of Dermatology" indicates that a "100 percent effective treatment

---

140 James G. Dinulos and Graham, Elinor A. "Self Teaching Module for the Influence of Culture and Pigment on Skin Conditions in Children, Category IV: Conditions Common in Adolescents and Young Adulthood, Photo 30: Pseudofolliculitis Barbae," accessed January 16, 2007 http://ethnomed.org/clin_topics/dermatology/pigment30html.

141 R.M. Halder, "Pseudofolliculitis barbae and related disorders," Dermatol Clin. 1988 Jul;6(3):407-12, PMID 3048823 accessed January 16, 2007 http://www.ncbi.nlm.nih.gov/entrez/query.fcgi?db=pubmed&cmd=Retrieve&dopt=AbstractPlus&list_uids...

is to let the beard grow."[142] Now that is a novel idea. Besides, a beard will not disfigure your face. It is far less expensive to maintain. And listen to this. In spite of the thousands of television commercials telling men to shave, surveys indicate an opposing view. Rook and Dawber report that most studies indicate that most people like beards. Even at a so-called "conservative university" in 1977, 55 percent of females prefer men with some facial hair.[143] Females have often commented to me personally, "what's the big deal about a little facial hair," and "I never understood why men are forced to shave." This later comment came from a woman who was also receiving pressure from a local "Christian" school to cut off her son's beautiful locks. Thankfully, for her son's sake and Jesus' sake, she told the shallow school "no." Based on personal experience, some females may prefer trimmed beards. But bare in mind, facial hair must be long enough so that the hairs are soft and do not stab your woman's face. Hairs ¼ of an inch or longer should suffice and feel soft enough for the touch.

Brian Thomas has understood that the "Creator God who appreciates beauty and wants others to appreciate His handiwork must be responsible for the origin of aesthetic features. Men have beards - some thick, some sparse - because it pleased God to adorn them so." It is the male brain that instructs the body to make the beard. "The hypothalamus produces surges of gonadotropin-releasing hormone, a small chemical that acts like a key to turn on the manufacture and export of follicle-stimulating hormone and leutenizing hormone (LH) from the pituitary gland." Hair follicles then build terminal hair in "certain areas of the body" including "beards."[144]

The Assyrians took away much that belonged to Israel - *cutting off the hair and shaving the beard* was used figuratively as a symbol for this destructive act (Isaiah 7:20). Not only did the ancients consider cutting off the hair as an act of destruction, it nearly always was associated with other forms of negativity. It is most interesting to note that in ancient times shaved heads or hair cut off short, akin to a shaved head, was the mark of a slave, criminal, mourner, or one who worshiped false gods (Table 4-1). In the latter, one could easily conclude that really short hair became a symbol of pagan idolatry.

---

142 "Pseudofolliculitis Barbae" Dermatologic Disease Database, American Osteopathic College of Dermatology, accessed June 22, 2010 http://www.aocd.org/skin/dermatologic_diseases/pseudofolliculitis.html.

143 Rook and Dawber, 462.

144 Brian Thomas, "The Apobetics of Aesthetics: A Hairy Problem for Evolution," accessed May 29, 2010 http://www.icr.org/article/apobetics-aesthetics-hairy-problem-for-evolution/.

Table 4-1: Reasons the Ancients Cut Off their Hair or Beards

Who/Where	Reason(s) Why
Egyptian Travelers	Shaved their heads as a thank-offering to their god at the end of a journey
Greek youths	Offered their hair to the local river upon reaching manhood
Arabia and Syria	Cut the hair as a puberty rite
Rome	Cut the hair as a puberty rite to some local deity
Roman sailors	Offered their hair to the sea god
Nero	Dedicated his first beard to Jupiter
Criminals and slaves everywhere	Cut hair to distinguish them from the free man
India and among the ancient Teutons	Cut off hair as a punishment for adultery
Assyro-Babylonians	Cut off hair as a punishment for several offences
Several Cultures as an act of mourning	Cut hair as an act of partial suicide

Information in **Table 4-1** was compiled from p. 244-245 of "Man Against Himself," (Menninger).

Who, in modern times, would have thought that in times past, ultra-short hair or a shaved head was the mark of a mourner or slave? Obviously, most seem to wear their hair as a matter of personal taste or style. Many young people today merely mimic pop culture and have no idea about the significance and importance of hair. The issue of unnaturally short hair and slavery is most interesting. There were two types of slaves, voluntary and involuntary. Voluntary slaves became servants out of their free will. For the most part this was the form of slavery in ancient Judaism. William Rafferty describes the situation: "the slavery of Judaism was not the cruel system of Greece, Rome and later nations."[145] For the purposes of this writing, "slave" refers to the Roman-type, those individuals forced into slavery without their consent.

---

145   William E. Rafferty, "Slave, Slavery," The International Standard Bible Encyclopaedia, ed. James Orr, Vol. IV. Hendrickson Publishers ed. 2nd Printing March 1996. 4 vols.

However, it should be stated at the offset: "Christ's life and teaching were against … any form of human slavery."[146] In short, Jesus came to free people from bondage, even slavery from themselves.

Ancient Egypt

Around 2000 B.C. the "upper classes" in ancient Egypt shaved their own heads and wore fake beards and wigs.[147] A little later, perhaps the 18th century B.C., when Joseph was released from the dungeon, he shaved himself and came before the Pharaoh (Genesis 41:14). But how or why did this Egyptian head shaving begin? It is well known that the Egyptians descended from Noah's son, Ham.[148] Proof of Ham's spiritual barrenness is well known (Genesis 9:20-27). Although speculative, it could be that Ham, after Noah cursed many of his descendents, cut off or shaved his own hair as an act of partial suicide or self-punishment, a symbol of self-destruction. This head-shaving idea would then naturally spread downward to Ham's descendents, the ancient Egyptians. But it is also evident that Egypt became a very religious culture of an idolatrous sort.

Long-haired scholar Albert Pike, in his "Morals and Dogma," informs us that the priesthood possessed one-third of the whole of Egypt.[149] Those who refused to be initiated were considered profane and unworthy of public employment. The Egyptians worshipped the goddess Isis, who is also known as Ceres, Venus, Diana, and Proserpine in other cultures. The goddess was considered to have "royal hair," which is described as "long thick hair hung in graceful ringlets."[150] The hair of female initiates was handled with great care by being perfumed and enveloped in a protective "transparent covering." However, males initiated into this goddess worship "were thoroughly shaven, and their bald heads shone exceedingly."[151] They must have looked like a collection of bowling pins, each one looking the same without any distinct identity. A belief that long hair is the glory of women only may stem from goddess worship.

---

146 Rafferty.

147 Ann Charles and Roger DeAnfrasio, The History of Hair (New York: Bonanza Books, 1970).

148 P.V.N. Myers, A General History for Colleges and High Schools (Boston and London: Ginn & Company Publishers, 1893), 7.

149 Albert Pike, Morals and Dogma of the Ancient and Accepted Scottish Rite of Freemasonry, 1871. The Supreme Council of the Southern Jurisdiction, A.A.S.R., U.S.A., 1906. (Richmond, Virginia: L.H. Jenkins, Inc., reprinted March 1947), 374.

150 Pike, 387.

151 Pike, 388.

So here we have male hair removal in an act of female worship, which is idolatry. This is nearly what is going on in America now. Apparently, when the long-haired Hebrews grew in population in Egypt they would not stoop so low as to worship the goddess or any other idol. The act of hair sacrifice to Isis would have been a move away from God the Creator. Naturally, the bald-headed Egyptian priesthood would have condemned the Hebrews as profane. After all, the Hebrews who lived in Egypt would have refused to worship their goddess. Part of the Egyptian plot then was to refuse the Hebrews fair employment, thus they became slaves (Exodus). But to the ancient Hebrews, it was the Egyptians who were really the ones in bondage with their worship of false gods and goddesses. Ironically, the Egyptians were even cursed with a plague of lice, which no doubt induced continued head shaving (Exodus 8:16-18).

Besides the Egyptians, it appears that all others in ancient times wore long hair, as God created it to be. It was not until several centuries later when forced hair elimination occurred on a larger scale. This is in conjunction with the rise of certain Greek and Roman tyrants. Up until this time, men of the West, just like those of the East, wore long hair and beards and their women enjoyed them too. As quite apparent, the beard did not hinder procreation otherwise, none of us would be here.

Speaking of the Hebrews, the only time God required some hair trimming was with a specialized group of priests, the sons of Zadok (Ezekiel 44:20). Here these men were told not to shave their heads or let their hair grow long. But if one would read the rest of the story, these guys were not to do anything that caused sweat (Ezekiel 44:18). They were told to trim their hair but no particular length is mentioned. Certainly the length would not have been unnaturally short (shorter than body hair), otherwise the head, ears and neck would not be protected. More than likely their hair was not allowed past the shoulders. The rule for these particular priests was never intended as a guide for all men at all places at all times.

The Rise of Greco-Roman Tyrannies

> Make thyself bald, and crop thy hair [cut off short] for the children of thy delight; make a wide baldness on thy head like a vulture; for they [your children] are exiled from thee (Micah 1:16).[152]

---

152 The Jerusalem Bible, (Jerusalem: Koren Publishers, 2000). This "Jerusalem Bible" version has the same name as, and must not be confused with the Roman Catholic's "Jerusalem Bible" (JB) quoted extensively in this book.

Long hair prevailed up until the 5th century B.C. or the time of Pericles, about 450 B.C. Then "it became customary for men [many in Athens and some other Greek cities] to wear their hair cut short and their beards trimmed."[153] But how did this change come about? In the 13th century B.C., Theseus, the legendary hero of Athens, clipped only the "fore part" of his head.[154] Presumably "fore part" means the bangs that fall upon the forehead. Theseus got this idea from another Greek tribe, the Abantes. Plutarch describes the Abantes as an exceedingly warlike brood used to close fighting above all other nations. Therefore, they cut their forelocks in this manner so their enemies could not grab them by the hair. Later, Theseus was accused of robbing men of their freedom by "having pent them all up in one city" and "using them as his subjects and slaves."[155] It is interesting to note that once the hair goes, so does the rest of freedom. Thus, from the beginning, Athens evolved into a society of great stress. This is in stark contrast to another Greek settlement, Sparta, under the leadership of Lycurgus, to be discussed in the following chapter. However, it should be pointed out that Theseus of Athens did not practice overkill against the scalp by cutting all his hair short, only the "fore part" or bangs were cut.

It even appears that Rome was founded by a long-haired individual. In the 8th century B.C. Romulus, the legendary father of the Romans, is described as having "flowing hair" crowned with a laurel garland.[156] Presumably, "flowing hair" means a full length, perhaps even long by scientific measurement. However, the Romans beginning with Romulus became very fond of sacred rites and divination. In their practice of divination, the vulture (a bird with a bald or naked head and neck – Figure 4-3) became the most highly regarded of all birds.[157] His successor, Numa Pompilius, was equally religious with respect to idol worship. He ordained many orders of priests. Among these were the "vestal virgins," whose hair was veiled and who were to remain virgin for 30 years. If that vow was broken, the females were "buried alive," a practice lasting centuries.[158] Besides forced celibacy, other not-so-friendly female customs were also handed down by Numa. Girls as

153 Howard F. Vos, Nelson's New Illustrated Bible Manners and Customs, (Nashville, Tennessee: Thomas Nelson Publishers, 1999), 571.

154 Plutarch, "The Lives of the Noble Grecians and Romans," Great Books of the Western World, vol. 14, ed. Robert Maynard Hutchins, (London: Encyclopaedia Britannica: William Benton, Publisher, 1952), 2.

155 Plutarch, 13.

156 Plutarch, 22.

157 Plutarch, 19.

158 Plutarch, 54, 149.

young as twelve years in age were simply delivered to their future husbands. Adult females did not have much of a life either. Another custom arose where women were not permitted to speak except in their husbands company only, even on the most ordinary subjects.[159] Then during one of his prayers a thought came to Numa concerning male hair.

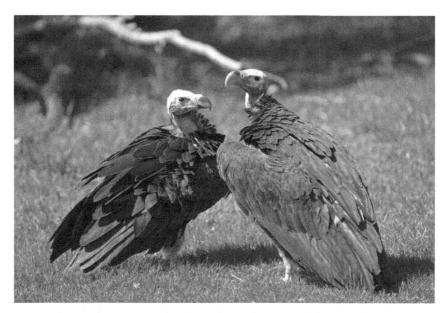

Figure 4-3: Vultures. The most highly regarded bird of the Romans. Look how the naked head and neck emerge from a well-clothed body. By their very nature these birds represent death. "Wherever the corpse is, there the vultures will gather" (Matthew 24:28, NEB).

The god, or demon, depending how you look at it, Jupiter was believed to tell Numa that "heads" are needed to "charm the thunder and lightning." Numa thought Jupiter meant "the hairs of men's heads."[160] Jupiter's answer was no, he wanted their heads literally. This was a way of telling Numa that blood must be shed. And the best way to come up with all these "heads" was to go out and conquer. In Numa's mind, the sacrifice of hair represented a symbolic act of death or partial suicide. So here we have, in the early history of Rome, 8th to 7th century B.C., hair being offered as a sacrifice to the gods as a substitute for the whole person. This is a most interesting sacrifice. While Roman leaders sacrificed their hair, Roman soldiers, pawns and conquered foe sacrificed their very lives for the sake of empire. Now let's turn back to Greece.

---

159 Plutarch, 63.
160 Plutarch, 57.

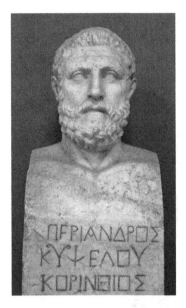

Figure 4-4: Periander, 627 - 585 B.C. He was the 2nd tyrant of Corinth. The advent of unnaturally short hair in Greece, probably due to ritualistic sacrifice, began in Corinth. Most other Greek cities at the time wore their hair naturally long, as per God's design.

Apparently, much hearsay and networking occurred between the Greeks and Romans. Although more prominent in Greek cities beginning in the 5th century B.C., short hair was already being worn in Corinth, not very long after Numa's idea of hair sacrifice. When the Bacchiadæ of Corinth fled to Lacedæmon in 657 B.C., the long haired Spartans were appalled at their appearance. In their view, these Corinthian men "looked mean and unsightly, having their heads all close cut."[161] Close-cropped short hair, similar to many modern men, can be seen in the stone image of Periander, the 2nd tyrant of Corinth (627 to 585 B.C.) (Figure 4-4). This short-haired idea eventually spread to Pericles, who usurped the Athenian throne from long-haired Cimon around 462 B.C.[162] Besides their unsightly appearance, many Greek men began to bald shortly after the new short-haired look spread during the 5th century B.C. The connection between short hair and rampant baldness is real, and close-cropped heads are quite appalling, some with oddly shaped skulls are even downright hideous as they disfigure their hair and even teach others to do the same. Hair hides a lumpy head.

Male hair elimination and treating women like property were contrary to the institutions of the long haired Spartans. Under the laws of Lycurgus, women were free to speak their opinions in public and openly, even on the most important subjects.[163] Many changes were taking place in Greece

161 Plutarch, 354.
162 Plutarch, 121.
163 Plutarch, 63.

during the 5th century B.C. under Pericles. Barber shops cropped up throughout the city. The Persians bribed Thebes and Athens inciting both states against Sparta. During this civil war, the Spartan, Gylippus, was mocked for his "staff and long hair."[164] Nevertheless, a great army followed Gylippus, for in him "they saw the badge and authority of Sparta, and crowded to him accordingly." The Spartans did not mind being out of style with the Athenians. Lysander of Sparta (~445 – 395 B.C.) upheld the customs instituted by Lycurgus and wore long hair and an ample beard even though it was suddenly "after the old fashion."[165] Although not in fashion with the Athenians and Corinthians, the Spartans resistance to short hair kept them from going bald. But the same cannot be said for those in other Greek cities.

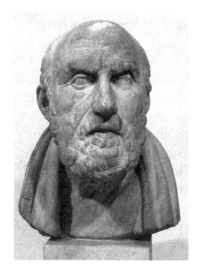

Figure 4-5: Chrysippos, 279 - 206 B.C.. As Short hair was introduced to much of Greek culture in the 5th century B.C., baldness followed. By 400 B.C., the study of baldness began with Hippocrates. © The Trustees of the British Museum, used with permission.

Baldness became more rampant. For example, the bust of Æschylus (525 - 456 B.C.) shows a bald crown.[166] Images of Socrates (469 – 399 B.C.) indicate thinning hair. And Chrysippos who lived during the third century B.C. is as bald as 21st century man (Figure 4-5). When their busts are examined all of these men appear to be in their 50s when their stone images were sculpted. Thus, it could be argued that perhaps their baldness was related to hormonal ravages or prostate issues. This is certainly possible. However, most archaeological finds of other men, young or old suggest that baldness was very rare in the centuries before the advent of short hair, or

---

164 Plutarch, 433.
165 Plutarch, 354.
166 Myers.

in those who still wore long hair. The truth is that baldness seems to have accelerated rapidly along with this new short-haired look.

Ironically, the "study of baldness" coincides with the advent of short hair! Valcović found that the "study of baldness dates from the observations of Hippocrates (circa 400 B.C.)."[167] This date is remarkable! For Hippocrates' "study of baldness" began only 50 years after short hair became more widespread in Greece, beginning with Pericles in 450 B.C.![168] Apparently, by 400 B.C., baldness became so prevalent in young and old that it was now a subject for "study." The simple solution to baldness was right before their very eyes - the long haired Spartans, the long haired Hebrews, the long haired Assyrians, the long haired Persians, and no doubt, some of their own citizens. Baldness was very rare with those long haired groups. As far as we know, Hippocrates and his students or companions never realized the connection between balding and short hair. Natural baldness occurs in conjunction with the advent of short hair, which naturally leads to scalp damage, even scalp death. After 2,400 years of baldness, is it not time to stop the ignorance? Hopefully by now, you understand that more is at work besides the common belief that baldness is caused by heredity.

Pressure against male hair continued to mount in the 4th century B.C. Plutarch says Archibiades, a general of Athens who preferred Spartan ways, had a "huge, overgrown beard." When he disagreed politically with Phocion (~402 – 317 B.C.), Phocion lashed out telling Archibiades that he "should shave."[169] Apparently, those who focus on one's outward appearance do not know how to deal with real issues of the heart. But at least leaders were not required to cut off their hair or shave at this time. However, shaving the beard began to be enforced to a higher level under Alexander the Great beginning in 328 B.C.

In James Ussher's "The Annals of the World," it is recorded that in 328 B.C. "Alexander assumed divinity and affirmed that he was the son of Zeus. He was no longer to be addressed in the Macedonian custom, but would be adored with prostration." Three years later, his apparent best friend Hephaestion died prematurely due to alcoholism. To lament the loss, Alexander shaved himself and ordered that "all the soldiers and even the horses and mules be totally shorn." He wanted everyone and everything

---

167 Vlado Valković, Human Hair. Vol. 1: Fundamentals and Methods for Measurement of Elemental Composition (Boca Raton, Florida: CRC Press, Inc., 1988), 25.
168 Vos, 571.
169 Plutarch, 608-612.

to "look poorly" as a sign "to lament and bewail his death."[170] It was the manes of the horses he had shaved, for the former beautiful appearance was to look "bald at his funeral."[171] Again, we see baldness instituted in times of grief - people were to look loathsome. Some say that in general, Alexander "had his Greek soldiers shave so that opponents could not grasp them by the beard."[172] Indeed, in 992 B.C. it is recorded that Joab grasped Amasa's long beard and killed him by the sword (2 Samuel 20:9-10). But why shave the face as smooth as a woman? A short beard cannot be grabbed.

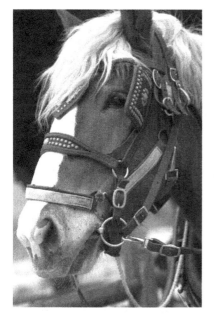

Figure 4-6: Clydesdale Horse with Long Beautiful Mane. The majestic mane was the primary target to be shaved off during Alexander's wrath while he mourned the death of Hephaestion. It is also a reminder that hair length has nothing to do with distinction between the sexes of any creature. Arguably, it is much easier to tell the difference between male and female humans, even if both have long hair, than it is to tell the difference between male and female animals at first glance.

Alexander and others in his service, such as Ptolemy I, wore hair down to the base of his neck or tops of the shoulders. Using the shoulder region as a dividing area between long and short hair is more in line scientifically than the prevailing modern view instilled in the minds of Americans via the military cut. Images of Alexander also show the hair around the face, the bangs, to be trimmed such as not to interfere with the eyes. Modernists, or better, those with shorn heads similar to the Corinthians, have erroneously called Alexander's shoulder-length hair "long." But in truth, long hair, by

---

170 James Ussher, The Annals of the World, ed. Larry and Marion Pierce (Green Forest, Arkansas: Master Books, 2003), paragraphs 2,305-2,312.

171 Plutarch, 245.

172 Joseph T. Shipley, "Barbarian." Dictionary of Word Origins, second ed. (New York: The Philosophical Library, 1945).

scientific measure, is that which hangs down the back, not merely to the shoulders. Alexander's hair was long enough to at least protect the head, ears and neck, but short enough so it did not interfere with his eyes during times of combat. On the other hand, a simple headband would keep long hair out of the eyes as it did with many long-haired warriors.

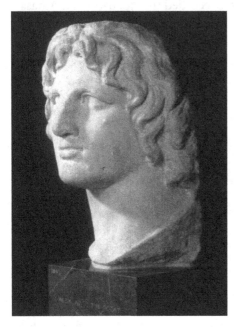

Figure 4-7: Alexander the Great, 356 - 323 B.C. Note the hair length over the ears but barely to the tops of the shoulders. His hair is called "long" by the accompanying description at The British Museum. Alexander's four-to-six–inch-length hairs shown here are hardly "long" by scientific measure at all. But at least his hair is at a sufficient length to protect the scalp, ears, and neck from damage. Obviously, he, like anyone who spends time outdoors, knew it was far better to have some hair rather than a scorched sunburned head. This leads to scalp damage, baldness and skin cancer, the consequences of a shorn head. © The Trustees of the British Museum, used with permission.

The present day, widespread practice of shaving the beard seems to have been handed down from Alexander. His so-called "clean-shaven" image, which implies that beards are dirty, became an object of worship. This idea contrasts greatly with the God of nature, who designed nearly all men to have some facial hair, albeit with various designs thereof. Not everyone is designed with the same type of beard, which is part of God's great variety amongst men. But as this new fashion spread, many men opted to let their beards show anyway. Some, like the ancient Persians, considered the shaven face an absurdity.[173] But the new, shaven Greek face could have been a symbolic cut against the Persians as "Persian garb" was being "displaced."[174] In reality, shaven Greek faces were physical cuts against themselves.

---

173 D.M. Podolsky, Skin: the human fabric (The Human Body) (Tarrytown, New York: Torstar Books, Inc., 1984), 94.

174 Victor Matthews, Manners and Customs in the Bible, third ed. (Peabody, MA: Hendrickson, 2006), 205.

Obviously, business-minded individuals saw this new, clean-shaven image as a way to make lots of money. So elimination of the beard caused barbering to expand even more. Barbering spread from Greece into Sicily, then to Rome. In 297 B.C., Sicilian barbers landed in Rome and started a "fashion of clean-shaveness."[175] Barbers lured men to their shops with food, wine, and female attendants.[176] Shipley informs us that a "conservative" named Cato attacked the Roman custom of shaving as being "foreign, and effeminate."[177] If you care to think about it, Cato is right. He saw the liberal use of the razor and shaving as a form of emasculation. Nevertheless, really short hair and shaved faces endured more than 400 years in Rome until about the second century A.D. Then, beginning roughly in the year A.D. 117, beards, and hair a little longer, were worn by the Romans.[178]

As all true scholars know, the ancient Israelites "extolled" long hair on males.[179][180] However, in the 2nd century B.C., Hebrew men felt pressured to cut off their hair. It is recorded in *1 Maccabees* of the "Apocrypha" that after Alexander died his officers began to rule, followed by their sons. "From them came forth a sinful root, Antiochus Epiphanes" (1 Maccabees 1:10) who reigned from 175 to 164 B.C. This murderer of women and infants (e.g., 1 Maccabees 1:60-61) wrote to "his whole kingdom that all should be one people, and that each should give up his customs" .... Or "die" (1 Maccabees 1:41-42;50). His whole kingdom included a vast amount of the Middle East, including Jerusalem. His "one people" were to be unified in language, religion, culture, and "even dress."[181]

To be perfectly in line with the image of their dictator, this no doubt caused many of the Jews to cut off their hair really short and shave. The image of Antiochus III, the father of Antiochus Epiphanies, depicts short hair, similar to many moderns, and no beard.[182] Jason, high priest at this

175 Podolsky, 94.

176 Charles and DeAnfrasio, 65.

177 Shipley.

178 Alf Henrikson, Through the Ages, An Illustrated Chronicle of Events from 2000 BC to the Present (New York: Crescent Books, 1983.)

179 Vergilius Ferm, ed., An Encyclopedia of Religion (New York: The Philosophical Library, 1945.)

180 H.L.E. Luering, "Hair," The International Standard Bible Encyclopaedia, James Orr, ed., Vol. II. (Hendrickson Publishers ed. 2nd Printing March 1996. 4 vols.)

181 Quotes from 1 Maccabees from The Oxford Annotated Bible with the Apocrypha, Revised Standard Version, Herbert G. May and Bruce M. Metzger, eds. (New York: Oxford University Press, 1965).

182 J.E. Harry, "Antiochus III," The International Standard Bible Encyclopaedia, James Orr, ed., Vol. 1 (Hendrickson Publishers ed. 2nd Printing March 1996. 4 vols.)

time, forced Jewish nobility to wear a "broad-brimmed hat" associated with allegiance to the Greek god Hermes.[183] Many Jews did succumb to the pressure and adopted the Greco-Roman custom of dress, including shaving and cropping the hair rather close, too close. God's protection, head hair, was removed and they were given a broad-brimmed hat as a cheap substitute. Apparently, the wide-brimmed hat, as a probable hair substitute, meant they were now under Hermes' protection, which is really man-made protection. As a result, many of these Jews go bald up to the present time. If you recall the scalp atrophy problem from the last chapter, baldness can affect anyone of any race or nation if the hair is cut too short. Their former healthy heads of long hair were now gone. This is how and when, 2nd century B.C., some of the Jews lost their hair and beards. Now let us turn our attention to Rome during the 1st century B.C. and learn what was happening there.

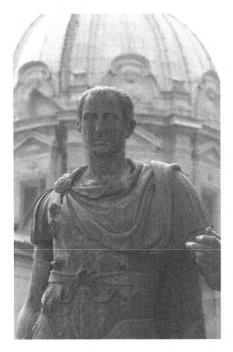

Figure 4-8: Julius Caesar, ~ 100 - 44 B.C. This statue is located in Rome, Italy. Note the short hair and receding hairline. He was going bald and the primary causes were, no doubt, short hair and stress due to fighting, warring, and his overall lust for power. The Romans often plucked out the beard … ouch! Who taught these guys to hate their own beards? Remarkably, in the 8th century B.C., the prophet Isaiah foretold that Christ would suffer at the hands of the beard pluckers, and this was long before beard-plucking became standard practice for many Roman men (Isaiah 50:6).

When Julius Caesar subdued the Gauls (~ 60 B.C.), "who esteemed long hair as a distinct honor," Caesar "required them to cut their hair as a token of submission."[184] The Gauls were right. Long hair is a distinct

183 Matthews, 205.

184 Raj Kumar Singh, "The significance of male hair – Its presence and removal," The Backlash! July 1998, Valparaiso University, accessed September 3, 2003 http://www. choisser.com/longhair/rajsingh.html.

honor, a blessing from God. All the historical evidence affirms this. But along with many other Romans, short-haired Julius Caesar himself became bald.[185] He very well may have lost his hair due to atrophy of the scalp caused by his short hair. Short hair naturally leads to unnecessary sun exposure, which probably caused additional damage to his pate (Figure 4-8). Perhaps Caesar felt that since he lost his hair, no one else should be allowed to have it. Ironically, Caesar got permission from the Roman senate to wear his laurel wreath at all times to hide his baldness. In effect the laurel wreath became his new hair (a wig?), part of his self.

There are other interesting accounts concerning Julius Caesar and the symbolism of hair. Cato, the younger, withstood the tyrant Caesar, who vied for world domination. He told the senate that "it was not the Britons or the Gauls they need fear, but Caesar himself, if they were wise."[186] Cato was like a lone prophet that foretold quite accurately Caesar's real intentions of tyranny. This act of political incorrectness caused Cato to be exiled. From that day Cato "never cut his hair, nor shaved his beard" … for he was "always full of sadness, grief, and dejectedness for the calamities of his country." In like manner, when Caesar joined Clodius to impeach Cicero from the Senate, Cicero grew out his hair as well. At least 20,000 young men followed Cicero in like manner as they supplicated to the people.[187] Thus, during the 1st century B.C. in Rome, untrimmed or long hair was an outward sign of grief or one ashamed. This is completely opposed to the view of ancient times when cutting off the hair or shaving the beard was the outward sign of mourning or one who was shamed. God never changed His plan for hair, man did. In fact, physically speaking, the new image (super short hair and a shaved face) forced on man is 180 degrees out of phase, for it diametrically opposes God's own design in nature.

In summary, long hair was designed for both sexes as a great ornament, was worn by all, and a great variety of hair types could be seen on individuals as unique persons. Cutting and shaving head hair began as a form of punishment, idol worship, mourning, and warring factions. For the military, only some hair cutting was done initially. Then, in the 7th century B.C., super short hair was seen on the men of Corinth. The practice of excessive hair cutting seems to have originated there. By the 5th century B.C., this idea became more widespread in Athens and elsewhere in Greece. Beards were still being worn. During the 4th century B.C.,

---

185 Podolsky, 95.
186 Plutarch, 640.
187 Plutarch, 716.

under Alexander the Great, shoulder length hair was worn but beards were shaved. Alexander's barely shoulder length hair could be called "long" by Corinthian standards, but was not "long" when compared to the ancients, and is not "long" by scientific measurement. Short hair and shaved faces spread to Rome at the start of the 3rd century B.C. By the 2nd and 1st centuries B.C. pressure against males to be shorn, or else, mounted. The weak-willed succumbed easily to this new system of uniformity, even though the new image is exceedingly unnatural.

Political nonconformists during 1st century B.C. Rome grew their hair long in an act of grief or shame against the rise of tyranny. No doubt, conformists began to see long hair as a symbol of rebellion against the State or empire. Unfortunately, Roman customs were passed throughout Europe, brought into the modern era, and into organized religion, even the churches. Much of the world now is of a Roman-type.

Everyone living in the so-called "civilized" Roman type worlds then come to believe that men are *supposed* to have short hair and women are *supposed* to have long hair. Beliefs like this are accomplished through coercive systematic education and training. Young boys and girls growing up would observe daily that males wore short hair, though by much force, even though they are designed with long hair, and females wore long hair. Suddenly, a man with his natural growth of long hair could have been pre-judged as a rebel, or uncivilized, or some other nonsense. So it was "by New Testament times, under the influence of the Greeks and Romans, hair was worn short".[188]

---

188 The Family Encyclopedia of the Bible, Pat Alexander, John W. Drane, David Field, and Alan Millard, eds. (London: Chancellor Press, 1988), 203.

Chapter 5: Our Long Haired Ancestors

///

For thou hast made him [man] a little lower than the angels, and hast crowned him with glory and honour (Psalm 8:5, KJV).

Ancient Times

Our long-haired ancestors had healthy heads of hair. "The International Standard Bible Encyclopaedia" informs us that the ancient Assyrians, Babylonians, and Hebrews "affected long and well-cared-for, bushy curls of hair as emblems of manly beauty" and the proofs of this occur frequently "in the Scriptures and elsewhere" (Figure 5-1).[189]

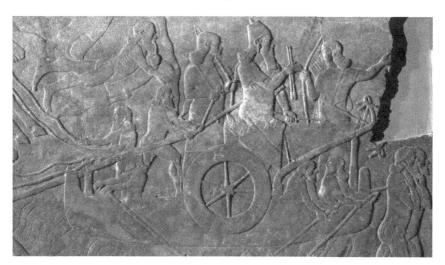

Figure 5-1: Long-Haired Assyrians. © The Trustees of the British Museum, used with permission.

---

189 H.L.E. Luering, "Hair," The International Standard Bible Encyclopaedia, James Orr, ed., Vol. II (Hendrickson Publishers ed. 2nd Printing March 1996. 4 vols.).

In fact, proof is found everywhere. All the evidence and beliefs passed along from the beginning of creation and down through all the centuries indicate that men wore long hair. As John Calvin said the ancients wore "long hair," and certain poets referred to them as the "unshorn."[190] The evidence is found in archaeology, various verbal legends, and in various ancient to more modern historical documents, including the many books which comprise the Bible. In ancient times cutting the hair was neither a consideration nor was it a priority in life. On the contrary, hair was considered a person's natural crown. According to Kapp, head hair has some spiritual connection "concerning the future life."[191] Recall, hair is built to last and is much tougher to destroy than bare flesh. In fact, it is so long-lasting that it seems to be an enduring symbol of eternity. The Creator has done everything possible to show that mankind is indeed the crown of creation. Our hair even "continues to briefly grow after death" symbolizing "a person's life-force and strength!"[192] We are designed to have a crown of long hair. In contrast, modern man has done everything humanly possible to destroy it.

Adam

In Louis Ginzberg's "Legends of the Bible," it says that Absalom had the hair of Adam, the first man. Later in this chapter we will discuss Absalom's hair in more detail. To summarize, after only one year of growth, Absalom's hair was greater than three feet in length and weighed nearly four pounds! It is believed Adam's hair could grow equally as fast and long. Apparently, both men had a long growth phase (anagen period). Thus, Adam had long hair and many other outstanding physical attributes that no other man of a later generation could compare.[193] After all, Adam was created directly by the Creator Himself. As all serious students of Scripture know, Adam was created as a mature young adult.[194] Even a cursory reading by a novice of the Book of Genesis, Chapters 1 and 2, would indicate that this is so.

---

190 John Calvin, Commentary on the Epistles of Paul the Apostle to the Corinthians, ed. Rev. John Pringle, Volume First (Grand Rapids, Michigan: Wm. B. Eerdmans Publishing Company, 1948).

191 J.W. Kapp, "Baldness," The International Standard Bible Encyclopaedia, ed. James Orr, Vol. I (Hendrickson Publishers ed. 2nd Printing March 1996. 4 vols).

192 David Fontana, The Secret Language of Symbols (London: Duncan Baird Publishers, 2001), 127.

193 Louis Ginzberg, Legends of the Bible, 1st paperback ed. 1992 (Philadelphia and Jerusalem: Jewish Publication Society), 31.

194 Henry M. Morris and John D. Morris, The Modern Creation Trilogy, Vol. 1 Scripture and Creation (Green Forest, Arkansas: Master Books, 1996), 87.

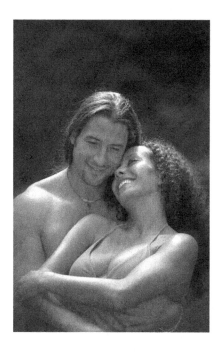

Figure 5-2: Couple in Paradise. This is a reminder of our first parents, Adam and Eve, in the Garden of Eden. A good, long natural head of hair or crown is what the Creator designed for both sexes.

In modern times, Adam is oftentimes depicted in children's books as a white, bare-faced man with very short cranial hair. Although we do not know what Adam looked like, it is doubtful that any of these physical attributes were true. Most people on earth today are mid-brown in color, not light brown, whites, and not dark brown, blacks. Since Adam was created with a mature adult body, then it naturally follows that his head hair would have been created at a mature functioning length just like the rest of his body hairs. A mature length of cranial hair would be quite long in fact, a length that far surpasses the length of his mature body hairs. By simple observation of long-haired men, a mature head of hair on Adam could have been one or two feet in length. And yet he is rarely shown as having hair even six inches in length, or even three inches in length. On the contrary, Adam is shown in some children's books as having hair shorter than even underarm hair, which grows to about two inches in length (Table 2-1). This unnaturally short hair, for the first man, is quite absurd and is based upon modern day ideas rather than reality. Ginzberg is right. Adam had long hair.

Noah

Several generations later, Noah, according to the Book of Enoch, a book mentioned and quoted in the New Testament (Jude 1:14-15), is said to have had long, white hair, like wool. He is depicted as resembling the angels of heaven.[195] As is well known, wool is thick hair and often curly. This is the same type of hair seen on Jesus when he appears to John several decades after the resurrection (Revelation 1:14). Hair, white as wool, symbolizes "Wisdom" or the "Ancient of Days."[196] Presumably, angel hair pasta is named after the hair of angels. And Noah was wise. For he listened to God and saved his family and all types of land-dwelling, air-breathing creatures from the Great Flood by building an enormous wooden ship, the ark (Genesis 6). The rest perished during the cataclysm while much marine life and other creatures and plants became fossilized in the geologic record.

A Few Centuries After the Flood

Several sculptures have been excavated in the ancient city of Ur at the time of Abraham (~ 2000 B.C.). The men are shown with shoulder-length hair, generally parted in the middle, and full beards. Near this time period, the Asiatic visitors to Egypt (19th century B.C.) depicted on the Beni-Hasan painting demonstrate the way hair was worn by some (Figure 5-3). Interestingly, the women did not wear veils. Only a headband was worn to keep their hair in place. Forced veiling seems to have occurred at some later period. Some of the men depicted on the painting wore full beards. These men also wore their hair over their foreheads, over the ears, and over the neck. A hairstyle like this actually protects the head, ears, and neck, as it is designed to do. Since the Egyptians called everyone from the Middle East "Asiatics," it is not known if the people are Moabites, Canaanites, or Hebrews.[197] However, the roundness of the cut may indicate that they were an Arab tribe rather than the Hebrews who were forbidden to round-off the corners of their head (Leviticus 19:27). Other men of a different nation, with darker skin, possibly Ethiopians or Egyptians, wore shoulder length hair, but these may have been wigs placed atop their shaven heads. The beards of both groups show them to be trimmed.

---

195 Richard Laurence, trans., Book of Enoch, 1821, ed. John Thompson 1882 (Muskogee, OK: Artisan Sales, 1980; Hoffman Printing, 1996 ed.), Part II, Chap. 105, p. 92.

196 Kevin J. Conner, Interpreting the Symbols and Types, completely revised and expanded edition. (Portland, OR: City Bible Publishing (formerly Bible Temple Publishing), 1992), 3. The "Ancient of Days" as in Daniel 7:9 describing God's glorious hair as also mentioned in Revelation 1:14.

197 Personal email communication with Todd Bolen (http://www.bibleplaces.com/) on February 27, 2006.

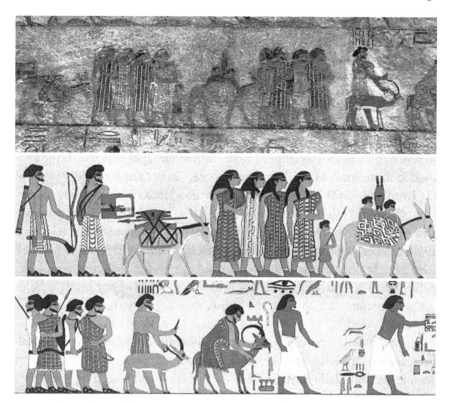

Figure 5-3: Beni-Hasan Painting - Visitors to Egypt from the Middle East (circa ~1890 B.C.). The upper image is an actual photograph by Todd Bolen showing a portion of the Beni-Hasan tomb painting. The center and lower images are paintings based on the original from *Lepsius, Carl Richard (hrsg.): Denkmäler aus Ägypten und Äthiopien : nach den Zeichnungen der vom Könige von Preussen Friedrich Wilhelm IV nach diesen Ländern gesendeten u. in den Jahren 1842 – 1845 ausgeführten wissenschaftlichen Expedition.* Used by permission courtesy Martin- Luther-Universität Halle-Wittenberg Universitäts- und Landesbibliothek Sachsen-Anhalt.

In the Beni-Hasan painting, compare the upper photograph with the painting (center and lower images) beneath it. The four females standing behind the mule and three boys in the upper photograph are the same four females repainted in the center image. They wore long hair extending to about the bottom of the shoulder blades. They did not wear veils to cover their hair, only a mere headband to keep their hair in place. The four men, to the right of the mule in the photograph, same as left side of bottom image, are probably the husbands of the four women based on their garment style and placement of the children. These men wore short hair, based on scientific measurement, but not unnaturally short. Their hair extended below the ears and was kept trimmed above the shoulders. Two other men, on the right side of the bottom image, have darker skin, small chin beards, and shoulder-length hair (medium length hair) and may have been Ethiopians or Egyptians.

Joseph

According to Rabbi Avrohom Davis, the English translation of the last sentence in Genesis 39:6 should read: "Yosief [Joseph] was well-built and good looking" or "well built and handsome" (as in "The Jerusalem Bible"). Dr. Brim and Rashi both relate that these good looks included long, curly, well-oiled hair.[198][199] Unfortunately, Potiphar's (Joseph's master) wife found him sexually desirable and pressed him daily to sleep with her (Genesis 39:7-20). The Book of Jasher (referred to in Joshua 10:13 and 2 Samuel 1:18) says her name was Zelicah. During one of her seductive attempts, Zelicah told Joseph, "How very beautiful is the hair of thy head, behold the golden comb which is in the house, take it I pray thee, and curl the hair of thy head."

Joseph would not commit adultery, nor did he permit the artificial altercation of his long hair, which would be a step towards the vile act.[200] She pressed him daily until one day she even grabbed Joseph by his tunic. But Joseph refused her advances and ran out of the house, but his tunic remained in her hand. So Zelicah yelled to her other servants and lied by telling them that it was Joseph who tried to seduce her and showed them the tunic as proof. Potiphar had Joseph imprisoned. "But Yahweh was with Joseph" and "made everything he undertook successful" (Genesis 39:21-23; JB).

God was with Joseph. With the consecration of God upon his head – his long hair – God gave Joseph the great gift of interpreting dreams while in prison (Genesis 40). The Pharaoh began to have strange dreams. Eventually he learns about Joseph, a true interpreter of dreams:

> Then Pharoah had Joseph summoned, and they hurried him from prison. He shaved and changed his clothes, and came into Pharoah's presence (Genesis 41:14).

---

198 Charles J. Brim, Medicine in the Bible (New York: Froben Press, 1936), 159.

199 Avrohom Bereishis Davis, The Metsudah Chumash/Rashi. A New Linear Translation, The Israel & Sara Fruchter Edition (Lakewood, New Jersey: Israel Book Shop, Judaica Distribution Center, 2002).

200 The Book of Jasher, 1840 (Muskogee, Oklahoma: Artisan Publishers, A Subsidiary of Hoffman Printing Co., 1988), Jasher 44:20-21.

As discussed earlier, the Egyptians, the sons of Ham, shaved their heads in those days. In Joseph's case it is not clear whether this meant the face only or the entire head. Some of the biblically inept have tried to use this as an example that men must constantly shave their beards; however, we will soon learn that this is not the case with God at all.

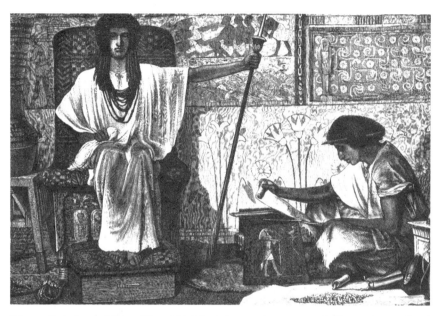

Figure 5-4: Long Hair of Joseph. More than a century ago, believers in our Lord recognized the importance of long hair. By Artist Lawrence Alma-Tadema sometime before 1908: from "The Bible and Its Story."

Joseph was now 30 years old (Genesis 41:46). After he interprets Pharoah's dream, Pharoah tells all: that Joseph possesses the spirit of God and makes Joseph governor of the whole land of Egypt. We also know of Joseph's long hair because the very first time the Hebrew term *nazir* (or N-Z-R) occurs in Scripture is in association with Joseph. *Nazir* is the same as *Nazarite* (this is how *nazir* is usually translated elsewhere), meaning consecrated of God, which includes no razor, but instead, long uncut hair. In Genesis 49:26, this same word, *nazir*, is usually translated *prince*, as being consecrated to God: he was a prince (i.e., nazarite) among his brothers.[201] This long hair, or consecration, may have been needed

---

201 William Gesenius, Gesenius' Hebrew and Chaldee Lexicon to the Old Testament Scriptures, trans. Samuel Prideaux Tregelles (Grand Rapids, Michigan: Baker Book House, 1979, reprinted November 1993).

to interpret Pharoah's dreams. His beauty, which always seems to have included long hair amongst the ancients, is adequately echoed in Jasher as well:

> … and all the women and damsels went upon the roofs or stood in the streets playing and rejoicing at Joseph and at his beauty.[202]

Moses writes concerning Joseph and his descendants in Deuteronomy 33:16:

> And with the best of the earth, and it's fullness; and the good will of Him who dwelt in the Bush – let it come on the head of Joseph, and on the crown of the consecrated one [nazir or N-Z-R] of his brothers ("The Interlinear Bible").

Or as "The Jerusalem Bible" puts it:

> May the hair grow thick on the head of Joseph, of the consecrated one among his brothers.

Here we see quite succinctly the words associated with long hair: best, fullness, good will of God, crown, and consecration! The Hebrews along with many, many other ancient peoples recognized the importance of a long, thick, full head of hair. Not only was it considered beautiful on men but the abundance thereof also represents an abundant life.

Deborah and Barak: The Loosing of the Locks

Deborah was judge of Israel (Judges 4:4) for 40 years (~1249 to 1209 B.C.). She was a great prophetess and inspired Barak, the military commander of Israel, how to be free of their oppressors, the Canaanites (Judges 4). Upon their defeat of the Canaanites, Deborah and Barak sang a song of praise beginning in Judges 5:2, mistranslated in the popular King James Version, but properly translated with the real meaning in other versions:

> That warriors in Israel unbound their hair, that the people came forward with a will, for this, bless Yahweh (JB)!

---

202 The Book of Jasher, Jasher 49:26.

For the loosing of locks of hair in Israel; for the willing offering of the people bless Jehovah (IB).

Or Charles Pfeiffer says it has been translated: "For that they let the long hair go loose in Israel."[203] This is said to mean that practically the whole nation of Israel were Nazarites. They enjoyed the freedom and strength associated with long hair. The Lord Himself instructed men from their youth to be Nazarites (Amos 2:11).

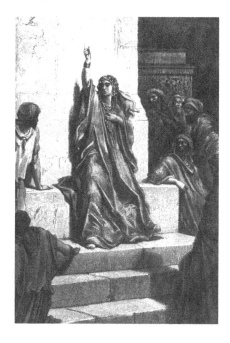

Figure 5-5: Deborah's Song. The Judge Deborah instructs the Israelites to let long hair prevail, a sign of freedom, health, eternal life, and for better looks. Artist Gustave Dore (1832-1883).

Samson

The history of Samson is quite remarkable and the entire account is recorded in the Book of Judges (13-16). An angel of the Lord appeared to Samson's parents before his birth. The first time he appeared to his mother only; the second time to both parents (again the angel appeared to the mother first who then went to get her husband). The mother was commanded to drink no wine or strong drink and not to eat any unclean thing (Judges 13:4, 7, 14), "for the child shall be a Nazarite to God from the womb to the day of his death" (13:7). Because she was about to carry a Nazarite in her womb, Samson's mother was commanded

---

203 Charles F. Pfeiffer, commentary on Judges 5:2 in Pfeiffer, eds. Charles F. and Everett F. Harrison, The Wycliffe Bible Commentary (Chicago: Moody Press, 1990).

not to drink wine (or strong drink), and eat anything unclean (Judges 13:4, 7, 14). Josephus says that Samson was to be content with water only.[204] Apparently, the health of an individual begins with the diet of his mother. As a result of optimal health, the Nazarite's hair would grow thick and long, well past the shoulders and down the back. Good health means healthy follicles to produce a full head of long hair built to last a lifetime. The specific command of the angel to Samson's mother was that no razor should come near his head:

> For, lo, thou shalt conceive and bear a son; and no razor shall come on his head (Judges 13:5).

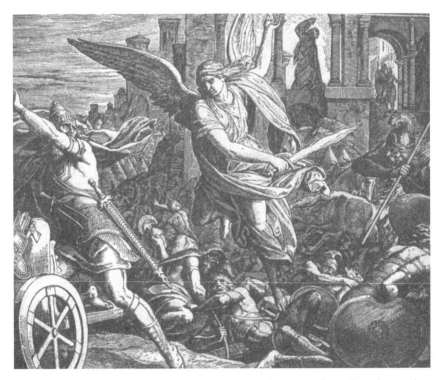

Figure 5-6: Long Hair of Angels. Historical accounts of angels indicate they look like young men, pre-beards. Their greatness and long hair, a symbol of divine strength, are some of their features. Artist Julius Schnorr von Carolsfeld (1794-1872), Die Bibel in Bildern.

---

204 Flavius Josephus, The Antiquities of the Jews (Book 5, Chapter 8, Paragraph 2 (278)), trans. William Whiston (Peabody MA: Hendrickson Publishers, The Works of Josephus: New Updated Edition, Complete and Unabridged in One Volume, 1987. Thirteenth printing – April 1998), 145, (Samson).

The angel saying "no razor" obviously means that some form of hair and beard trimming was being practiced on other men at the time. It was perhaps the trimmed hair styles depicted on the Beni-Hasan painting, but certainly not the real short hair of the Corinthians or certain Romans, who appear later in history. Josephus describes the angel thus: he "resembled a young man, beautiful and tall, and brought her the good news."[205] The angel, no doubt being "beautiful," has long hair as an example to Samson's mother. Long hair was indeed admired especially "in the case of young men."[206] We find that Solomon's royal guard were also young men, beautiful, tall, and wore long hair, to be discussed shortly. Apparently, they too resembled the appearance of angels.

So Samson grew up with a head of hair that was never ever cut. The Lord blessed Samson and the Spirit of the Lord came upon him (Judges 13:24-25). He had no fear of wild animals. Samson slew a lion with his bare hands, and he caught 300 foxes, attached torches to their tails, and sent them running through the crops of his enemies (Judges 14:5-6; 15:4-5). Sometime after this, Samson's own people had him bound and delivered to the Philistines. As he was being led away captive he came to the place, Lehi. Here "the Philistines shouted against him: and the Spirit of the Lord came mightily upon him" so much so that Samson broke his bindings and killed 1,000 men with the jawbone of an ass (Judges 15:13-16). Then Samson met the woman, Delilah (Figure 5-7).

Delilah was sent by the Philistines to find out where Samson got his great strength. It was a trap in which many men have fallen. Knowing how much he loved her, Delilah pressed him daily to tell her the secret of his strength (Judges 16:4-16). Finally, Samson said, "There hath not come a razor upon mine head; for I have been a Nazarite unto God from my mother's womb: if I be shaven, then my strength will go from me, and I shall become weak, and be like any other man" (Judges 16:17).

Once she discovered his secret, Delilah wasted no time. While Samson was sleeping upon her knees, she called for a Philistine man to rob Samson of his crown. Delilah told the man to "shave off the seven locks of his head" (Judges 16:19). When this happened, "the Lord was departed from him," thus Samson's strength was gone. The Philistines captured him and put out his eyes and caused him to grind grain in the prison (Judges 16:20-21). Samson went from a long-haired servant of God to a shorn prisoner in the Philistine

205 Josephus, "The Antiquities of the Jews" (Book 5, Chapter 8, Paragraph 2 (277)), 145.
206 "Hair," The Illuminated Bible, King James Version (Columbia Educational Books, 1941), (Text previously published as the New Indexed Bible, John A. Dickson Publishing Co., 1901, 1909, 1913, 1923, 1929, 1940), 91.

economy all because a female sent him to a barber. This is precisely how some men are being reduced today. Psychiatrist Karl Menninger relates, saying cutting off hair represents a partial renunciation of virility and power.[207]

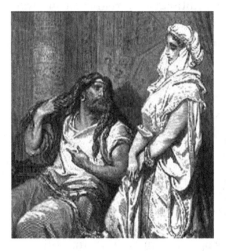

Figure 5-7: Samson and Delilah. Judges 16:17 ...There hath not come a razor upon mine head; for I *have been* a Nazarite unto God from my mother's womb: if I be shaven, then my strength will go from me, and I shall become weak, and be like any *other* man. Artist Gustave Dore (1832-1883).

During his time in prison, Samson's hair grew back (Judges 16:22). Apparently, the Philistines either forgot or did not believe that somehow Samson's strength was connected to his hair. Eventually, the Philistines made sport of him in a sanctuary of idol worship. While there, they placed him between two pillars, which supported the temple. Samson pushed apart the pillars, killing himself along with 3,000 Philistines when the structure collapsed (Judges 16:23-30).

So Samson received strength from Lord when his hair was long. But when his hair was cut off, the Lord left him and he became weak (Judges 16:20). Thus, it could be said that hair has some spiritual connection. Besides this, there are at least four ways hair is strong from a natural perspective. As discussed earlier, we already learned that hair is as strong as copper wire, but much lighter in weight. Secondly, long hair adds strength to the individual's appearance. Third, long hair helps to keep the scalp strong, healthy and more durable. Finally, long hair demonstrates the power of God in creation. It is a symbol of His divine strength.[208] For angels, this symbol of divine strength is apparently displayed as angel hair, long and strong.

---

207 Karl Menninger, Man Against Himself (New York: Harcourt, Brace & World, Inc., 1938), 247.
208 Luering, "Hair."

Here is another fascinating detail concerns the "seven locks" of Samson's head (Judges 16:13,19). Some Rastafarians believe "locks" mean that Samson had dreadlocks, or better, dredlocks. This could be possible. Noah Webster informs us that "lock" could mean either a tuft of hair or a ringlet, or curl, of hair. Furthermore, H.L.E. Luering says that the Hebrew word translated "locks" with regards to Samson's hair is *mahlāphāh*, meaning plaited, braided, or interwoven hair.[209] The number seven mentioned in conjunction with locks may represent the amount of locks Samson had. If so, then how were these locks arranged? On the other hand, numbers also have symbolic meanings.

Kevin Conner informs us that seven is the number for "perfection" and "completeness,"[210] which seems to have more to do with hair length rather than an exact number of braids. Samson's hair was allowed to grow to completion, perfection or maturity as determined by his own genetic code. Luering believes that his appearance was probably akin to a Bedouin warrior.[211] All we know for certain is that he had long, probably curly, hair which was plaited, braided, or interwoven in some unknown arrangement.

Nevertheless his long hair is considered perfect by God's standards. In contrast, the number eleven is the number for "incompleteness" or "disintegration," like the modern haircut, and also is a symbol for the "Antichrist."[212]

Samuel and the Time of King David

In the case of Samuel, it was his mother who was unable to conceive, so she cried out to God and vowed, "O Lord of hosts, if thou wilt indeed look on the affliction of thine handmaid … and give unto thine handmaid a man child, then I will give him unto the Lord all the days of his life, and there shall no razor come upon his head" (1 Samuel 1:11). Her prayer was answered. Samuel went on to become the great prophet who anointed Israel's first King, Saul, and later anointed King David (Figure 5-8).

So, like Samson, Samuel was a Nazarite from the womb. Those consecrated to be Nazarites by their parents from birth are called "perpetual Nazarites."[213] Can anyone imagine uncut hair from childbirth? Yes,

209 H.L.E. Luering, "Locks," The International Standard Bible Encyclopaedia, ed. James Orr, Vol. III (Hendrickson Publishers ed. 2nd Printing March 1996. 4 vols).
210 Conner, 54.
211 Luering, "Locks."
212 Conner, 54.
213 Advanced Bible History in the Words of Holy Scripture, 14th Printing (St. Louis, MO: Concordia Publishing House, 1936.)

probably some Native Americans and Rastafarians know, and certainly the Sikhs.

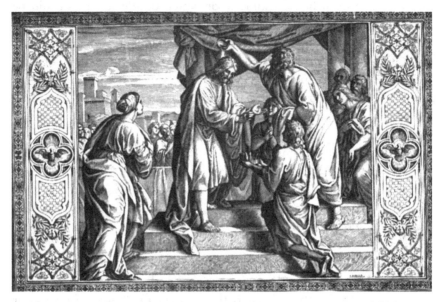

Figure 5-8: Crowning of King David. Artist Julius Schnorr von Carolsfeld (1794-1872), Die Bibel in Bildern.

Unfortunately, prejudice still ranks high in America. Just like the Native Americans before them, Sikhs growing up in America are often the targets of discrimination. Diana Eck mentions one particularly disturbing story, though there are many, probably thousands. One young Sikh man related that he could not find a job for five years! He finally succumbed to the pressure by cutting his hair and shaving his beard. Even Sikh women are judged for having "really super long hair."[214] Eck goes on to say that "stereotypes and prejudice have a long history in America," and the most important thing to Americans seems to be the "visible difference" between people. She is absolutely correct. For the record, Jesus opposed this predominating American view completely (e.g., Matthew 6; John 7:24).

Actually, it is not too hard to imagine uncut hair from childbirth, as all types of hair, including head hair, are genetically programmed to reach a certain length, and remain at that overall completed length. On the other hand, it is hard to imagine, especially if one had the ability to grow super-long hair greater than three feet. Nevertheless, at the time of King David, the "longer" a man's

214 Diana L. Eck, A New Religious America (New York: HarperSanFrancisco, 2001), 297-298.

hair was, "the more it was esteemed."[215] This long hair somehow transmits the strength of the Creator. David's men were described as having faces like lions (1 Chronicles 12:8), which denotes long hair and full beards. As for David himself, his long hair is known from the time when Micah saved his life from Saul. She placed a dummy beneath the blankets of his bed and used a "tress of goats hair" to mimic his long hair (1 Samuel 19:13-17; JB).

Adino the Eznite, one of David's mighty men, displayed the incredible power of Samson as he slew 800 men in a single battle (2 Samuel 23:8). Clearly, Yahweh was with him, for long hair is a symbol of devotion to God. What the world needs are more parents like Samson's and Samuel's mothers, who both came to recognize the significance and importance of male hair. At the same time we need to be aware of adulteresses and prostitutes such as Zelicah and Delilah, who wish to either alter the texture of our natural long hair or just cut men short.

The importance of the beard is also demonstrated during the time when King David's servants were accused of being spies. A man named Hanun humiliated them. Hanun caused half of their beards to be shaved, probably one side of their faces. When they returned, King David granted his men leave of absence from duty until their beards grew back (2 Samuel 10:4-5). Imagine, being sent home from work until your beard grew back! The world certainly has changed, the natural being replaced by the artificial, in this case the daily ritual of the razor.

God spoke highly of his long-haired Nazarites. The long-haired Nazarites (also spelled Nazirites) of Holy Scripture were described thus:

> Her Nazarites were purer than snow, they were whiter than milk, they were more ruddy in body than rubies, their polishing was of sapphire (Lamentations 4:7).

Conner says the word "white" means "pure, righteous and holy," not skin color. On the other hand, the last part of the verse has to do with the appearance of their body and the most visible part, the skin. By definition, ruddy means "tinged with red; especially having a healthy glow; rosy." "Sapphire" is symbol of beauty and hardness.[216]

What does this all mean? Well, the Nazarites were beacons of health as evidenced by their rosy complexion. They were long-haired men of iron.

---

215 Ann Charles and Roger DeAnfrasio, *The History of Hair* (New York: Bonanza Books, 1970), 51.
216 Conner, 165, 180.

Lifelong Nazarites, like the Sikhs of today, never cut their hair. However, individuals who took a Nazarite vow on a temporary basis did shave off (probably crew cut) their hair at the end of the vow in accordance with the rules listed in Numbers 6. Besides keeping a metal blade away from the head, they abstained from wine and strong drink, and were to stay away from the dead. At the end of this temporary vow, they were permitted to drink wine and the new emerging hairs symbolized a new beginning of life.[217] Lifetime Nazarites had special calls in life, as unique individuals, and did not seem to adhere too strictly to the rules of Numbers 6. For example, both Samson and Samuel were in direct contact with dead bodies (Judges 14:8-9; 15:14-16; 1 Samuel 15:33). Neither shaved their head nor did they lose their power from the Most High. Their healthy long hair was an outgrowth of their healthy skin, which was an outgrowth of their healthy lifestyle including a healthy Old Testament diet. Proper nutrition for hair health will be discussed later.

Absalom

The story of Absalom occurs in 2 Samuel 13-19. This young man was praised in all of Israel due to his great beauty. Absalom was extraordinarily handsome in physical appearance like Adam. He surpassed the beauty of his father, King David: who was also known for his handsome appearance, being described as ruddy with auburn hair and a fair complexion.[218] But all this incredible outward beauty added little to his heart for eventually Absalom led a revolt against his own father. His physical beauty is described thus:

> But in all Israel there was none to be so much praised as Absalom for his beauty: from the sole of his foot even to the crown of his head there was no blemish in him. And when he polled his head [cut his hair], (for it was at every year's end that he polled it: because the hair was heavy on him, therefore he polled it:) he weighed the hair of his head at two hundred shekels after the king's weight (2 Samuel 14:25-26).

In this passage the Lord informs us that Absalom was perfect in outer appearance. The problem was that he was praised for his outward beauty rather than a good heart. It is most interesting that he cut his hair at

---

217 Luering, "Hair."

218 Fred Young, commentary on 1 Samuel 16:12 and 2 Samuel 14:25 in Pfeiffer, Charles F. and Everett F. Harrison, eds., *The Wycliffe Bible Commentary* (Chicago: Moody Press, 1990).

the end of every year. The Hebrew year ended sometime in our modern February or March,[219] basically at the end of winter. If one was to cut his hair once a year that would indeed be the perfect time. The long hair would protect the head from cold throughout the winter, and be long enough to protect the head from over-exposure to the sun's rays by summer.

One day Absalom encountered certain servants of King David. Absalom fled on his mule and his head got caught in a great oak tree and the mule that was under him went away. David gave strict orders not to kill Absalom, but ten young men killed him while he hung in the tree (2 Samuel 18:9,15). Neil believes Absalom was probably caught in the tree "by the neck rather than by his legendary long hair."[220] This could be true because Absalom did cut his hair off once a year. It would depend on when his last haircut was. But the story detailed by the first century historian and military leader Josephus was quite different: Absalom "entangled his hair greatly in the large boughs of a knotty tree that spread a great way, and there he hung, after a surprising manner."[221] So whether true or not, the story that was handed down through the centuries was that Absalom's long hair got caught in a tree during battle. A story this profound would eventually catch the ears of later military leaders. It is not hard to imagine some general telling his young troops "see what can happen to you in a military conflict if you have long hair?"

Some have used the story of Absalom as proof that God does not want men to have long hair. As already proven, they all wore long hair in those days. Head hair is created to be long or at the very least, long enough to do its job, which is to protect the head. Absalom's hair did not make him evil. He became wicked in his heart. The truth about his appearance as Walter Wilson said: Absalom's outer beauty was "perfection," just as the Scriptures indicate.[222] This perfection of appearance included his long hair, which was created that way. But how long was Absalom's hair?

The length of Absalom's hair can be estimated by its weight of 200 shekels. Different scholars have estimated this weight to be roughly between four and six pounds. The study notes in "The 1599 Geneva Bible" claim six

---

219 Jack Finegan, Handbook of Biblical Chronology, revised ed. (Peabody, MA: Hendrickson Publishers, 1998), 35.

220 William Neil, Pocket Bible Commentary (Edison, New Jersey: Castle, 1997. Hodder & Stoughton, 1962).

221 Josephus, The Antiquities of the Jews (Book 7, Chapter 10, Paragraph 2 (239)), 199 (Absalom).

222 Walter L. Wilson, "Absalom," Wilson's Dictionary of Bible Types (Grand Rapids, Michigan: William B. Eerdmans Publishing Co.).

pounds, but Eugene Merrill says "about five pounds."[223] [224] On the other hand Porter believes that the shekel of the King's weight, or royal shekel, was most likely the "light shekel."[225] If we consider the "light shekel," it corresponds to 130 grains (grain not gram), which equates to 8.42 grams per shekel. By multiplying the 8.42 grams/shekel by 200 shekels, Absalom's hair weighed 1,685 grams or about 3.7 pounds! No wonder his head hair felt heavy on him. Four to six pounds of hair would feel heavy on anyone. But at least his heavy long hair trained his scalp to be strong and healthy, rather than to atrophy into cell death, thinning hair, and nothingness.

To be as conservative as possible, the weight of 3.7 pounds can be used to estimate Absalom's hair length. According to the U.S. Environmental Protection Agency a single human hair 4.0 cm (about 1.575 inches) in length weighs about 312 micrograms.[226] However, we are not told if this is a fine, medium, or coarse diameter hair. Since most people have medium diameter hair, the weight of 312 micrograms probably corresponds to that. And we are not told if this hair was stripped of all natural oil, which adds weight to hair. Nevertheless, from this data we can approximate the length of Absalom's hair.

Let's assume that Absalom had a real thick density of hairs, say 150,000 hairs on his head. If his hair was truly medium diameter hair, then his hair would have been well over 1.0 meter long, even approaching 1.5 meters or nearly five feet. This assumes perfectly straight hair, which is highly doubtful. Thus the curling locks he probably had along with his natural oils (which also add weight), then his hair would have been shorter than five feet. Nevertheless, with all things considered, Absalom's hair probably hung in curling locks about three feet or about 1.0 meter down the full length of his back.

The other remarkable thing is that this length was achieved in one year. Assuming he cut his hair really short, his hair growth rate was quite impressive. No matter how you slice it, this growth rate must have been greater than 8.0 cm or three inches per month. This is an extraordinary growth rate well beyond the norm. Now it is true that some men have

223 Commentary notes on 2 Samuel 14:26 indicate that Absalom's hair weighed "6 pounds 4 ounces" in The 1599 Geneva Bible. (White Hall, West Virginia: Tolle Lege Press, 2006).

224 Eugene H. Merrill, "2 Samuel," The Bible Knowledge Commentary, Old Testament, eds. John F. Walvoord and Roy B. Zuck (Victor Books, 4th printing 1987).

225 H. Porter, "Shekel of the King's Weight, or Royal Shekel," The International Standard Bible Encyclopaedia, ed. James Orr, Vol. IV (Hendrickson Publishers ed. 2nd Printing March 1996. 4 vols.).

226 "U.S. Environmental Protection Agency, Laboratory and Field Operations – PM 2.5," accessed May 13, 2006 http://www.epa.gov/region4/sesd/pm25/p5.htm.

achieved the length of Absalom's hair, not in one year, but more like three to five years. But then again, Absalom's physical body is described as being "perfect." This would include all the processes in his cells including the rapid cell division within the follicles of his scalp.

Solomon and His Soldiers

Solomon became King of Israel after his father, King David, passed away. Again, they all wore healthy long hair in those days. Adam, Noah, Samson, Samuel, King David, King Solomon and many others are considered "types" of Jesus Christ.[227] The Shulammite sings of the locks of her beloved which are "bushy and black as a raven" (Solomon's Song 5:11). Gesenius informs us that she is comparing Solomon's long "flowing locks" to "pendulous branches of palms."[228] She adored his long curly locks, which hung loosely about his head. The world today needs more Shulammite women who admire men with long hair, and less Delilah's who wish to emasculate men. Walter Wilson says that Solomon's type of hair is exactly what the Lord Jesus Himself would have about 1,000 years later.[229]

Females who admire long hair on men have often commented as follows:
- Long hair is fun!
- Long hair is really cool!
- Long hair is beautiful or exquisite!
- Long hair makes you look like a "somebody"!
- There's just something about a man with long hair!

Like a breath of fresh air, is a woman who admires a man with long hair. All this reminds me of a film-clip when longer hair on males became popular in the 1960s with the arrival of British rock bands like The Beatles. At that time, women apparently grew tired of the ultra-short boring hair of the early part of the 20th century, and loved the longer hair look. Of course scientifically, The Beatles' hair was short. It was barely over the tops of the ears when their career began. It was only long when compared to ultra-short modern military standards. Charles and DeAnfrasio put it quite well: "The

---

227 Conner.
228 William Gesenius, Gesenius' Hebrew and Chaldee Lexicon to the Old Testament Scriptures, trans. Samuel Prideaux Tregelles (Grand Rapids, Michigan: Baker Book House, 1979, reprinted November 1993), 865, Strong's number 8534.
229 Walter L. Wilson, "Hair."

beginning of the 20th century, was probably one of the dullest periods in the history of men's hair fashions".[230] The beginning of the 21st century seems to be equally abysmal with all the close-cropped heads running about.

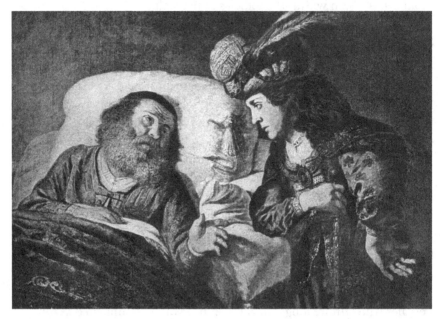

Figure 5-9: King David's last counsel to his son: Long-haired King Solomon. The Shulammite female adored Solomon's long curly locks (Solomon's Song 5:11) as some modern women who appreciate God's artwork still do. Painting by Jan Victoor, an early Dutch Master (died in 1673), from "The Bible and Its Story."

Great fame went around all the neighboring countries, which proclaimed Solomon's virtues and wisdom. All the men of Solomon's royal guard had great long hair and rode magnificent horses. Josephus records it as follows:

> This addition then he [Solomon] made to those chariots and horses which he had before from those that were sent him, augmented the number of his chariots by above 400, for he had a thousand before, and augmented the number of his horses by 2,000, for he had 20,000 before. These horses also were so much exercised, in order to their making a fine appearance, and running swiftly, that no others could, upon the comparison, appear either finer or

---

230 Charles and DeAnfrasio, 165.

swifter; but they were at once the most beautiful of all others, and their swiftness was incomparable also.

Their riders also were a further ornament to them, being, in the first place, young men in the most delightful flower of their age, and being eminent for their largeness, and far taller than other men. *They had also very long heads of hair hanging down*, and were clothed in garments of Tyrian purple. They had also dust of gold every day sprinkled on their hair, so that their heads sparkled with a reflection of the sunbeams from the gold. The king himself rode upon a chariot in the midst of these men, who were still in armor, and had their bows fitted to them [emphasis mine].[231]

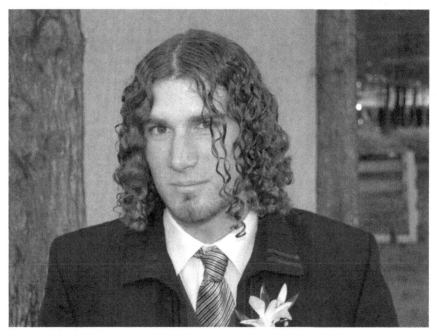

Figure 5-10: Young Man with Long, Dark, Curly Hair. This is the type of hair Solomon and Jesus may have had, although theirs was no doubt longer than this. Notice how the hair is designed to protect the head and frame the face. Photograph by the author, April 28, 2007.

Solomon's men are described as having very long hair "hanging down," but hanging down from where? Obviously, this means their "very

---

231 Josephus, "The Antiquities of the Jews" (Book 8, Chapter 7, Paragraph 3, (183-186)), 225, (Solomon's Long-Haired Men).

long" hair hung down well past the shoulders and down the back. Their bows being "fitted to them" indicate how each man was respected as an individual. Their natural long hair, which is unique to each individual, and their custom fitted armor allowed these men to be themselves. And they faithfully and wholeheartedly served the king. The king riding "in the midst" of these long haired men is actually a picture of the Lord's second coming along with thousands of His holy ones (Jude 1:14). By the looks of things, modern militaries are quite opposed to this Christ-like model. It is most unfortunate for scalp health that a man is not even allowed to have enough hair to protect his own head, ears and neck. A good military leader should go after a man's heart, not after his hair.

Elijah the Tishbite

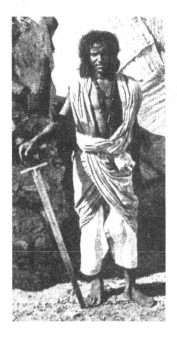

Figure 5-11: Bedouin Strongman of the Bisharin Tribe, Nubian Desert. His long hair, no doubt, hangs down the back. The appearance of Elijah, Samson, and other prophets and judges were similar to this man. Photograph from "The Secret Museum of Mankind," late 19th to early 20th century. Image courtesy of David Stiffler.

Elijah the Tishbite prophesied from about 883 to 868 B.C. in the days of King Ahab. He was a "hairy" man (2 Kings 1:8), meaning hair being tossed about like a whirlwind or tempest.[232] In 1856, William Smith in his "A Concise Dictionary of the Bible" remarks that Elijah lived in the

---

232 James Strong, Strong's Exhaustive Concordance of the Bible (Gordonsville, TN: Dugan Publishers, Inc.). The Hebrew dictionary explains the Hebrew *saʾar* (Strong # 8181) is from Strong # 8175 in the sense of "disheveling" as being "tossed" or hurled about as in a "storm," tempest, or "whirlwind," all denoting great length of hair.

"wild loneliness of the hills and ravines of Gilead." Indeed, he spent a great deal of time in the wilderness where he drank water from the streams and ravens brought him food (1 Kings 17:2-6). There are no barber shops in the wilderness.

About the appearance of this desert Prophet Elijah, William Smith remarked thus:

> Of his appearance as he "stood before" Ahab, with the suddenness of motion to this day characteristic of the Bedouins from his native hills …. His chief characteristic was his hair, long and thick, and hanging down his back; which if not betokening the immense strength of Samson, yet accompanied powers of endurance no less remarkable.[233]

When Jesus Christ was transfigured on the high mountain rising from Caesarea Philippi (Matthew 16:13), Peter, James, and John witnessed this event, along with the sudden appearance of Elijah and Moses (Matthew 17:1-8; Mark 9:2-8; Luke 9:28-36). After this, and as they came back down the mountain, Jesus informed these disciples that John the Baptist is the "Elijah" that was to come at this time in history (Matthew 11:14; 17:9-13). Both John the Baptist and Elijah were similar in appearance with long uncut hair hanging down their backs.

Physical Proof

The ancient Hebrews, as opposed to most of their modern counterparts, understood the importance of hair. Because of the prohibition against graven images, actual images of ancient Hebrews are rare. However, archaeology gives us snapshots of world history in action. After Solomon's reign, long hair continued. Thanks to the artists of Assyria, we have physical evidence carved in stone that displays what the Assyrian and Hebrew men looked like during the 9th century B.C. (841 B.C.). On the Black Obelisk displayed at The British Museum, the Hebrews are shown paying tribute to the Assyrians. From this and much other archaeological evidence we know exactly how these men looked. Both people groups are shown with majestic shoulder-length hair.

---

233 William Smith, ed., "Elijah," A Concise Dictionary of the Bible, Comprising its Antiquities, Biography, Geography, and Natural History (Boston: Little, Brown, and Company, 1865), 236.

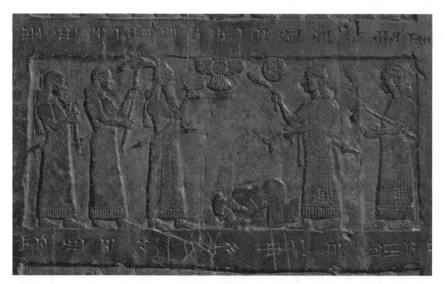

Figure 5-13: Black Obelisk, King Jehu kneeling before King Shalmaneser III. The Assyrians are on the left, the Hebrews on the right. Note the fine detail that shows the different facial characteristics of each man. Their shoulder-length hair is shown to be curly, a probable physical trait of both people groups (e.g., the bushy curls of Solomon – see Solomon's Song 5:11). If their hair was straight, a common trait of Native Americans and Asians, it would naturally extend below the shoulders. God makes both curly long hair and straight long hair according to His will. © The Trustees of the British Museum, used with permission.

The Spartans

It is well known that the ancient Spartans of Greece wore long hair. One of the great leaders of these long-haired men was Lycurgus. He is said to have established harmony, simplicity, and strength in Sparta around the 9th century B.C. Lycurgus believed in a proper diet and exercise – their warriors endured extremely tough and rigorous training. He was considered very well educated and has been called a "creative genius."[234] A good diet and exercise are good for healthy long hair, of which the Spartans took care in arranging, particularly before battle. Lycurgus understood that long hair enhances a person's appearance. He said long hair adds beauty to a handsome man, and makes an ugly face even more terrible.[235] Since hair is decorative, it could

234 P.V.N. Myers, A General History for Colleges and High Schools (Boston and London: Ginn & Company Publishers, 1893) 113.

235 Plutarch. "The Lives of the Noble Grecians and Romans." Great Books of the Western World, vol. 14, ed. Robert Maynard Hutchins (London: Encyclopaedia Britannica: William Benton, Publisher, 1952), 43-44; 354.

be added that more beauty is also brought to those who are plain or average looking. Therefore, for most people, long hair increases beauty overall.

The great strength of the Spartans is reminiscent of Samson. This strength was remarkably displayed when King Leonidas, along with 300 of his Spartan soldiers, stayed to defend the pass at Thermopylæ in 480 B.C.[236] Of all men, the long-haired Spartans were the manliest. In fact, when Spartan King Agesilaus took prisoners from Phrygia, he was appalled by their "white and tender-skinned" bodies "want of all exposure and exercise."[237] These soft, white, tender bodies were completely opposite of the Spartans, who in appearance were similar to the Hebrew Nazarites described as ruddy (Lamentations 4:7). The long hair and ruddy appearance has ancient connections. It is believed that the Spartans and Hebrews were brothers, both people groups descending from Abraham.[238]

Indeed, it is worthy to note that the wisdom of Lycurgus appears to originate in the ancient Scriptures. The similarities are striking. Under Lycurgus (like the ancient Hebrews) men were encouraged to grow and display their long hair as individuals. Teamwork to men like King David, King Solomon, and Lycurgus meant that men were respected as individuals. Each man has his own type of hair, which is designed to be displayed. The modern idea that all men must look the same, like robots, to be on the team is foreign to nature, individuality, the ancients, and God. Plutarch also informs us that the women were free to speak their opinions in public and openly, even on the most important subjects (see Numbers 27:1-8). Lycurgus was a kind man of peace and quiet. He promoted equality among men, had few laws, and dealt fairly with enemies. Beginning with Lycurgus, the Spartan people were forewarned that the love of money would ruin them, a great truth he apparently acquired from long-haired King Solomon (Proverbs 8; 16).

Life under the mandates of Lycurgus was far better than the fathers of other Greco-Roman cities. For comparison see Table 5-1. "The Laws of Plato" summarizes it well. He says that the Spartans "filled the stage of Greek history with noble and unforgettable exploits," and that early men were more peaceful, trusting, simpler, courageous, moderate and "in every way more just."[239] The Spartans were not drunken revelers because they

236 Myers, 132-133.
237 Plutarch, 484.
238 Herbert G. May and Bruce M. Metzger, ed., "1 Maccabees 12:19-21," The Oxford Annotated Bible with the Apocrypha, Revised Standard Version (New York: Oxford University Press, 1965).
239 Thomas L. Pangle, trans., The Laws of Plato (Chicago and London: The University of Chicago Press, 1980), 425-430.

wished to always be ready and sober if attacked.[240] Luis Navia informs us that the followers of Socrates had such a high regard for Sparta that they all wore long hair.[241] And this was at a time when short hair came in style.

Table 5-1: Life Under Long-Haired Lycurgus vs. the Cropheads[242]

Subject	Long Haired Lycurgus/ Spartans	Numa Pompilius (8th-7th century B.C. Rome) Theseus (founder of Athens)
Women	Allowed to speak freely even on important subjects in public.	Numa: Were not to speak at all except in the company of their own husbands. Daughters as young as 12 years were delivered to their future husbands.
Forced Celibacy	None known	Numa: Forced many women to become Vestal Virgins (a 30 year vow). If the vow was broken, even by rape, they were buried alive without mercy.
Idolatry	?	Numa: Worshiped idols continually; formed priesthoods who wore special caps and who called upon strange & horrible deities (demons).
Tyranny	Punished lawless and cruel tyrants	They were tyrants
Freedom	Promoted freedom and equality for all men	Theseus: Robbed men of freedom by having them pent up in one city and using them as his subjects and slaves.
Male Hair	Men encouraged and free to grow long hair and arrange it as per individual for each person has their own type of hair as designed. Adds beauty to a handsome man.	Theseus: Warlike like the Abantes, so the forepart of the hair (bangs) was cut. Numa: offered hair as a sacrifice to the gods.

---

240 Pangle, 17.

241 Luis E. Navia, Socrates: A Life Examined, (Amherst, New York: Prometheus Books, 2007), 69.

242 Table 5-1 is compiled from information gathered in Plutarch's The Lives of the Noble Grecians and Romans, 2, 13, 33-57, 61-63, 149.

The laws of Lycurgus were followed for some 500 years, and as a result the Spartan people prospered. The beginning of Spartan corruption began with their conquest of Athens. By the time of Agis (264 to 241 B.C.), the love of money had virtually destroyed the laws of Lycurgus. It was the highest wish of Agis to restore Sparta to its ancient glory. He stirred quite a controversy. In the end, most of his people would not turn from their wicked ways, and for his valiant efforts, Agis was slain.[243] Could it be that short hair, corruption, and loss of freedom are interrelated?

Both the Spartans and Hebrews wore long hair, even their respective militaries. And this long hair was worn at a time when men actually fought hand-to-hand combat. Why are enlisted men practically scalped when hand-to-hand combat in modern warfare is rare?

Hair, the Spiritual Connection

So it seems long hair was admired on men, as well as women. As Nekhena Evans correctly surmises in her book, "Hairlocking, Everything You Need to Know," "The ancients as opposed to modern man, understood that hair has a much deeper meaning."[244] She suggests that long, naturally spiraled hair, typical of those primarily of African decent, "becomes a receiver and transmitter of divine emanations."[245] Who could argue with that, especially in light of Joseph's or Samson's hair? In other places in her book, Evans remarks that "your hair is your crowning glory" and gives the Creator the glory for such a great blessing. She dismisses the notion that hair is "dead matter, a waste product that serves no significant purpose," which she attributes to certain writers of European decent. "Europeans attempt to divide things into distinct, measurable, compartmentalized entities."[246] Is she right or what? Well, she is right about many of them, but there are also many of us of European descent who feel the way she does. Another way of putting it is that certain people groups, those who think like Romans, like to place others in a box or cage. Over several centuries, the Native Americans saw this same problem with many, but not all, of their white conquerors, especially in the later part of the 19th century.

---

243 Plutarch, 499.
244 Nekhena Evans, Hairlocking, Everything You Need to Know (Brooklyn, NY: A&B Publishers Group), 44.
245 Evans, 63.
246 Evans, 43.

Of course Evans wishes blacks to wear their hair naturally. But she is clearly wrong in one matter. Tightly spiraled hair is not more spiritual than straight hair. However, long hair, no matter what type of hair you have, (straight, wavy, large curls, or tight curls) seems to definitely have spiritual significance. Two most interesting historical accounts bear this out. In 592 B.C. the prophet Ezekiel had quite an experience:

> He put forth the form of a hand, and took me by a lock of my head, and the Spirit lifted me between heaven and earth… (Ezekiel 8:3).

According to Charles Dyer, Ezekiel was not moved physically from the spot. So then why grab his hair? If Ezekiel was not transported physically, then apparently, there is some spiritual connection between God and mankind through long hair. Dyer goes on to tell us that it was a "vision" where Ezekiel was flown from Babylon to Jerusalem.[247]

Another story involves the prophets Habakkuk and Daniel, who lived contemporaneously including the time when Cyrus conquered Babylon (Daniel 1:21; 6:28; 10:1; Habakkuk 2:3; 3:16). This event would have occurred possibly around 539 B.C. It is recorded in the book "Bel and the Dragon." In this account, "the angel of the Lord took him [Habakkuk] by the crown of his head, and lifted him by his hair and set him down in Babylon, right over the den [where Daniel was], with the rushing sound of the wind itself."[248]

Several facts can be ascertained in these two accounts. Since a man's hand (or form of a hand) is about four inches wide, the hair of their (Ezekiel and Habakkuk) heads must have been longer than this, otherwise the hand would have nothing to grab. Short hair would slip out of the hand. They were probably unshorn Nazarites, or at the very least they had shoulder-length hair. The accounts also, once again, demonstrate the strength of hair itself and its anchoring strength in the skin. A person can be lifted up and carried about by the very hairs of their head.

---

247 Charles H. Dyer, "Ezekiel," The Bible Knowledge Commentary, Old Testament, eds. John F. Walvoord and Roy B. Zuck (Victor Books, 4th printing 1987). In his commentary on Ezekiel 8:3 he says "In the vision Ezekiel was lifted … up between earth and heaven and transported to Jerusalem."

248 Herbert G. May and Bruce M. Metzer, eds. "Bel and the Dragon, v. 36," The Oxford Annotated Bible with the Apocrypha, Revised Standard Version. (New York: Oxford University Press, 1965). Please note that "Bel and the Dragon" is the same as chapter 14 of the Book of Daniel (14:36) in many Catholic Bibles.

Based on these accounts it appears that head hair certainly is a neurotransmitter as recently discovered by science.[249] This new discovery, along with the historical accounts about Joseph, Samson, Ezekiel, Habakkuk, and Solomon, do seem to indicate some deep spiritual connection as Nekhena Evans indicates. Thus, one should not take his or her natural crown lightly.

---

249 Desmond J. Tobin, "Biochemistry of human skin – our brain on the outside," Chemical Society Reviews. 2006, 35, 52-67.

Chapter 6: The Long Hair of Jesus

Yet there shall not one hair of your heads perish (Luke 21:18).

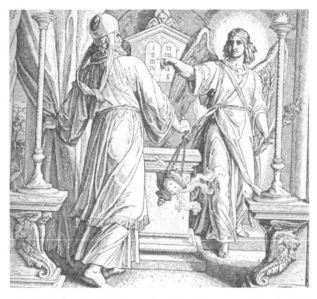

Figure 6-1: Angel Gabriel with Majestic Shoulder-Length Hair. He foretells the birth of John the Baptist to Zechariah. Artist Julius Schnorr von Carolsfeld (1794-1872), Die Bibel in Bildern.

People are always interested in what other people look like. Jesus himself was no exception. All the evidence mandates that Jesus wore long hair. There are several lines of evidence in the Scriptures when properly understood and other historical sources. First of all we must remember that hair is a person's natural crown (Genesis 49:26; Leviticus 21:12; Deuteronomy 33:16) and it is created to be long by the Creator Himself.

This chapter shows that long hair is holy, a consecration or blessing from God.[250]

Evidence from Scripture

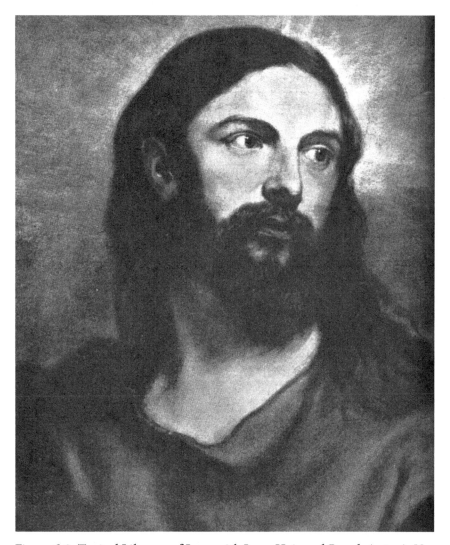

Figure 6-2: Typical Likeness of Jesus with Long Hair and Beard. Artist A. Van Dyck (1599-1641) where Jesus teaches about tribute money.

---

250 W.M. Christie, "Nazirite," The International Standard Bible Encyclopaedia, ed. James Orr, Vol. III (Hendrickson Publishers ed. 2ⁿᵈ Printing March 1996. 4 vols.).

Not only did Jesus wear natural long hair, but of His certainty of being a Nazarite will also be shown. As mentioned earlier, Jesus was foretold to have long curly hair, black as a raven similar to King Solomon's hair (Solomon's Song 5:11). Black does not necessarily mean pure or pitch black. It could also mean very dark, or brown, like how skin color is described then (Solomon's Song 1:5) and now. Thus, when it is said that a person is black, it should be obvious to the observer that the person's skin is actually brown. On the other hand, ravens are fairly black with hues or highlights of other colors. Therefore, Jesus hair was either, or somewhere between, very dark brown or nearly black or some combination of the full spectrum of colors in that range.

His unsurpassed beauty was also foretold in Psalm 45:2 and Solomon's Song 1:16, which is part of the reason multitudes of people were attracted to him (Matthew 8:18).[251] Some have erred with Isaiah 53:2 thinking Jesus not to be handsome from "no comeliness;" however, the meaning of this is that Jesus would "lack the earthly grandeur that allures the admiration of the world."[252] Jesus could care less about keeping pace with modern fashions and did not wear kingly or uppity attire. Solomon's Song 5:11 is the most detailed passage concerning the type of hair Jesus has. Although He has long curly hair, does this mean Jesus is a Nazarite, even from the womb?

Like Samson and Samuel, all scholars recognize that John the Baptist was a Nazarite from birth.[253] The angel commanded his father, Zacharias, that John was to drink no wine or strong drink; and he would be filled with the Holy Ghost; and his purpose was to prepare people for the Lord's coming (the promised Messiah or Christ) (Luke 1:11-17). As stated in the last chapter, John was the Elijah that was to come. John, like Elijah, spent much time in the wilderness where he ate locusts and honey (e.g., Mark 1:4-8). An interesting tidbit concerning John's appearance comes from the "Archko Volume: Herod Antipater's Defense before the Roman Senate in Regard to the Execution of John the Baptist." In this report Herod cleverly ridicules the appearance of John the Baptist before the short-haired Romans:

---

251 As he was the "type" of Christ in this regard, Solomon's beauty in these passages is also a prophecy of Christ's beauty.

252 Gleason L. Archer, commentary on Isaiah 53:2, eds. Charles F. Pfeiffer and Everett F. Harrison, The Wycliffe Bible Commentary (Chicago: Moody Press, 1990).

253 Christie.

[John] had no authority from God for what he was doing ....
And there is nothing better qualified than the course he took to
make an impression upon the ignorant and unlearned – to go
away out into the wilderness by himself, get a few friends from
Jerusalem to go out and hear him, and come back and tell of the
great wonders which they had seen .... Then John's appearance
– his long, uncombed hair and beard, his fantastic clothing, and
his food, nothing but bugs and beans – such a course and such a
character are well qualified to lead the illiterate astray. [254]

Obviously, Herod thought by condemning John's long hair before the
senate would somehow convince the senate of his innocence and John's
guilt. John did not have merely shoulder-length hair as depicted in most
Hollywood movies. As one who never cut his hair, he looked rather like
Elijah with hair hanging down his back. No doubt Herod was acquitted
for killing this innocent man, who was made to look like a rebel. Herod
pulled a bait and switch tactic. He switched the focus to John's outward
appearance rather than the heart of the matter. In truth, Herod may have
looked like a model citizen, but he was a wicked, evil man. Long-haired
John is in Heaven. The angel in similar fashion said to Mary, the mother
of Jesus:

The Holy Ghost shall come upon thee, and the power of the
Highest shall overshadow thee: therefore also that holy thing
which shall be born of thee shall be called the Son of God (Luke
1:35).

Jesus, being the Son of God, means He was the holiest person to ever
walk the earth. The word "holy" always carries with it the idea of being
separated unto God, consecrated. Consider what Mary knew. Who would
be more blessed or consecrated than the one born of the virgin, Mary, by
the power of God? Even Mary herself was probably a Nazarite with virgin
hair. As already stated, long uncut hair is a symbol of devotion to God.
Her devotion and separation unto God is revealed in the New Testament.
Because of this humble devotion Mary was considered highly favored by

---

254 McIntosh and Twyman, trans. The Archko Volume or, The Archeological Writings of
the Sanhedrim and Talmuds of the Jews. These Are The Official Documents Made in
These Courts in the Days of Jesus Christ. From manuscripts in Constantinople and the
Records of the Senatorial Docket taken from the Vatican at Rome. (New Canaan, CT:
Keats Publishing, Inc. 1975), Chapter X, 157-158.

God (Luke 1:28). Soon after the angel Gabriel gave her the announcement of Jesus' birth, Mary went to visit Elisabeth, the mother of John the Baptist (Luke 1:39-56). Surely Elisabeth, pregnant with John, would have told Mary that John is to be a Nazarite. Plus, Mary knew the holiness of what was in her womb. The angel only needed to say the words "holy thing" and "Son of God," thus Mary would have known what to do and what not to do. With this being said, would she have dared to bring a razor against his holy head? The idea of such a thing is unconscionable. On the contrary, Mary would have done as Samson's and Samuel's mothers, who never brought a razor to their holy sons' heads.

The Prophetess Anna, who was well over 100 years old, "went not out of the Temple, but served God with fastings and prayers night and day" was obviously a Nazarite (Luke 2:36-38). She had great strength for she practiced her faith in this way for an astounding 84 years after she became a widow. For her devotion to God, she was blessed to affirm the Christ child Jesus. For these reasons alone makes Jesus a Nazarite from the womb. But there is more, much more. Now let us examine the case of Matthew's Gospel, as translated from "The 1599 Geneva Bible."

> Then Herod, seeing that he was mocked of the Wise men, was exceeding wroth, and sent forth, and slew all the male children that were in Bethlehem, and in all the coasts thereof from two years old and under, according to the time which he had diligently searched out of the Wise men. Then that was fulfilled which is spoken by the Prophet Jeremiah, saying, in Ramah was a voice heard, mourning, and weeping, and great howling: Rachel weeping for her children, and would not be comforted, because they were not. And when Herod was dead, behold, an Angel of the Lord appeareth in a dream to Joseph in Egypt, Saying, Arise, and take the babe and his mother, and go into the land of Israel. But when he heard that Archelaus did reign in Judah instead of his father Herod, he was afraid to go thither: yet after he was warned of God in a dream, he turned aside into the parts of Galilee. And went and dwelt in a city called Nazareth [Gr. Ναζαρετ: *Nazaret*] that it might be fulfilled which was spoken by the Prophets, which was, That he should be called a Nazarite [Gr. Ναζωραιος: *nazoraios*] (Matthew 2:17-23, "The 1599 Geneva Bible").

In Matthew 2:23 the village of Nazareth is not mentioned in any ancient records other than the New Testament. Matthew goes on to inform us that the fulfillment of prophesy, from the Old Testament prophets, was that he would be called a *Nazoraios*. Argyle says there is an intended allusion to the birth of and long hair of Samson, both called to be unshorn: no razor.[255] *Nazor* seems to be a shortened form of *no razor*. In modern versions *Nazoraios* is usually translated Nazarene, which is actually from a similar Greek word to be discussed later.

So Jesus was to be called a *Nazoraios* who grew up in Nazareth, apparently a town of like-minded people. Ancient notes on Matthew 2:19-23 state that "Jesus is the Lord's true Nazarite."[256] All the ancient English translations (compiled in "The English Hexapla") prior to the King James Version translated Matthew 2:23 in like manner (see Table 6-1).[257] The better translation of *Nazoraios* is indeed "Nazarite."

Table 6-1: Translation of *Nazoraios* from Matthew 2:23

Ancient English Versions compared to Greek Bible and Latin Vulgate	
Greek Bible	ναζωραιος = *nazoraios*
Latin Vulgate	Nazaraeus (or Nazareus) [1]
Wiclif -1380	nazarey
Tyndale - 1534	Nazarite
Cranmer - 1539	Nazarite
Geneva – 1557 & 1599	Nazarite
Rheims – 1582	Nazarite
King James Version -1611	Nazarene

1   Leo F. Stelten, "Dictionary of Ecclesiastical Latin," (Peabody, Massachusetts: Hendrickson Publishers, Inc., 1995)

---

255 A.W. Argyle, "The Gospel According to Matthew," The Cambridge Bible Commentary on The New English Bible (London: Cambridge University Press, 1963).

256 Commentary notes on Matthew 2:19-23 in The 1599 Geneva Bible (White Hall, West Virginia: Tolle Lege Press, 2006).

257 The English Hexapla, Exhibiting the Six Important English Translations of the New Testament Scriptures. Includes the Wycliffe, Tyndale, Cranmer, Genevan, Anglo-Rhemish, and Authorized English versions (Reprint of the 1841 ed. published by Samuel Bagster and Sons, London. New York: AMS Press, Inc., 1975).

Table 6-2: Various Greek Forms of Jesus' Title in Context

Passage	Transliterated Greek Word	Comments
Matthew 2:23	Nazoraios	Fulfillment of Prophecy
Mark 1:24; Luke 4:34	Nazarene	Demons identify Jesus
Mark 10:47	Nazoraios	Blind man @ Jericho when he heard it was Jesus
John 18:5,7	Nazoraiou	Arrest of Jesus: I am He
Mark 14:67	Nazareno	Peter accused: you too were with Jesus the Nazareno
Matthew 26:71*	Nazoraiou	Peter accused: you too were with Jesus the Nazoraiou
John 19:19	Nazoraios	Pilate had a sign written on the cross: Jesus the Nazoraios
Mark 16:6	Nazarenon	The Angel's message to the women who came to Jesus' tomb
Luke 24:19	Nazoraiou	After Jesus resurrection on road to Emmaus
Acts 2:22	Nazoraion	Peter addresses a crowd
Acts 3:6	Nazoraiou	Peter heals in the name of Jesus the Nazoraiou
Acts 4:10	Nazoraiou	Peter addresses the Sanhedrin
Acts 6:14	Nazoraios	Jewish leaders accuse Stephen of saying: Jesus the Nazoraios is going to destroy this place
Acts 22:8	Nazoraios	Jesus introduces Himself to Saul (Paul): I am Jesus the Nazoraios
Acts 24:5*	Nazoraion	Paul accused of being a ringleader of the sect of the Nazoraion
Acts 26:9	Nazoraiou	Paul originally thought his duty to oppose Jesus the Nazoraiou

* In Matthew 26:71: The Rheims – 1582 version translate Nazoraiou as Nazarite; likewise, in Acts 24:5: Tyndale – 1534; Cranmer – 1539; and Geneva – 1557 Bibles all translated Nazoraion as Nazarites.

Besides Matthew 2:23 of the Greek Bible, the town of Nazareth itself is only mentioned eleven other times: in Matthew 4:13, 21:11; Mark 1:9; Luke

1:26, 2:4, 39,51, 4:16; John 1:45,46; and Acts 10:38). But in "The English Hexapla," the six ancient English versions translate *Nazoraios* as Nazareth: "Jesus of Nazareth" instead of "Jesus the Nazarite" in many other passages of the New Testament. Apparently, since Matthew is the first book of the New Testament these translators believed that to say "Jesus of Nazareth" meant the same as "Jesus the Nazarite." Although there certainly is a rich variety words with the letters N-Z-R, to be consistent, should not the same Greek word be translated into the same English word? Besides, many of these words have the definite article in Greek (ο or του). This would indicate the title of Jesus rather than where he was from (see Table 6-2).

Today, some attempt to deny that Christ was a Nazarite with long hair, and these people further show a Jesus with relatively short hair in their books. They also think Nazarene is merely someone from Nazareth. These claims fall well short of the facts of Holy Writ. Besides, the main reason some modern Protestant theologians claim such has little to do with word relationships and more to do with the lifestyle of the Saviour.[258] They cannot seem to understand that Nazarites *for life* had special callings. For example when Samson, Samuel, and Jesus came near and even touched dead bodies, none of them lost their status as a Nazarite. Likewise, Samson and Jesus mixed with the sinners of society, and neither lost their Naziriteship. We must remember that God cannot be placed into some rigid manmade system of theology. He is the God of great variety, individuality, diversity, and thus special callings in life. Now John the Baptist was one of those lifelong Nazarites who may have separated himself completely from the ways of the world, just like those under the vow on a temporary basis (Numbers 6). In truth, Dosker and those like him are wrong and Jerome did get it correct along with all the ancient English versions as well. Jesus is a Nazirite.

One reason they believed Jesus is a Nazarite may be due to the fact that the Greek word *Nazoraios,* which occurs five times in the New Testament (Table 6-2) is very similar to ancient Greek translations of the Hebrew term for *nazir* (or Nazarite) in the Old Testament. Sometime between 285-247 B.C., the Hebrew Scriptures (i.e., Old Testament) were translated into Greek. This Greek version is called the Septuagint (LXX). Three manuscripts of the Septuagint or LXX have been handed down to us:

---

258 Henry E. Dosker, "Nazarene." The International Standard Bible Encyclopaedia, ed. James Orr. Vol. III (Hendrickson Publishers ed. 2nd Printing March 1996. 4 vols.). Dosker thinks Jesus' lifestyle did not match that of a Nazarite. However, this idea is a short-sighted, narrow view of what a Nazarite is suppose to do or be. Each individual Nazarite has his own calling or purpose.

Codex Alexandrinus; Codex Vaticanus; and Codex Sinaiticus.[259] From Lamentations 4:7 of the Codex Vaticanus used by Brenton,[260] Nazarite was translated from the Greek word *Naziraioi*, which is remarkably similar to *Nazoraios* and *Nazoraiou* of the New Testament. The slight difference of vowel choices is probably due to spelling or pronunciation changes from the time the LXX was penned to the time of the various New Testament authors' writings, some 300 years later.

Tables 6-3 and 6-4 indicate how the New Testament terms are traced back into the Old Testament. These also show the relationship between the Greek ναζωραιος, *nazoraios* (as in Matthew 2:23) and the Greek term ναζαρηνε, *Nazarene*, (as in Mark 1:24). Nazarene too is used as a title of Jesus and is synonymous with Nazarite.[261] Again, the word Nazarite (or Nazirite) means "holiness," "devotion," "consecrated one," and one who took "a vow of separation."[262] Thus, Nazarene is not just someone from the town of Nazareth, it is also a title of Jesus confirmed by the spirit world. "The Interlinear Bible" gives us a very literal translation of Mark 1:24, in which a demon-possessed man said:

> What is to us and to You, Jesus, Nazarene? Have You come to destroy us? I know You, who You [Jesus] are, the Holy One of God

Just after the demons identify Jesus as a "Nazarene," they call Him the "Holy One of God." This cannot be just a coincidence ... Jesus, Nazarene: Jesus, Holy One of God! Here in Mark 1:24, Nazarene is defined as Holy One of God, which is one of the definitions of Nazarite. As Table 6-3 shows, the Greek translators of the Codex Vaticanus version of the LXX, actually paraphrased what the title Nazir (or Nazirite, Nazarite) meant. In most cases they paraphrased the meaning of the Hebrew rather than a word for word translation. On the other hand, the Codex Alexandrinus (LXX) did a literal word for word translation in most cases (Table 6-4).

---

259 Edwin Hatch and Henry Redpath, A Concordance to the Septuagint, In Three Volumes (Grand Rapids, Michigan: Baker Book House, 1987).
260 Sir Lancelot C.L. Brenton, trans., The Septuagint with Apocrypha: Greek and English (reprint of the 1851 ed. Published by Samuel Bagster and Sons, London. Peabody, Massachusetts: Hendrickson Publishers, Inc., Fifth Printing, 1995).
261 Robert Eisenman, The New Testament Code (London: Watkins Publishing, 2006), 52.
262 Christie.

Table 6-3: Tracing the Connection between Various N-Z-R Forms of the New Testament back to the Greek Septuagint (LXX) Old Testament based on the Codex Vaticanus.

OLD TESTAMENT			
Scripture	**Prophet**	**Old Testament Word, Nazarite**	**Greek Translations of Nazarite as recorded in the LXX: Codex Vaticanus**
Numbers 6:2		Nazarite*, to separate	Vow to separate oneself
Numbers 6:13	Moses	Nazarite	Him that has vowed
Numbers 6:19		Nazarite, consecrated hair	Holy hair
Judges 13:5		Nazarite	*Nazir* translated Nazarite
Judges 13:7	Samuel	Nazarite to God	Holy to God
Judges 16:17		Nazarite unto God	Holy one of God
Amos 2:11	Amos	Young men for Nazarites	Young men for consecration
Amos 2:12		Nazarites	Consecrated ones
Lamentations 4:7	Jeremiah	Nazarites	Nazarites from the Greek *Naziraoioi*
NEW TESTAMENT			
Scripture	**Comment**	**Greek Translations**	
Matthew 2:23	Above Prophets fulfilled in Jesus	The Greek *Nazoriaos* translated Nazarite in the following ancient English versions: Tyndale 1534; Cranmer – 1539; Geneva – 1557; Rheims – 1582; and Geneva – 1599. But is translated Nazarene in modern versions beginning with the King James Version - 1611.	
Mark 1:24	Jesus confirmed by the spirit world	Jesus, Nazarene from the same in Greek: *Nazarene*, Holy One of God	

* Nazarite (or Nazirite) in English is simply *Nazir* in Hebrew or better: NZR or N-Z-R since Hebrew originally had no vowel markings but consonants only.

Table 6-4: Greek Septuagint (LXX) Old Testament based on the Codex Alexandrinus

Greek Old Testament		
Scripture	Transliterated Greek	Comments/Meaning of N-Z-R form
Leviticus 21:12	*nazer*	For the ***crown[nazer]*** of the anointing oil of his God is upon him (KJV). In Lev. 21 the sons of Aaron are called to be Nazarites.
Leviticus 25:5	*nazaraios*	used of the *untrimmed* **vine**
Numbers 6:18-19	*nazeraios*	For those taking a temporal nazarite vow: no razor
Judges 13:5	*naziraion*	Parents instructed that Samson was to be a nazarite from the womb; no razor to touch his hair
Judges 13:7	*nazeiraion*	
Judges 16:17	*nazeiraios*	Samson informs Delilah that the secret of his strength is in his long hair
Scripture	Greek Translations of New Testament Again	
Matthew 2:23	The Greek *Nazoriaos* translated Nazarite in the following ancient English versions: Tyndale 1534; Cranmer – 1539; Geneva – 1557; Rheims – 1582; and Geneva – 1599. But is translated Nazarene in modern versions beginning with the King James Version - 1611.	
Mark 1:24	Jesus, Nazarene from the same in Greek: *Nazarene*, Holy One of God	

Several things become apparent as shown in Tables 6-2, 6-3, and 6-4. First of all, (see Table 6-3) if Nazarite unto God means "Holy one of God" (Judges 16:17), and Nazarene means "Holy one of God" as Mark indicates (Mark 1:24), then Nazarene is a synonym of Nazarite. And who was ever more holy than Jesus? Now we can see plainly why Matthew (in Matthew 2:23) referred to Prophets, plural. Thus, Matthew 2:23 is not a direct quote from any single prophecy by one Prophet. It is rather a fulfillment of the entire idea of the Lord's Holiness – the ultimate Nazarite based on several Prophets represented by several "types" of Christ within the Old Testament, including King Solomon as mentioned earlier. Next, the word spellings of three main forms in the Greek Old Testament (LXX) are directly comparable to the three main forms in the Greek New Testament (Table 6-5).

Table 6-5: Word Spellings of the translators of the Greek Old Testament (Septuagint, 3rd century B.C.) compared with the Greek New Testament (1st century A.D.).

Greek Septuagint (LXX) Old Testament Words	Corresponding Greek New Testament Terminology
Nazaraios; nazeraois; nazeiraios	Nazoraios
Naziraion; nazeiraion	Nazoraion
Naziraoioi	Nazoraiou

Table 6-5 compiled from Tables 6-2 and 6-4.

In consideration of the fact that the Hebrew language in its pure form had consonants only, and no vowels, the word relationship between Nazarite, Nazirite, Nazaraios, Nazeraois, Nazieraios, Nazoriaos, Naziraion, Nazieraion, Nazoraion, Naziraoioi, Nazoraiou, Nazarene, Nazareno and so forth becomes even more obvious. In the first place, the English word Nazarite, or Nazirite, is transliterated from only three consonants of the Hebrew. These correspond to the English letters NZR. Some prefer N-Z-R, the dashes meaning where vowels are supposed to be inserted. But which vowels do we add? And what suffix do we put on the end of the word? As far as suffixes go, this is something done in Greek (e.g., aios, aion and so forth), Latin (e.g., aeus, eus) and English (e.g., ite as in Nzr-ite), but again, the original transliterated Hebrew merely corresponds to the English letters NZR with no suffix.

Vowel markings were added to the Hebrew Bible (Old Testament) sometime around A.D. 600 to standardize pronunciation.[263] This is nearly 900 years after the Septuagint and about 500 years after the books of Matthew, Mark, Luke, John, and Acts were written. The readers at that time had to supply the vowels, and thereby the vowel sounds. The vowel sounds must have varied greatly within the many different sects of people, especially over this vast amount of time. To believe otherwise would be a preposterous notion. It is interesting to note that all translators, modern and ancient, believe the letter 'a' is the first vowel: Naz-r. The difference

---

263 John J. Parsons, "Hebrew Vowels," accessed June 30, 2008 http://www.hebrew4christians.com/Grammar/Unit_Two/Introduction/introduction.html.

occurs only with the second vowel choice in the pronunciation of the second syllable.

Some modern scholars may insist the vowels of N-Z-R are thus: nazir. This form does occur in Lamentations 4:7 (LXX-Codex Vaticanus) and also in Judges 13:5 (LXX-Codex Alexandrinus). However, the Codex Alexandrinus also gives us nazer (Leviticus 21:12; Numbers 6:18-19) and nazar (Leviticus 25:5).[264] The most logical reason for these slight differences in spelling is the way that people of different dialects pronounced the same word. Even Peter was recognized as being from Galilee based upon the way he spoke (Mark 14:70). Apparently, the Galileans preferred nazar (as in Nazarene), and nazor (as in Nazoraois). The Jewish Virtual Library puts it this way: "Transliteration is more of an art than a science, and opinions on the correct way to transliterate words vary widely .... Each spelling has a legitimate phonetic and orthographic basis; none is right or wrong."[265] What honesty, none is right or wrong! It is good to know that such honest scholarship still exists in our day.

The *crown of the anointing oil* (*nazer*) is long hair (Leviticus 21:12; see Table 6-4). The sons of Aaron were not to make bare any part of their heads. The oil extruded by each follicle is designed to protect both the scalp (crown) and the hair. In Leviticus 25:5, where the Greek (LXX-Codex Alexandrinus) *nazaraois* (nazar) is translated as the "untrimmed vine," is most interesting. Of course in the Hebrew it is simply N-Z-R. For Jesus identifies Himself to his apostles as the vine:

> I am the true vine .... I am the vine, ye are the branches (John 15:1,5).

The *untrimmed vine* corresponds to the real long hair of a *nazarite* being unshorn from the womb. In like manner Jesus even introduces Himself this way to the apostle Paul, saying *I am Jesus the Nazoraois* (Acts 22:8). The long hair of God signifies that His kingdom of eternal life is extended to all nations and people who truly believe in Christ. So what do the Scriptures teach? Jesus wears long virtuous majestic hair, uncut from the womb.

---

264 Edwin Hatch and Henry A. Redpath, A Concordance to the Septuagint. See this work for all the various N-Z-R forms used in the Greek translation of the Hebrew Bible (or Old Testament).

265 Mitchell G. Bard, ed., "Hebrew Alphabet," Jewish Virtual Library, The American-Israeli Cooperative Enterprise 2008, accessed August 3, 2008 http://www.jewishvirtuallibrary. org/jsource/Judaism/alephbet.html.

Table 6-6: Comparison between Samson and Jesus

Nazarite Rules (Numbers 6)	Samson	Jesus
No going near dead bodies	Touched a dead lion's body (Judges 14:8-9) and was in contact with 1000 Philistines who he killed (Judges 15:14-16).	Touched and healed a young girl's dead body (Mark 5:35-43); came near Lazarus' tomb who He raised from the dead (John 11); but also called people still alive (in body only) "dead": "let the dead bury their dead" (Matthew 8:22); "God is not the God of the dead, but of the living" (Matthew 22:32)
No Wine/ Strong Drink	Samson probably drank at his wedding feast (Judges 14:10), he did make love out of wedlock (Judges 16:1-4), which Josephus says included "drinking."	Turned water into wine at a wedding feast (John 2:11); and mixed with various people including the drinking of wine, which He did with "wisdom" (Luke 7:34-35); and shared a cup of wine* with His disciples at the last supper. A little wine was okay, but not drunkenness. The "wisdom" Jesus used was that He did this with "wisdom" – sparingly.
Hair / No razor to come upon the head	Samson's hair was never cut until Delilah betrayed him (Judges 16:17-19)	He relayed that every head hair is numbered (Matthew 10:30); and as He addressed a large crowd (Luke 20:45) Jesus forewarned that His followers would be hated, betrayed, and persecuted "Yet there shall not one hair of your heads perish" (Luke 21:18).
Result of cut hair	His strength left him for the Lord departed from him (Judges 16:19-20)	Soldiers struck His head after they placed a crown of thorns on His head (Matthew 27:29-30). This act damaged / cut some hairs and follicles. The Romans may have plucked some beard hairs as well (Isaiah 50:6). After this they crucified Him: Jesus said "My God, my God, why hast though forsaken me?," which means God departed from Jesus.
Long Hair grows back	The Lord hears his prayer, and his strength is restored (Judges 16:22-28)	Jesus was resurrected after three days (Mark 16:6-9; Luke 24:1-7), and not one of His long hairs perished (or will ever perish again) as a result of His resurrected body.

*wine – probably "new wine" being only lightly fermented.

As stated earlier, some claim that Jesus could not have been a Nazarite due to his lifestyle. This confusion arises over the rules stated in Numbers 6. The vow in Numbers 6 was written for those who were already adults, and who took the vow on a temporary basis.[266] W.M. Christie also recognizes this fact. Numbers 6 was written for those taking the Nazarite vow for a "limited time," usually 30, 60, or 100 days.[267] Therefore, a strict following of the rules applied only to those taking the vow temporarily. This temporal vow was for individuals who would separate themselves unto the Lord, perhaps to seek His will for their life, without any distractions from the world. Even if the temporary devotee's family members died during his vow, he was not to go near them. Otherwise the vow was null and void (Numbers 6:7-8). But lifelong Nazarites had special individualized callings and did not adhere to any strict rules like those taking the vow for a small amount of time. We can further show this to be the case by comparing the life of Christ to one of His forerunners or "types," the lifelong Nazarite, Samson.

As indicated in Table 6-6, neither Samson nor Jesus lost their power from the Most High when they touched dead bodies or drank wine. In both cases they lost their power when the Lord departed them. And this forsaking or departing by God occurred only after their consecrated hair, the most high part of the body, was ruined. Thankfully, their cut, damaged or ruined hair grew back (Samson), or was made virgin again (Jesus in the resurrection). In eternity, no man (or woman) will ever force us to cut our long hair and thereby bring damage to our heads (Luke 21:18).

Other Historical Writings

The next evidence that Jesus wears long hair and a beard concerns more detail about Him being a Nazarite. This source is a book titled "Yehoshua Nazir, Jesus the Nazarite" by Dr. Otoman Zar-Adusht Hanish. According to Hanish, his book summarizes much larger works about Jesus' (or Yessu) life and mission as found recorded in Oriental Temples, especially from Johannitan communities and Coptic monasteries. Much of this work fills the vacuity of Jesus time as a young man prior to His works written by the Gospel writers. Hanish relates that Jesus greatly disliked bigotry and false interpretations of etiquette and customs. He "enjoyed perfect freedom."[268]

---

266 William Smith, ed., "Nazarite," A Concise Dictionary of the Bible, Comprising its Antiquities, Biography, Geography, and Natural History (Boston: Little, Brown, and Company, 1865).

267 Christie.

268 Otoman Zar-Adusht Hanish, Yehoshua Nazir, Jesus the Nazarite: Life of Christ (Los Angeles, CA: Mazdaznan Press, 1917), 29.

Jesus' heart and mind went out toward the oppressed and downtrodden, so He intended to be a Nazarite, dedicating His life to the sole purpose of redemption.[269] Again, Nazarite means no razor, thus He wore long natural hair. Jesus also showed that the ruling priesthood did "nothing" to liberate the masses. In fact, Jesus believed that neither the religious system nor the state was engaged in the interest of humanity, except in so far as their own gain was concerned. He strongly advanced the idea of individualism:

> As an avowed individualist, recognizing in every man the potentialities of infinite possibilities, Yessu decried any and every measure that impeded the growth or development of individual souls, and for this reason refused identification with any form or system calculated to uphold one certain class at the expense of another.[270]

The reader should understand that the Gospel writings declare much of what Hanish is saying. Jesus often gets a bad rap for what certain ignorant religious people do. His way is diametrically opposed to any system of religion which destroys individuality. Forced male head shearing is one of these reductions in individuality. Hanish goes on and says that Jesus believed that "all the immoral, degrading, and destructive tendencies in man had grown or developed because of despotic practices by those in authority."[271] And what destroys or despoils individuality more than the continual removal of the hair and beard by steel blades?

There are even first century descriptions about the likeness of Jesus. Some of these occur in "The Archko Volume" or "The Archeological Writings of the Sanhedrim & Talmuds of the Jews." These writings are considered to be "The Official Documents Made in These Courts in the Days of Jesus Christ." Chapter V in "The Archko Volume" is called "Gamaliel's interview with Joseph and Mary and others concerning Jesus." These holy writings were found in the St. Sophia Mosque at Constantinople, now the Hagia Sophia, Istanbul, Turkey, made by Gamaliel, in the Talmuds of the Jews, 27B. Gamaliel, mentioned in Acts 5:34; 22:3, was a chief priest of the Pharisees from A.D. 30 – 60 and instructor of the Apostle Paul. In this account the Sanhedrim sends out Gamaliel to find out more about Jesus. In a small part of his detailed report Gamaliel describes Jesus' appearance:

---

269 Hanish, 33-34.
270 Hanish, 48, see also pages 46-49 about Jesus' ill feelings about the ruling priesthood and state.
271 Hanish, 49.

He is the picture of his mother, only he has not her smooth round face. His hair is a little more golden than hers, though it is as much from *sunburn* as anything else. He is tall, and his shoulders are a little drooped; his visage is thin and of a swarthy complexion, though this is from *exposure*. His eyes are large and a soft blue, and rather dull and heavy. The lashes are long, and his eyebrows very large. His nose is that of a Jew. In fact, he reminds me of an old-fashioned Jew in every sense of the word (emphasis mine).[272]

This description was given by Gamaliel when Jesus was 26 years old. When he says that Jesus' hair was "more golden" than Mary's does not mean Jesus had blonde hair, for he said it was from "sunburn," what we would call sun-bleached hair. Mary's hair remained darker because when outdoors her hair would have been veiled as customary for women in those days. If Jesus regularly had His hair cut, then it would never have appeared sun-bleached. Sun-bleaching of hair occurs after much time in the sun with long uncut hair. His long hair would appear much lighter on the surface and towards the ends, the oldest part of the hair, when compared to the darker hair first emerging from the follicles of the scalp. Obviously, Jesus spent much time outdoors in the sun with His head uncovered. This fact combined with His tanned skin called "swarthy," and his being "old-fashioned" like one of the ancients fits the copies of the portraits of Jesus handed down to us.

Physical Images and Icons of Christ

In Rome, early Christian art prior to the 4th century pictured Jesus "as an ideal type, a type of the classical Roman."[273] This was until believers in that far away land came to realize that the likeness of Jesus was not Roman. If the early Roman church had a copy of the Scriptures and studied them they may have been able to discern the fact of Jesus' long hair and beard. However, the first three centuries of Christianity were quite

272 McIntosh and Twyman, trans. The Archko Volume or, The Archeological Writings of the Sanhedrim and Talmuds of the Jews. These Are The Official Documents Made in These Courts in the Days of Jesus Christ. From manuscripts in Constantinople and the Records of the Senatorial Docket taken from the Vatican at Rome. (New Canaan, CT: Keats Publishing, Inc. 1975). Quote from Chapter V: *Gamaliel's interview with Joseph and Mary and others concerning Jesus*, 92-93.

273 Orazio Marucchi, Manual of Christian Archeology, Fourth Italian Edition revised by Giulio Belvederi, secretary of the Pontifical Institute of Christian Archeology, Rome 1933. Hubert Vecchierello, trans. (Patterson, NJ: St. Anthony Guild Press, Franciscan Monastery, 1935), 312.

brutal, and other matters such as the resurrection of Christ and His Gospel message were much more important than Jesus' appearance. Along with the message, avoiding persecution and death from their fellow citizens was also more of a concern. And then there were schisms amongst believers over the issue of idolatry or the worship of images, a great problem in those days. The worry about images stems from an interpretation of Exodus 20:4-5:

> Thou shalt not make unto thee any graven image, or any likeness of anything that is in heaven above, or that is in the earth beneath, or that is in the water under the earth: Thou shalt not bow down thyself to them, nor serve them …

The context of this passage means that one is not to make images for the purpose of worship. You are not to "bow down" before them. God is not against art or artists. The main thing is that pictures, statues, and other works of man, like modern photographs, are not to be worshiped, as is clear in this passage. As all know, a picture saves a thousand words. As long as a person can avoid idolatry, pictures, whether ancient or modern, are perfectly fine.

The pictures or icons of Jesus Christ handed down through the centuries are based upon two images originating in the first century: (1) a statue of Christ erected in Philippi (also called Paneus or Paneas, modern day Banias); and (2) a painted portrait of Christ brought back to Edessa, Syria, modern Urfa, Turkey. Eusebius (A.D. 260-340) wrote about the statue and pictures of Jesus in existence at the time along with many other facts and events of early Christianity in his "Ecclesiastical History."

While at Caesarea Philippi, Eusebius and his companions saw the statue of Jesus Christ there with the woman kneeling before Him.[274] Tradition held that the woman diseased with a hemorrhage, who was healed by touching the hem of the Lord's garment (Matthew 9:20-22; Mark 5:25-34; Luke 8:43-48), erected it to honor Christ. Eusebius says this was a typical practice of the Gentiles who "were accustomed to pay this kind of honor." He also says that before the kneeling woman's feet, "there is a certain strange plant growing, which rising as high as the hem of the brazen garment, is a kind of antidote to all kinds of diseases." In the "Manual of Christian Archeology," Marucchi says:

---

274 C.F. Cruse, trans, Eusebius' Ecclesiastical History, Book 7, Chapter 18. Complete and Unabridged, New Updated Edition (Peabody, MA: Hendrickson Publishers, 1998, Fifth Printing – June 2006).

This statue, which was held in great veneration .... must had a certain resemblance to the real type of the Saviour, and served as a model for the Oriental pictures and those introduced into the Occident toward the end of the same century. In these paintings, the Saviour is represented as having a beard .... From these types the ancient iconographic pictures of Christ were derived – bearded images with long, flowing hair, such as may be seen in some paintings dating from the time of peace.[275]

There can be little doubt that word about the statue of Jesus Christ spread quickly to the known Christian world. This would inspire pilgrimages to view the statue, for most people are very interested in the appearance of others, especially the Son of God. John Francis Wilson in his book "Caesarea Philippi" relates that a powerful orthodox Christian community is believed to have worshiped there and was an "aspiring place of pilgrimage."[276] Then Julian the Apostate came along.

According to Wilson, during Julian's reign (Roman emperor from A.D. 361 – 363), the pagans pulled down the statue and dragged it through the streets with ropes fastened around its feet.[277] Local Christians recovered the head and other fragments. Julian thought very highly of himself and had a statue of himself erected in its place, which was his plan all along. He ordered the rebuilding of the Jewish temple in Jerusalem and set out to conquer Persia where he died at the age of 32. On May 19, 363 a great earthquake occurred that "ripped up the Jordan valley." It was this catastrophic event that probably triggered nearby eruptions, "fire from heaven" and lightning, which destroyed Julian's statue of himself.[278] A third part of Caesarea Philippi was destroyed and the rebuilding of the Jewish temple in Jerusalem ceased. The statue of Christ was rebuilt after Julian was gone.

Two witnesses, Philostorgius (who wrote from A.D. 425 – 433), and Sozomen (who wrote in A.D. 445), both say the statue was placed inside the church at Caesarea Philippi after the Julian catastrophe. But after the 5th century the statue is merely mentioned by various authors who never visited the area. These, Wilson says, only cited older sources. By the 6th century the city became completely abandoned for reasons not

---

275 Marucchi, 312.
276 John Francis Wilson, Caesarea Philippi (Banias, The Lost City of Pan). (London (or New York): I.B. Tauris & Co Ltd, 2004), 96.
277 John Francis Wilson, 99.
278 John Francis Wilson, 99, 102.

fully understood.[279] The final fate of the statue is unknown. Although the whereabouts of the statue are unknown, a 4th century artist appears to have visited the site and sculpted a likeness of the statue. In 1591, a 4th century Christian sarcophagus was discovered beneath the floor of the basilica of St. Peter in Rome. Wilson concurs that this artist must have based his work on the actual statue. This image can be seen in Figures 30 and 32 of Wilson's book, or online. It is called the Lateran sarcophagus and is now in the Pio Christian Museum in the Vatican.[280] Although Wilson compares the image on the sarcophagus with the possibility of it being the Roman emperor Hadrian, the comparison falls short on several counts. Hadrian's bust is well known and looks nothing like the man on the sarcophagus except for his full beard. Hadrian's facial features are much different and he did not have hair as long as the man on the sarcophagus. Furthermore, the Roman Christians at the time could easily have seen the various statues and busts of Hadrian that were made. If they even thought for a moment that it was Hadrian, the carving of Christ on the sarcophagus would not have been made. They believed it represented Jesus Christ as handed down by the church at Caesarea Philippi. Even the Roman emperor Julian clearly would have seen images of Hadrian in Rome. He knew it was not Hadrian's image that he had dragged through the streets. By his instigation, it was the statue of Christ dragged through the streets.

The next image created during the first century was a painting made of Christ while he was alive. The story begins with an ancient Syriac document called "The Doctrine of Addai, The Apostle," which is a very scholarly detailed account concerning the history of Addai, also known as Addæus or Thaddaeus, a disciple of Christ, in Edessa.[281] The writer identifies himself as "Labubna, the son of Sennac, the son of Abshadar, the king's scribe." In this manuscript is a record of a correspondence between King Abgar V (Abgar Ukkama) and Jesus. It all began when Abgar, who had a disease for some time, heard about the miracles and healings done by Jesus. Apparently, many from Syria travelled to Palestine to be healed by Jesus:

And his [Jesus] fame went throughout all Syria: and they brought unto him all sick people that were taken with divers diseases and

279 John Francis Wilson, 109.
280 John Francis Wilson, 93-94. Figures 30 and 32 in this book are photographs of the Lateran sarcophagus showing the image of Christ.
281 "The Doctrine of Addai, The Apostle," The Doctrine of Addai (1876), English Translation, accessed August 15, 2008 http://www.tertullian.org/fathers/addai_2_text.htm.

torments, and those which were possessed with devils, and those which were lunatic, and those that had the palsy; and he healed them (Matthew 4:24).

Even though Jesus was controversial, and crucified, in His own country, in Syria it was quite the opposite. Syria is where Jesus became famous. "The Doctrine of Addai" informs us that in October (of the 343rd year of the Seleucian era, probably A.D. 32) Abgar sends two nobles Marihab, Shamshagram, along with Hannan, who was the tabularius or keeper of the city archives on a long journey. Hannan is also known as Ananias, considered to be the same man who helped Paul (Acts 9:10-18).[282] This included a ten day stay at Jerusalem. As the tabularius, it was Hannan's job to record all things of import during their travels. He wrote down everything "he saw that Christ did" as well as the other things already done by Him. They returned to Edessa probably before winter, sometime in December. Hannan reads his report about Christ to the king and his princes. Upon hearing such things, Abgar said "These mighty works are not of men, but of God" for only God can "make the dead alive." Eventually Abgar writes a letter to Jesus. In it Abgar testifies that Jesus must be the Son of God due to the miracles, and he then invites Jesus to Edessa to heal his disease. So in the following spring, on the 14th day of Adar (February/March), Abgar sends Hannan back to Jerusalem with the letter to deliver it to Christ.

Hannan arrives back in Jerusalem on the 12th day of Nisan (March/April) and finds Jesus at the house of Gamaliel. When Jesus received the letter he did not write back but told Hannan His reply. Jesus said He could not come to Edessa because His work "here is now finished, and I am going up to my Father, who sent me, and when I have gone up to Him, I will send to thee one of my disciples, who will cure the disease which thou hast." Thus Hannan wrote down all the things Jesus said and returned to Edessa with a portrait of Christ, which he painted:

> by virtue of being the king's painter, he took and painted a likeness of Jesus with choice paints, and brought [it] with him to Abgar the king ... when Abgar saw the likeness, he received it with great joy, and placed it with great honour in one of his palatial houses [palaces].[283]

---

282 Also see Eisenman, 80.
283 The Doctrine of Addai, The Apostle.

We know from Jesus' words that His "work here is now finished," along with the date of Hannan's arrival that spring, meant that this event occurred within days of the crucifixion. After Christ was resurrected and ascended to heaven the Apostle Thomas (Judas Thomas) sent Addai, one of the seventy, also known by the name Thaddeus, to Abgar. These seventy, or seventy-two, disciples were already trained by Christ and had great success healing others (Luke 10: 1-17). In fact, Addai, also being from Caesaria Philippi,[284] obviously knew the woman with the issue of blood who was healed by touching Christ's hem (Luke 8:43-48). If he was not a disciple already, Addai must have become one instantaneously after that miracle. As part of the seventy, Christ empowered him with the gift of healing. Soon after his arrival in Edessa, Addai, in the presence of several others, put his hand on Abgar in Jesus' name, and immediately Abgar was healed from the disease. Because of this miracle and others in the king's court and elsewhere in Edessa, Addai was commissioned by Abgar to build the first church there as well as other churches in the region.

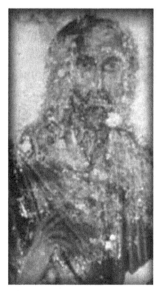

Figure 6-3: Incredibly Lifelike Painting of Christ from the Catacombs. This catacomb image appears to have been painted directly onto a plastered wall. It is very realistic and looks like an actual portrait. Could this painting be based on Hannan's portrait? Observe that there is no halo about the head. The halo began to be placed on Christ's head in mid 4th century and became a fixed symbol by late 4th century. For this reason this painting is probably early 4th century or even older! Some later images like the 6th century icon at St. Catherine's Monastery in Sinai seem to be based upon the two dimensional image on the Shroud of Turin.

During his research, Eusebius also traveled to Edessa and documented the account of King Abgar, Jesus, and Thaddeus (i.e., Addai) in his "Ecclesiastical History," early 4th century. Eusebius said he translated the

---

284 Kevin Knight, ed., Extracts from Various Books Concerning Abgar the King and Addæus the Apostle," New Advent featuring The Catholic Encyclopedia, Ed. 2. www. NewAdvent.org, 2007.

Syriac epistle directly from the archives of Edessa and also related that this document was already quite "ancient," even at the time he wrote.[285] He does not mention the picture of Christ painted by Hannan (Ananias), but is occupied with the more spiritual matters: words of Christ and the healing of Abgar (or Abgarus) by Thaddeus (or Addai). In fact, because Abgar and many more were healed along with other events, the "whole city of Edessa" became "devoted to the name of Christ." Eusebius does not mention the title of the Syriac epistle he used. However, Kerr understands that both Thomas and Thaddeus were connected with Edessa and indicates that "The Doctrine of Addai, The Apostle" was indeed the document Eusebius "made use of" in his translation.[286] The "made use of" comment obviously means Eusebius summarized what he felt were the most important portions of this ancient document, which came to be called "The Doctrine of Addai, The Apostle."

Concerning paintings of Christ, Eusebius simply mentions that portraits were "still preserved" in his time (again early 4th century), which testifies how ancient these portraits really were.[287] He attributes their making to the customs of the Gentiles. There is little doubt that one of these must have been the first century portrait of Christ brought to Edessa. Eusebius' mission to record early church history inspired the whole Christian world. It was Eusebius who was the chief bishop presiding at the right hand of the Roman Emperor Constantine at the Council of Nicea in A.D. 325. This world-changing event included 250 bishops from various cities of the world.[288] Among these was Philokalos, bishop of the church at Caesaria Philippi.

Although the likeness of Christ was not a top priority, most people, especially Gentiles, would have wanted to know what Jesus looked like. It was Philokalos who had firsthand knowledge about the statue at Caesaria Philippi, which Eusebius saw and wrote about while he himself resided there. They recognized that these things testified that Jesus had long flowing hair and a beard. Images aside, by this time many in the Council would have realized by then that this is what Scripture has always taught. Thus, as Constantine brought peace to the church, the true likeness of Christ showing long hair and beard became knowledge to all. News about

285 Eusebius' Ecclesiastical History. Book 2, Chapter 1.
286 C.M. Kerr, "Thaddaeus," The International Standard Bible Encyclopaedia, ed. James Orr, Vol. IV (Hendrickson Publishers ed. 2nd Printing March 1996. 4 vols.).
287 Eusebius' Ecclesiastical History, Book 7, Chapter 18.
288 Kevin Knight, ed., "Life of Constantine," New Advent featuring The Catholic Encyclopedia, Ed. 2. www.NewAdvent.org, 2007.

the statue and portraits spread abroad quickly. Concerning King Abgar and Jesus in "The Lost Books of the Bible," it relates that "the common people in England have this Epistle in their houses, in many places, fixed in a frame, with the picture of Christ before it."[289]

Late in the 5th century the correspondence between Abgar and Jesus was under consideration by the Roman church to be placed among the canon of Scripture. Unfortunately, in a council under Pope Gelasius in 494, it was declared apocryphal.[290] So it did not make it into the Bible. However, the highly respected conservative scholar and church father Eusebius believed the record as real history, for he translated portions of the account from "ancient" historical records in the city archives of Edessa. The church of the west did not place it in the canon of Scripture, but did the church of east, where Armenia and Edessa are located? This is just an interesting side note. But the main point is that both the church of the east and of the west agreed that all the evidence showed that Jesus has long hair and a full beard regardless of their other differences. They all knew the true likeness of Jesus – long, uncut hair as God Himself created it to be for all people.

Edessa is the place of yet another discovery. After decades of scientific and historical research, the Shroud of Turin is fascinating in every way.[291] It may very well be the burial cloth of Christ. In the year 730 St. John Damascene refers to a grave cloth now called the "Cloth of Edessa."[292] Daniel R. Porter explains how this oblong burial cloth was discovered hidden behind some stones of one of the city gates in the 6th century Edessa. The correlation between the Edessa cloth and the Shroud is good.

The thousands of scientific tests conducted by scores of scientists have demonstrated that the Shroud image is authentic. It shows a long haired bearded man who was crucified Roman style. The blood is real. The marks on this man's body depict the same marks Jesus received as described in the Gospels. Dr. John Heller and his colleagues found that he was beaten by two men, one taller the other, with a flagrum. There are blood flows

289 "The Epistles of Jesus Christ and Abgarus King of Edessa." The Lost Books of the Bible (World Bible Publishers. Alpha House Inc., 1926), 62.
290 Marucchi, 312.
291 John H. Heller, Report on the Shroud of Turin (Boston: Houghton Mifflin Company, 1983).
292 Daniel R. Porter, "The Shroud of Turin for Journalists, Where Have All the Skeptics Gone,?" accessed August 7, 2008 http://www.factsplusfacts.com/carbon-14-now-we-know.htm

from numerous puncture wounds on the "top and back of the scalp and forehead," the wounds in his left wrist and side are both visible, "a spike had been driven through both feet," and his legs were not broken.[293] This particular crucifixion matches precisely how Jesus was crucified.

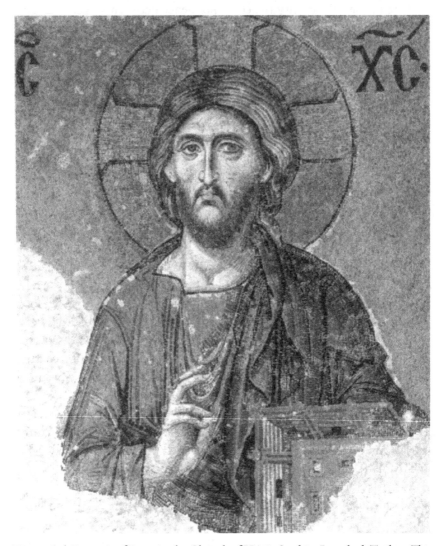

Figure 6-4: Portrait of Jesus in the Church of Hagia Sophia, Istanbul, Turkey. This mosaic icon of Christ is dated between the years 1185 to 1204. Beneath the surface was an earlier mosaic that appears to be of a 6th century date, which probably coincides with the re-construction of the Hagia Sophia dedicated in 537 A.D. This 12th or 13 century mosaic is more than likely an overlay replica of the 6th century image.

---

293 Heller, 2-4.

Images of the Shroud can be seen all over the internet. The most interesting work to date was just recently aired on the History Channel.[294] Ray Downing of Studio Macbeth, Inc. spent an extraordinary amount of time to produce a three dimensional illustration of the man in the Shroud. This remarkable work may be the most accurate image of Jesus yet. Portraits are available from his studio where you can see the images.[295]

The portraits of Jesus are based upon his age of somewhere between 30 to 33 years based on his earthly ministry. But his healthy long hair was an outgrowth of his healthy skin. He showed us the way hair should be worn – the natural way as it was created to be. If hair is cut too short then a young man may thin, go bald, become prematurely gray, or, in essence, lose his crown. Short hair exposes the skin and is a good way to look old and wrinkled due to the weathering effects of the elements especially the sun.

294 http://www.history.com/shows/the-real-face-of-jesus, accessed February 26, 2011
295 http://www.raydowning.com /, accessed February 26, 2011

Chapter 7: A LONG HAIResy

For I am the Lord, I change not ... (Malachi 3:6).

Paul's Haircut: A Rare Event Indeed

Is it a heresy (or better HAIResy) for a man to wear long hair as per God's own design in nature? If not then why are males in modern society forced to be shorn? Oftentimes the Apostle Paul's life and letters are often misread and used to promote constant head shearing, as if God Himself invented the razor. Paul and his haircut are mentioned in the "The Acts of the Apostles," a book that covers a time span of more than three decades.[296] Some time after his conversion to Christianity, Paul arrives in the metropolitan city of Corinth (Acts 18:1). According to chronologist Jack Finegan, this occurred in the year A.D. 51.[297] While there, Paul demonstrated that Jesus is the Christ, but the Jewish leadership resisted the message. So Paul said "from henceforth will I go unto the Gentiles" (Acts 18:6). He boldly preached at Corinth for a year and a half (Acts 18:9-10). The church that resulted consisted of mainly non-Jews.[298] Paul then sailed for Syria (Acts 18:18). But before doing so he had his head shorn in Cenchrea, or Cenchraea, a seaport of Corinth. The text (Acts 18:18) says that the reason Paul cut his hair is because he had a "vow":

> And Paul after this tarried there yet a good while, and then took his leave of the brethren, and sailed thence into Syria, and with

---

296 A.T. Robertson, "Acts of the Apostles," The International Standard Bible Encyclopaedia, ed. James Orr. Vol. I (Hendrickson Publishers ed. 2nd Printing March 1996. 4 vols.).

297 Jack Finegan, Handbook of Biblical Chronology, Revised ed. (Peabody, MA: Hendrickson Publishers, 1998), 396.

298 J.E. Harry, "Corinth," The International Standard Bible Encyclopaedia, ed. James Orr, Vol. 2 (Hendrickson Publishers ed. 2nd Printing March 1996. 4 vols.).

him Priscilla and Aquila; having shorn his head in Cenchrea: for he had a vow.

Most scholars agree that the "vow" was indeed a Nazarite vow.[299][300][301] On the other hand, the vow, perhaps in part, was made to the Corinthians who generally wore short hair at the time - it was a Roman controlled military city. For Paul's motto was to become "all things to all men" (1 Corinthians 9:22). However, if this was the case, then why did he wait until he departed Corinth? Rather it does seem likely that this was indeed a Nazarite vow because Paul served the Lord for a year and a half at Corinth. That was Paul's vow, his consecration, his mission to reach the Gentiles (Acts 18:6). During the 18-month vow, no razor would have touched his hair while under the Lord's protection to teach the Corinthians. Upon completion of this vow, he had his hair cut off. Head hair is not to be touched by cutting tools while under a temporal Nazarite vow. Therefore, his hair was untouched for at least 18 months. This means 18 months or longer without a haircut!

Four years after his haircut at Corinth, Paul arrives in Jerusalem.[302] Believers at Jerusalem could see plainly that Paul was a Nazarite by his hair and beard. So they compelled Paul to have his head shorn with four others also under the "vow" (Acts 21:18-29). These men were all under a temporary Nazarite vow. In accordance with this ritual of purification, described in Numbers 6, the head was shaved on the seventh day. But sometime before the seventh day ended, certain Jews from Asia saw Paul in the temple. They shouted and stirred up a great crowd against Paul who was seized and dragged out of the temple (Acts 21:27-30). This may have occurred prior to the head-shaving ritual. Therefore, as far as Paul's Nazarite vows are concerned, the Scriptures evidence only one or maybe two haircuts, one at the Corinthian seaport of Cenchrea, and possibly four years later at Jerusalem. What is certain is that Paul took temporal Nazarite vows on a regular basis.[303][304] He rarely cut his hair. On the contrary, Paul's

---

299 W.M. Christie,"Nazirite," The International Standard Bible Encyclopaedia, ed. James Orr, Vol. 3 (Hendrickson Publishers ed. 2nd Printing March 1996. 4 vols.).

300 C.H. Irwin, ed., The International Bible Commentary (Philadelphia: John C. Winston Co., 1928.).

301 Paul Levertoff, "Vow," The International Standard Bible Encyclopaedia, ed. James Orr, Vol. 4 (Hendrickson Publishers ed. 2nd Printing March 1996. 4 vols.).

302 Finegan, 397. He says this occurred in the year A.D. 55, four years after his haircut in Corinth.

303 Robert Eisenman, The New Testament Code (London: Watkins Publishing, 2006), 70.

304 The Catholic Bible, Personal Study Edition: New American Bible (New York: Oxford University Press, 1995, 73.

Nazarite vows seem to be tied to missions, he cut his hair at the end of one mission, which was the beginning of another. This is similar to Absalom's haircut at the end of every year, which marked the beginning of a new year (2 Samuel 14:26). In short, the Scripture teaches that Paul was a Nazarite who seldom cut his hair. He let it grow most of the time and was not addicted to the razor.

Never does Scripture teach anywhere that men were to constantly cut themselves as most do in these days. Those addicted to hair cutting tools could be called razorites or cropheads, the complete opposite of a long-haired Nazarite (i.e., no razor). On the contrary, as argued earlier, God forbade head shaving in general. The only exceptions to this rule were in cases of leprosy (Leviticus 13:32-33), and those under a temporal Nazarite vow (Numbers 6). A full head of hair and beard, for men who can grow beards, the amount of hair, length, texture, and color (being highly diversified) is all per God's instruction and design in the genetic code (see also Leviticus 19:27).

The Misinterpretation of a Single Verse

"Can you judge a man by the way he wears his hair ..."[305]

It has been most unfortunate for the health of a man's scalp that one verse of Paul's writings has been completely misunderstood, 1 Corinthians 11:14. This verse is part of a larger statement, which also includes verse 15. And then 1 Corinthians 11:14-15 is part of a larger paragraph, 1 Corinthians 11:2-16. Although the paragraph is about whether unveiled women should be allowed to pray to God in church,[306][307][308] the single verse of 1 Corinthians 11:14 continues to be used to argue by unlearned men that God does not want men to have long hair. In fact verse 14 made its way into "The Big Book of Bible Difficulties": "This is a difficult passage, and commentators are not in agreement on it."[309] With this in mind we

305 "Mr. You're A Better Man Than I," songwriter Mike Hugg, producer Giorgio Gomelsky, performed by The Yardbirds, 1966.
306 W.A. Criswell, ed., The Believer's Study Bible, New King James Version (Nashville: Thomas Nelson Publishers, 1991). 1 Corinthians 11:2-16 is about whether unveiled women are allowed to pray in church; Irwin and Shaw (below) agree on this fact as well.
307 Irwin.
308 R. Dykes Shaw, "Corinthians," The International Standard Bible Encyclopaedia, ed. James Orr, Vol. 2 (Hendrickson Publishers ed. 2nd Printing March 1996. 4 vols.).
309 Norman L. Geisler and Thomas Howe, The Big Book of Bible Difficulties (Grand Rapids, Michigan: Baker Books, 1992). If there is no agreement then why are men forced to be shorn? This is never what Christ had in mind.

will delve into the passage a little deeper to determine if it really is true that God does not want men to have long hair. First let the reader understand that 1 Corinthians 11:2-16 is one of many answers to several questions the Corinthians wrote to Paul about:

Now concerning the things whereof ye wrote unto me ... (1 Corinthians 7:1).

In fact, Paul's answers to their questions are recorded from this point forward to the end of the book of 1 Corinthians. Although Paul begins his answer in 1 Corinthians 11:3, he tosses the question back to the Corinthians in verse 13 and says:

Judge in yourselves: is it comely that a woman pray unto God uncovered?

Many interpreters and commentators have struggled with 1 Corinthians 11:2-16, and for good reasons. For example Erdman says:

It seems to be a tendency of human nature to retain and exalt insignificant forms and petty rules and disregard or abandon important principles which should abide.[310]

Apparently, Erdman has experience with many American church people and especially the male head scalping instituted in the Christian education system early in the 20th century. A case in point is the nationally renowned "preacher" who forced haircuts on the men in his choir, but left his wife for another woman.[311] It is bad enough that Paul had to deal with such petty things. But it is far worse, even appalling, that many so-called "preachers" do not understand that true Christianity has always been about the heart, not petty customs. This is especially true when Jesus said not to worry about things like outward apparel, which trains people to be judgmental (Matthew 6:25-7:5). R. Dykes Shaw concurs and says that Paul dealt with the issue "in a manner quite his own." He then passes on to more important matters beginning in

---

310 C.R. Erdman, The First Epistle of Paul to the Corinthians, An Exposition (Philadelphia, PA: Westminster Press, 1929), 100.

311 Joe Stowell, "Get A Haircut," From Strength for the Journey, RBC Ministries, accessed October 22, 2010 http://www.rbc.org/bible-study/strength-for-the-journey/2010/10/22/daily-message.aspx.

verse 17.[312] Likewise, the "Mercer Commentary on the Bible" informs us for what Paul "attributes to nature is merely human fashion, reflecting culture, not necessarily God."[313] And "The Oxford Bible Commentary" says that the entire passage (1 Corinthians 11:2-16) is "full of awkward argumentation," so awkward that a few scholars even consider it "a later addition by another hand" and further remarks that Paul has confused nature with custom.[314]

Yes, the issues and problems with this passage have proven to be difficult as evidenced by differing translations and interpretations, customs, culture, and nature or what is natural. More than likely, the confusion between natural head cover we call hair, and a piece of clothing to cover the hair, was brought about by the Corinthians in their written questions to Paul. It was the Corinthians who made an attempt to confuse between the artificial, such as a veil, hood or head attire, and the natural hair, not Paul. Because of this lack of understanding some have made the passage more difficult than is necessary. The main issue is the placement of some sort of artificial covering over the head. The question is who, what, where, when and why? Here is what 1 Corinthians 11:4-6 says about what, who and when:

[4]Every man praying or prophesying, having his head covered, dishonoureth his head. [5]But every woman that prayeth or_ prophesieth with her head uncovered dishonoureth her head: for that is even all one as if she were shaven. [6]For if the woman be not covered, let her also be shorn [hair cut very short]: but if it be a shame for a woman to be shorn or shaven, let her be covered.

The 'when' is while praying or prophesying. The 'what' is clearly an artificial head covering or type of clothing called *peribolaiou* in Greek (1 Corinthians 11:15). Thayer calls it a "wrapper," "mantle" or "veil" with the idea to cover or conceal.[315] In Hebrews 1:12, *peribolaiou* is translated

312 Shaw.
313 Watson E. Mills and Richard F. Wilson, eds., Mercer Commentary on the Bible (Macon, Georgia: Mercer University Press, 1995).
314 John Barton and John Muddiman, eds., The Oxford Bible Commentary (New York: Oxford University Press, 2001), 1,125-1,126. Concerning the "awkward argumentation" comment, could it be that Paul was being deliberately ambiguous?
315 Joseph H. Thayer, Thayer's Greek-English Lexicon of the New Testament (Peabody, MA: Hendrickson Publishers, first printing June 1996). Thayer translates *peribolaiou* (Strong's # 4018) properly as a covering thrown around, a wrapper, mantle, or veil. He also says Euripides translated it "down," therefore, what is being described is a large piece of outer clothing to conceal.

"vesture" (KJV) or "robe" (ESV). Apparently, the outer garment worn by both sexes had a sort of a hood that could be easily drawn forward from behind the neck to cover the crown of the head.[316] With all things considered, Paul is talking about a very large piece of clothing.

What about 'where'? While anyone can pray, the gift of prophesying was given to certain males and females for the edification of others in the church (1 Corinthians 14:4). So the wearing or not wearing a head covering was during the assembly in church. Prophesying is speaking in front of others in the congregation. During those times of public prayer or prophesying in the Corinthian church, Paul says a woman ought to cover her head. Specifically, to cover the hair of the head, and a man should not (1 Corinthians 11:7-10). Whether others in the congregation did so as they listened to those preaching is not clear. Now it very well may be that the others in the congregation followed suit, but not necessarily.

So what is the deal about shaving a woman's head? Many women, particularly married women, of that time and in that region were required to cover their hair both in worship and in public.[317] The covered or veiled head in that era symbolized a woman's submission to her own husband (her head); as Criswell puts it:

> To fail to acknowledge publicly this headship was a disgrace of such magnitude as to be equal to having a shorn head, which in antiquity was the symbol of a shameless, dishonored woman.[318]

Traditions of veiled women came down from ancient times. For example, in the Assyrian code of laws, wives were to be veiled to distinguish them from prostitutes who were to remain uncovered.[319] David Stern relates that a woman's head was uncovered when accused of adultery and refers to Numbers 5:18.[320] Loose, flowing hair was also an outward sign of a widow in some cultures (Figure 7-1). In the first century, cutting off a woman's hair was the punishment for prostitution.[321] Therefore, short hair on a woman at that time and place would have been a great shame.

---

316 Barton and Muddiman, 1,125-1,126.

317 Irwin.

318 Criswell, see study notes on 1 Corinthians 11:2-16.

319 George A. Barton, Archæology and the Bible 7th ed. (Philadelphia: American Sunday School Union, 5th printing, 1949), 431.

320 David H. Stern, "1 Corinthians 11:5," Jewish New Testament Commentary 5th Ed. (Clarksville, Maryland: Jewish New Testament Publications, 1996), 474.

321 Eerdmans Handbook to the Bible (Grand Rapids, Michigan: Eerdmans Publishing in conjunction with Lion Publishing, England, 1992, Reprinted 1993).

People would have assumed her short hair, even in the first few months of growing back after punishment, meant that she was one who was punished for prostitution, adultery, or some other crime. Likewise, Craig Keener says that not only prostitutes, but Greek virgins as well, were not to cover their hair because they were seeking men.[322] In fact, it seems that any available woman wore loose, flowing hair. Many of these customs are still being enforced today in various cultures.

Customs change. Women did not always have to wear a veil or shawl over their head in public. In the ancient Near East, women "did not ordinarily wear a veil except at the time of their wedding."[323] This custom is similar to weddings of our time. The women in the Beni Hasan painting around 1900 B.C. shows only a headband to hold the hair in place, and that is all. Furthermore, these women appear to be married and are shown without a veil in public. It becomes quite clear that veiling a woman's hair is a manmade custom. Even worse, the idea that women must wear a virtual tent with only her eyes exposed is utterly preposterous. Even though veils are a manmade custom, they were expected in Paul's day especially in metropolitan cities like Corinth.

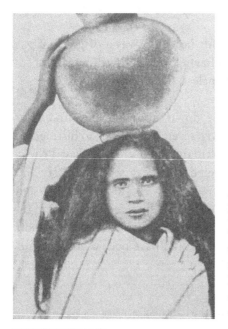

Figure 7-1: Unveiled Hair Flowing Loose. In ancient times single women, virgins, prostitutes and widows wore their hair hanging loose. In the case here, this woman is a widow from Madagascar. Photograph from "The Secret Museum of Mankind," late 19th to early 20th century.

---

322 Craig S. Keener, "Women II," The IVP Dictionary of the New Testament, ed. Daniel G. Reid (Downers Grove, Illinois: InterVarsity Press, 2004).

323 Jack S. Deere, "Song of Songs," The Bible Knowledge Commentary, Old Testament, eds. John F. Walvoord and Roy B. Zuck (Victor Books, 1987).

In the first century Keener says that Greek women did not ordinarily wear a veil, but Roman women did during worship, and Hebrew women and those of the east did even in public.[324] Since Corinth was located near a major seaport made it an international city. Thus, Paul encourages the Greek women to cover their hair during worship while assembled with others. Peter and Paul both acknowledge that 1st century Greek women did not ordinarily wear a head covering in public. This is why the Apostles instructed them not to go about with braided hairstyles laced with gold or plaited hair (1 Timothy 2:9; 1 Peter 3:3). Again, the idea for Christian females is to be modest.

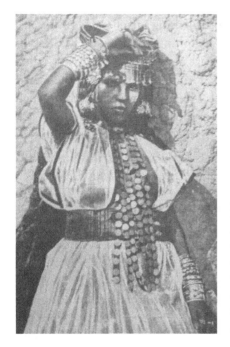

Figure 7-2: Beautiful Woman with Plaited Hair and Gold Attracts Attention to Herself. The manner of dress is no doubt quite similar to those of the 1st century who the apostles had to deal with. This photograph was taken in Biskra, Algeria, late 19th to early 20th century, from "The Secret Museum of Mankind." Courtesy of David Stiffler.

To summarize, Paul gave three reasons why women should wear a veil over her hair while in the company of men in church: (1) it respected the man's (or husband's) headship (v. 3,5); (2) it respected herself so that no one would think she was available (v. 4-6); and (3) for the sake of the angels present during church gatherings (v. 10). Some have alluded that a woman's beautiful hair, if exposed, could cause angels to lust similar to those in the years before the Great Flood (Genesis 6:2). Or perhaps "angels" is used figuratively with regards to young innocent males in the congregation, who could be tempted to lust. After all, if only a few women, in a congregation

---

324 Keener.

of many, remained unveiled would that not be a distraction to the men in those days?

Another problem in the passage is that a man should not place a covering on his head while praying or prophesying (1 Corinthians 11:4;7). Keener informs us that Roman men did wear head coverings during their worship of idols.[325] Likewise, it appears that Hebrew men also wore head coverings. George Eager says the "universal custom among ancient Orientals was to cover the head."[326]

According to Eager two types of head coverings are now in use, the turban and kufiyeh. However, when the Hebrews emerged as a people they did not wear head coverings, but the hot scorching sun changed this. Thus, many customs emerge from a practical beginning, but after a generation or two the reasons why people do this or that may become lost to antiquity. Who would not want to shade themselves from the sun or cover their head when cold? As shown earlier, the Black Obelisk shows the Hebrew men with long hair, but with no head coverings over their hair (Figure 5-12). On the other hand, Scripture indicates that certain men were instructed to wear head coverings. One of these coverings is the *tsaniyph* from Hebrew root word meaning to *wind around* (Strong).[327] Depending on translation, this has been called a royal diadem (Isaiah 62:3), miter, or the turban as in Zechariah 3:5:

> Let them set a clean turban on his head. And they sat a clean turban on his head ... (I.B.).

In fact, Eager thinks that no Jewish teacher of Jesus' day would appear in public without the head covered. He says Jesus "probably" wore the customary white linen napkin called a *sudarium (or soudarion)*, wound around the head as a turban (Figure 7-3).[328] A cloth like this is mentioned in the tomb of the resurrected Christ in John 20:7:

> And the napkin [i.e., *sudarium*], that was about his head, not lying with the linen clothes, but wrapped together in a place by itself (KJV).

---

325 Keener.

326 George B. Eager, "Dress," The International Standard Bible Encyclopaedia, ed. James Orr., Vol. 2 (Hendrickson Publishers ed. 2nd Printing March 1996. 4 vols.).

327 James Strong, Strong's Exhaustive Concordance of the Bible (Gordonsville, TN: Dugan Publishers, Inc.). "*tsaniyph*": Strong's # 6797 is from #6801 meaning a head-dress or piece of clothing wrapped around.

328 Eager.

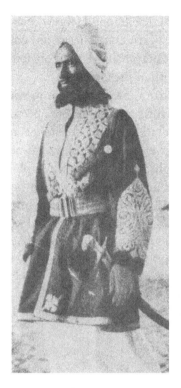

Figure 7-3: Man with Turban, India.
Most of his noble long hair is protected
beneath the turban, but some flows out to
protect the neck. Many with long hair from
India and elsewhere have great difficulty
finding employment in America. They
are forced to be shorn, or else no work,
no money. This photograph was taken in
Southern Baluchistan, India, late 19th
to early 20th century: from "The Secret
Museum of Mankind." Courtesy of David
Stiffler.

So was this just some burial cloth or was it the cloth Jesus used as a turban? If Jesus did wear a turban, did He wear it all the time? For one thing, these types of cloths served many purposes. They could be worn as a turban, headband, or used to wipe sweat of from the face, and other things. The historical evidence of Jesus' sun-bleached hair suggests that Jesus did not wear a turban most of time (see Chapter 6). On the other hand, Jesus may have worn a turban occasionally, for example, when He taught in the temple.

The other issue is with regards to outer garments. Rabbi Lerner says this is called a *tallit* or *prayer shawl*, which appears to go back to ancient times where tassels were to be attached to this outer garment (Numbers 15:38-41).[329] Originally *tallit* meant gown or cloak, which is apparently called *himation* in the Greek New Testament.[330] This was a rectangular mantle that looks like a blanket and was worn by men in ancient times, and is still worn today by the Bedouins for protection against the weather.[331]

---

329 Rabbi Lerner, Origin of Tallit – History of Jewish Prayer Shawl, accessed January 30, 2009 http://judaism.about.com/library/3_askrabbi_c/bl_tallit_history.htm.
330 Eager.
331 Lerner.

So the question is, was there a common practice among Hebrew men to cover the hair during prayer with this outer garment? If Jesus did cover his long hair during prayer with a turban or prayer shawl, then obviously Jewish customs were indeed much different than the Greeks.

But Paul said in 1 Corinthians 11:4;7 that a man ought not to cover his head during prayer and prophesying (teaching, preaching, etc.) because he is "the image and glory of God." Since all men are the image and glory of God, would this indicate that Jesus removed the outer garment from off his head when he prayed and taught? Or did this just apply to a Corinthian custom? Obviously, Jesus or anyone would wear a head covering for practical reasons such as weather conditions. Baruch, the Prophet Jeremiah's secretary, seems to indicate that Hebrew men did wear head coverings in worship and further supports the notion that shaved heads and shaved beards are associated with the worship of false gods:

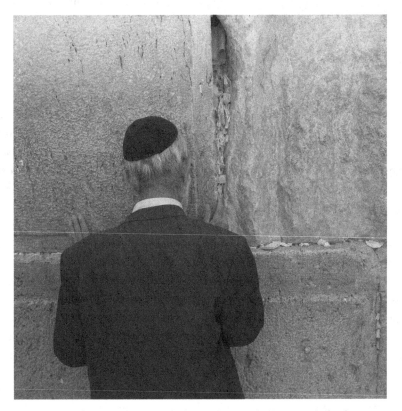

Figure 7-4: Jewish Man Praying with a Cap. Jewish customs differ from present-day European customs who remove all types of caps while praying, even though Paul was talking specifically about a large cloth used as a veil to conceal all.

In their temples, the priests stay sitting down, their garments torn, heads and beards shaved and with heads uncovered; they roar and shriek before their gods as people do at funeral feasts (Baruch 6:30, JB).

The bottom line regarding head coverings is as David Stern says: Paul was talking about "wearing something down over his head ... he was talking about wearing a veil, not a hat."[332] For men then, skullcaps, headbands, caps, and bandanas which do not conceal all are perfectly fine for prayer and worship (Figure 7-4). Just the outer garment, veil, or hood was to be removed.

The Resolution of 1 Corinthians 11

Commentators, who do not address translation issues, merely think that Paul was just dealing with what was customary in the first century and not at other times.[333] This is certainly possible. As we have already learned, the Corinthians cut their hair short, before and after the Romans took over the city. However, commentators have not realized that even translators have had great difficulty with 1 Corinthians 11:14. This is important because commentaries are commenting on what has been translated by others. If the translation is wrong, then the commentary is worthless. With that in mind we can begin our analysis. The reader must understand that 1 Corinthians 11:14-15 is part of a larger paragraph: 1 Corinthians 11:2-16. Verses 14 and 15 are packaged between verses 13 and 16:

[13] Judge in yourselves: is it comely that a woman pray unto God uncovered?

[16] But if any man seem to be contentious, we have no such custom, neither the churches of God (KJV).

This is the main question of the whole issue: "is it comely that a woman pray to God uncovered?" Nearly every translator interprets verse 13 in essentially the same way.

---

332 Stern, "1 Corinthians 11:4," 474.

333 John Calvin, Commentary on the Epistles of Paul the Apostle to the Corinthians, trans. Rev. John Pringle, Volume First (Grand Rapids, Michigan: Wm. B. Eerdmans Publishing Company, 1948).

But there are three ways verse 16 can be interpreted. First, what is the custom? Paul said, "we have no such custom" *that allows* "a woman" to "pray unto God uncovered." Alternatively, "we have no such custom" *to force* "a woman" to wear a veil while praying to God. Or we have no such custom one way or the other as Paul passes the issue back to them: "Judge for yourselves …" These are the choices regarding "we have no such custom."

Nearly all Bible versions translate verse 13 the same, and all ancient English versions and modern literal translations (e.g., ESV; IB; NKJV) translate verse 16 essentially the same as the KJV. However, the reader should understand that some popular modern versions such as the NIV and NASB have changed the word "such" to "other" in verse 16, a grievous error making it sound as though the church required these manmade customs! Thankfully, other translations have not erred in verse 16. But, out of the whole paragraph (i.e., 1 Corinthians 11:2-16), the translations of verses 14 and 15 are the most problematic. Keep these things in mind while we analyze the passage at hand. The following are several literal English translations of 1 Corinthians 11:14-15 (Table 7-1).

The early English translations of Wicliff, Tyndale, Geneva, and Rheims are from "The English Hexapla."[334] The only difference in Table 7-1 is that the spelling of words in these early versions has been updated to modern usage.

As you can see in Table 7-1, there are stark differences in punctuation, insertions of new words, deletions of other words, and even disagreements amongst the meanings of certain words, in all of these various literal translations of this particular text. Translation can be a very daunting task. This is one of those passages particularly difficult to translate because certain assumptions and interpretations are involved. So, to begin our quest for the truth, the reader must understand that the original Greek books of the New Testament had little punctuation.[335] For that matter, even the accents above the Greek letters were not added to the text until after A.D. 600.[336] These accents, if wrong, could cause the statement to be

---

334 The English Hexapla, Exhibiting the Six Important English Translations of the New Testament Scriptures, Includes the Wycliffe, Tyndale, Cranmer, Genevan, Anglo-Rhemish, and Authorized English versions (Reprint of the 1841 ed. Published by Samuel Bagster and Sons, London. New York: AMS Press, Inc., 1975).

335 Thomas Hartwell Horne, An Introduction to the Critical Study and Knowledge of the Holy Scriptures (New York: Robert Carter and Brothers, 1854), 213-214.

336 Herbert Weir Smyth, Greek Grammar (Cambridge, MA: Harvard University Press, 1920. Revised by Gordon M. Messing, 1956. Renewed 1984), 38.

misread forcing the insertion of the English word "doth" or "does" usually placed as the first word in verse 14.

Table 7-1: Ancient and Modern Literal Translations of 1 Corinthians 11:14-15

Version - Year	1 Corinthians 11:14-15
Wiclif* - 1380	[14] neither the kind itself teacheth us, for if a man nourish long hair: it is schenschip to him, [15] but if a woman nourish long hair: it is glory to her, for hair is been given to her for coverage,
Tyndale - 1534	[14] Or else doth not nature teach you, that it is a shame for a man, if he have long hair: [15] and a praise to a woman, if she have long hair? For her hair is given to cover her with all.
Geneva - 1557	[14] Doth not nature itself teach you, that it is a shame for a man, if he have long hair? [15] And a praise to a woman, if she have long hair? For her hair is given her to cover her with all.
Rheims - 1582	[14] Neither doth nature itself teach you, that a man indeed if he nourish his hair, it is an ignominie for him: [15] but if a woman nourish her hair, it is a glory for her, because hair is given her for a veil?
King James Version - 1611 (KJV)	[14] Doth not even nature itself teach you, that if a man have long hair, it is a shame unto him? [15] But if a woman have long hair, it is a glory to her: for her hair is given her for a covering.
The Interlinear Bible (Green, Ed.) – 1985 Main translation	[14] Or does not nature herself teach you that if a man indeed adorns the hair, it is a dishonor to him; [15] but if a woman should adorn the hair, a glory to her it is? Because the beautified hair instead of a veil has been given to her.
The Interlinear Bible (Green, Ed.) – 1985 Secondary sidebar translation	[14] Or does not nature herself teach you that if a man indeed adorns the hair, it is a dishonor to him? [15] But if a woman should adorn the hair, it is a glory to her; because the long hair has been given to her instead of a veil.

*also spelled Wycliffe.

Concerning punctuation, Horne informs us that the stroke we call a comma was invented in the 8th century, although Jerome began to add something like our comma, and also the colon, in the 4th century:

> The numerous mistakes of the fathers, or their uncertainty how particular passages were to be read and understood, clearly prove that there was no regular or accustomed system of punctuation in use, in the fourth century.[337]

The Greek note of interrogation (;) was first used in the 9th century. Of course the mark of interrogation (;) became the question mark (?), and the (;) is now used as a semi-colon. Roger Gryson puts it rather succinctly: punctuation has "enabled editors to apply their own interpretation."[338] Gryson also believes it is imperative to return to an unpunctuated text.

Another vital issue as evident in 1 Corinthians 11:14-15 concerns the verse numbers. The verse numbering system in which the New Testament is now divided was introduced by Robert Stephens in the 16th century, the year 1551. Verse numbers are great as a quick reference guide, but have caused much "injury of its interpretation, as many passages are now severed that ought to be united, and *vice versa*."[339] The best interpretation is that verses 14 and 15 are one long sentence, or question, and should have never been severed. Other concerns include what Paul meant by his use of the Greek words, particularly κομα (koma) and κομη (kome): usually translated long hair (see Appendix I for additional information). Are you beginning to see why the passage is very difficult, as Geisler and Howe say?

John Wycliffe (Wiclif – 1380) (Figure 7-5) is considered the first to translate the whole Bible into English from the Latin Vulgate, which on the whole is an accurate version based on the original Greek.[340] At least it seems so in the verses at hand. Notice how Wycliffe considers the whole passage to be one long continuous sentence with no question marks. In fact, he does not even place a period until well after verse 15, at the end of verse 17! He begins verse 14 with "neither" (L. *nec*; Gr. *oude*) and did not insert the word "does" or "doth."

---

337 Horne, 214.

338 Roger Gryson, "Preface to the Fourth Edition," Biblia Sacra Vulgata (Stuttgart: Deutsche Bibelgesellschaft, 1994).

339 Horne, 215.

340 Both the commentary in The English Hexapla, p. 9-10, 20; and Horne, p. 212 believe the Latin Vulgate to be an accurate version based on the original Greek.

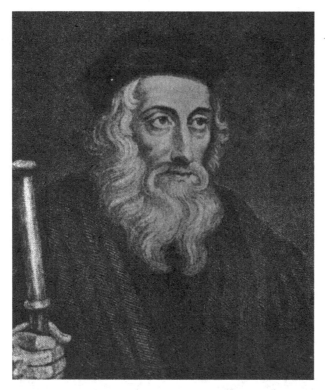

Figure 7-5: John Wycliffe (also spelled Wiclif), ~ 1320 - 1384. He was the first to translate the Bible into English. Notice the full head of hair and full beard. His hair is somewhat long. At least it is long enough to protect the ears and neck. He saw no reason to be stripped of his hair or be shorn.

The first to introduce "doth" (modern "does") into verse 14 was William Tyndale (Tyndale – 1534). He inserted it as the first word of the sentence. This insertion has been followed ever since in most versions, but perhaps more by tradition. This is because most translators compare what former translators have done, and they also think it poses an additional question beyond the question asked in verse 13. But where to place the question mark has varied: Tyndale – 1534, Geneva – 1557, The Interlinear Bible -1985 (Green), ESV, and a host of other modern versions all place the question mark half-way through verse 15; the King James Version (KJV) – 1611 and several modern versions place a question mark after verse 14, and the KJV also considers verse 15 a complete sentence. However, Rheims -1582 considers verse 14 and verse 15 as one continuous statement and places a question mark at the end of verse 15. So how can we tell which versions are better than others?

Placing a question mark after verse 14 has erroneously severed verse 14 from verse 15. Placing the question mark after verse 14 began to appear in the Geneva – 1557 version, which also places a question mark halfway through verse 15, and subsequently in the Authorized Version – 1611. The Geneva – 1557 and the KJV - 1611 translations are from what came to be called the Greek "Textus Receptus" and they both appear to have been influenced by the new verse numbering system of Stephens in 1551. This is how verse 14 became severed from verse 15. But in spite of this, Miles Coverdale, who was involved in the Geneva Bible translation, saw no reason to bring the blade to his head and wear unnaturally short hair (Figure 7-6).

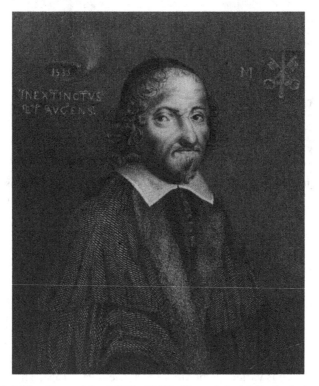

Figure 7-6: Miles Coverdale, 1488 - 1568. One of the biblical scholars involved in the Geneva Bible. Apparently he did not think it a shame for a man to have long hair, if shoulder length hair can even be considered long.

The Rheims -1582 was apparently not influenced by this new verse numbering division. Furthermore, the mark of interrogation or question mark was obviously inserted in the Greek Received Text (TR) prior to the

Tyndale – 1534 translation, perhaps as early as the 9th century.[341] Thus, the question mark being placed either after verse 14 or halfway through verse 15 depends upon which Greek textual variant was being used by the various translators. Most modern versions follow suit by translating from punctuated Greek texts. They, in turn, are literal translations. However, they are based on Greek texts punctuated by some grammarian of the middle ages rather than the true original Greek.

Based on the Greek analysis in Appendix I, we can now see why differences occur in English translations (Table 7-1). Essentially, there are three quite different types of translations of 1 Corinthians 11:14-15: (1) the King James Version – 1611; (2) Rheims – 1582; and (3) The Interlinear Bible.

The King James Version (KJV) – 1611

Overall, this translation is good in that it translates each Greek word and considers verse 15 a complete statement. However, the insertion of the word "Doth" prior to "not even" and the severance of verse 14 from 15 is an interpretation. The question mark being placed after verse 14 places the emphasis on men, rather than the women, who were the ones who wanted approval to discard the veil and is what the entire paragraph (1 Corinthians 11:2-16) is all about. Even though most modern versions sever verse 15 by placing a question mark half-way through it, they also make it sound like long hair on a man is a shame, but it is permissible for a woman to use her long hair as a veil.

The problems with these type translations are the contradictions involved. If Paul really said a woman's long hair is her glory and can be used instead of a veil, then this contradicts what he already said earlier in the same paragraph! Even worse, did Paul really say long hair on a man is a shame? If so, then this contradicts practically the entire Old Testament, the life, long hair and teachings of Jesus Christ, Paul's teaching about circumcision, and even Paul's own Nazarite vows discussed earlier. It makes Paul appear ignorant about his own long-haired ancestry in which long hair was a man's strength and glory, not just a woman's glory. The Old Testament is clear about this. KJV-type translations including the ESV and several other modern versions all state it that way. The only way this translation is possible is that Paul refuted with irony, his way to suggest the opposite of what he wrote. While it is true that many first century men who lived in cities wore their hair short, did all men?

---

341 Horne, 215.

Obviously, the answer is a resounding no! Besides, hair grows all the time and can attain great lengths per the genetic code. So how can God be against his own design?

While it is true that Corinth was one of the early origins of unnaturally short haircuts, do you really believe that Paul was elevating their customs above all others? And that this custom was to be applied to every man around the globe? This would be an assault against many other people groups, even those Paul himself knew. If it was simply a Corinthian custom, then it was to stay in Corinth and not be applied to all men at all times in all places. Paul was not inventing some sort of new hair law, a law that contradicts Old Testament law, which Jesus upheld (Matthew 5:17-19). In reality, this would have been Paul's opportunity to challenge the Corinthian custom of unnaturally short hair by saying nature itself teaches that long hair is not a shame, which coincides even with his own Nazarite vow.

The big problem is the use of the punctuated and accented Greek texts. If we avoid these later additions and the verse numbering system, perhaps the King James translators could have translated the passage this way:

> [14] Not even nature itself teaches you that if a man have long hair is a shame to him, [15] but if a woman have long hair, it is a glory to her: for her hair is given her for a covering.

All that was done herein was the removal of interpretive punctuation and the word "doth," both of which were not in the original Greek, but an interpretation based on translating from accented Greek texts. This translation is very similar to the Rheims – 1582 version, but would probably be better with a question mark at the end of verse 15. The translation of 1 Corinthians 11:14-15 of the International Standard Version (ISV) is along similar reasoning:

> [14] Nature itself teaches you neither that it is disgraceful for a man to have long hair [15] nor that hair is a woman's glory, since hair is given as a substitute for coverings.

The ISV translation uses the word "long" before hair in verse 14 but in their study notes it says that the Greek "lacks *long*."[342] The ISV

---

342 The Holy Bible, International Standard Version, New Testament with Psalms and Proverbs. Version 2.0 (Paramount, CA: Davidson Press, 1996-2010 The ISV Foundation). This Bible can be downloaded for free @ http://isv.org/downloads/index.htm

translators are right. They obviously used an untainted Greek text and have thoroughly thought through the issues as well. Long hair on a man is not disgraceful and furthermore, it is not just a woman's glory. If one would take the time to carefully look at the passage, the idea that hair is a woman's glory is being questioned as the Rheims-1582 says in the later half of verse 15: "because hair is given her for a veil?" In other words, hair would be a glory to her if she covered it during prayer. Or, if her hair is too glorious to behold by men, then it would be better to cover it.

Rheims – 1582 (The Anglo – Rhemish Version)

Although the translators of Rheims - 1582 version insert the word "doth" (does), they do so not at the beginning of verse 14, but place it as the second word. They also consider verses 14 and 15 as one complete statement with a question mark at the very end of verse 15. They understood that they were translating a complete sentence or question. It is very apparent that they handled this difficult passage of Scripture with more care as the translators of the International Standard Version (ISV) have. Although they translated from the Latin, they diligently conferred with the Greek and other editions in diverse languages, and by doing so, discovered "corruptions of diverse late translations."[343] Modern Catholic Bibles such as the "New American Bible" and "The Jerusalem Bible" both translated from the Greek agree with the Rheims - 1582 version in the following regard: that the question mark belongs at the end of verse 15. So most Roman Catholic scholars agree that overall, verses 14 and 15 are presenting a question. However, placing "does" at the beginning of verse 14 as done in most other versions is unnecessary. Verses 14 and 15 are a long sentence and the question part of the passage comes at the end, not at the beginning (Table 7-1).

The other interesting thing about the Rheims - 1582 version and Wicliff -1380 is the use of the word "nourish." Wicliff says, "if a man nourish long hair" and Rheims says "if he nourish his hair," the word "long" not in the Rheims. Recall these translations are from the Latin, which is from the Greek. Nourish is from the Latin *nutrio*, meaning nurse. It seems evident that the Latins originally felt that the context of the passage is describing something besides length, something being done to the long hair. There are all sorts of things this could mean. For one, to nurse the hair could mean feed (add to), caress, fondle, arrange, or constantly worry about, things nurses do. To nurse the hair would mean to apply an inordinate amount of care. So really what does "nature itself" teach us:

343 The English Hexapla, 144.

1. Is it natural for a man to have long hair? Yes
2. Is it natural for a woman to have long hair? Yes - most can grow it longer than men.
3. Is it natural for a woman to constantly worry over, fondle, and arrange her hair? Yes
4. Is it natural for a man with long hair to constantly fuss about it? No

Thus, for a man to spend a great deal of time nurse-maiding his hair in some elaborate way would be seen as what many women tend to do. On the other hand, for a man to allow his long hair to simply hang naturally or to have it pulled back in a ponytail or to hold it in place with a headband is certainly not nourishing or nursing the hair. In Acts 19:12, Paul also used the *soudarion* cloth that Jesus did. Usually translated as handkerchief, it was actually a multi-purpose napkin similar to a modern-day bandana. Paul used them as "head bands" to keep his long hair in place.[344]

In context, Paul seems to be saying that there is no real comparison between a man's long hair and a woman's long hair unless the man intentionally beautifies his hair like a woman. For this reason, it was recommended that a woman's intentionally beautified hair be covered, as a humble gesture during prayer. This interpretation matches the science of a woman's hair, which is by nature chemically different than a man's hair (see Chapter 2). There is manly long hair and there is womanly long hair.

The Interlinear Bible

The translators of this version insert the word "does" at the beginning of verse 14, but interpret the Greek term κομα, *koma* as *adorn the hair* rather than *long hair*. In this regard, the question we should be asking is: what is meant by *koma*? Does it mean *long hair*? Or does it have more to do with what is done to the long hair as this version implies? Is it strictly length? And, if so, what length? And if there is a restricted length for men, what is that length? But, if there is some restricted length, then why is hair designed by God Himself to grow long – especially among certain races of men than others? Did God make a mistake? No length specifications

---

344 Igumen Luke, "Concerning the Tradition of Long Hair and Beards," reprinted from Orthodox Life – Vol. 46, No. 5 – October 1996, accessed May 24, 2010 http://www. holycross-hermitage.com/pages/Orthodox_Life/longhair.htm, or Orthodox Christian Information Center, http://www.orthodoxinfo.com/praxis/clergy_hair.aspx.

are ever given in Scripture. Specifically, if length is the issue, then this contradicts Leviticus 19:27, Numbers 6:5d, Amos 2:11 and a host of other passages. It is clear in this version that the translators believe that *koma* means to intentionally beautify the long hair like women. This is very similar to the early Latin translations just mentioned. Thus, if a man grows his hair long that is alright. However, he should not manipulate it like women do, in elaborate female fashions of tresses.

Way back in the 2nd century, this is precisely how early Church father Clement of Alexandria (A.D. 150 – 215), who was very familiar with Paul's epistles, felt about it. He was appalled by those who lived unnatural luxurious lifestyles. This included "cutting their hair in an ungentlemanlike and meretricious way" [to falsify the looks, like a prostitute] ... and "adorning their locks like women." He called them "haters of hair" and "destitute of hair" for they were "addicted to base passions whose body is made smooth by the violent tugging of pitch-plasters ... for those who are men to shave and smooth themselves, how ignoble!" He said the towns were full of shops that removed male body hair and beards. The men who frequented these places, he called "degenerate" and "effeminate." Clement of Alexandria also had the following to say:

But for one who is a man to comb himself and shave himself with a razor, for the sake of fine effect, to arrange his hair at the looking-glass, to shave his cheeks, pluck hairs out of them, and smooth them, how womanly!

But I approve the simplicity of the barbarians [this simply meant a foreigner]: loving an unencumbered life, the barbarians have abandoned luxury. Such the Lord calls us to be....

Of the nations, the Celts and Scythians wear their hair long, but do not deck themselves. The bushy hair [recall Solomon's locks] of the barbarian has something fearful in it; and its auburn colour threatens war, the hue being somewhat akin to blood. Both these barbarian races hate luxury... the Scythian man leads a frugal life.[345]

---

345 **Clement of Alexandria,** The Instructor (Book III), Chapter 3 Against Men Who Embellish Themselves, trans. William Wilson, From Ante-Nicene Fathers, Vol. 2. eds. Alexander Roberts, James Donaldson, and A. Cleveland Coxe (Buffalo, NY: Christian Literature Publishing Co., 1885.) accessed June 8, 2010 Revised and edited for New Advent by Kevin Knight, http://www.newadvent.org/fathers/02093.htm.

Clement of Alexandria approved the simple, "frugal life" of the long haired foreigners because they avoided the luxury of materialism. The issue was not long hair by length, but rather a man who forces himself to look like a woman through inordinate hair care, adorned or stylized hair, a shaved face, and hairless body. A life addicted to close-cropping the head is also in mind, the "unencumbered" or unburdened simplicity of the long-haired barbarians, a life approved by God. For Jesus said "my yoke is easy, and my burden is light" (Matthew 11:30). And how much a burden and addiction it is to shave and rush to the barber constantly as if male hair is a mistake, a waste product.

For more proof, the Eastern, also called Greek, Orthodox Church, which is the direct continuation of the Church from the time of the apostles, believed the same. As proven earlier, the sacred tradition of long hair and beards originates in the Old Testament. Jesus and the apostles passed the tradition to the early church, which was originally one Holy Catholic (meaning universal, not Roman Catholic) and Apostolic Church. Once peace was brought to the Church, all the bishops of equal authority met to discuss and agree on meanings of difficult passages. These meetings are called Ecumenical or General Councils. Igumen Luke understands that Paul's choice of words for hair indicates hair as an ornament with length being only a secondary and suggested issue. This same approach to hair as that of St. Paul was restated in the 96th canon of the Council of Trullo in A.D. 691 or 692 sometimes called Quinisext Council, or the completion of the Fifth and Sixth General Councils:

Those who by baptism have put on Christ have professed that they will copy his manner of life which he led in the flesh. Those therefore who adorn and arrange their hair to the detriment of those who see them, that is by cunningly devised intertwinings, and by this means put a bait in the way of unstable souls, we take in hand to cure paternally with a suitable punishment: training them and teaching them to live soberly, in order that having laid aside the deceit and vanity of material things, they may give their minds continually to a life which is blessed and free from mischief, and have their conversation in fear, pure, [and holy]; and thus come as near as possible to God through their purity of life; and adorn the inner man rather than the outer, and that with virtues, and good and blameless manners, so that they leave in themselves no remains of the left-handedness of the adversary.

But if any shall act contrary to the present canon let him be cut off [excommunicated].[346]

Clearly the issue was adorning the hair by "cunningly devised intertwinings." It was giving the natural long hair a falsified look. Obviously, this was always more of a female problem than with the men (1 Timothy 2:9; 1 Peter 3:3; Figure 7-2), with certain women wanting to ornament their long hair like Cleopatra. It is bad enough that modern women constantly change the color, texture, and other unnatural means to alter, stylize or feminize their hair, but for a man to do that is a disgrace. But we see by the use of the word "him" that men are in mind. For a man to alter his hair or have hair interlaced with gold or other ornaments is not natural. Really, the apostles wished for both men and women to look natural. This is why Christian men of the Orthodox Church are encouraged to copy the manner of the life which Christ lived in the flesh. This includes long hair and beards, as long as little is done to the hair to alter its natural disposition.

Nicodemos the Hagiorite's comment on the 96th canon says that a man should not grow his hair "long enough to reach the belt like that of women," "bleach their hair," alter the hair's natural texture, and nor should they destroy the beard, because it is the beard that distinguishes a man from a woman.[347] In "Concerning the Tradition of Long Hair and Beards," out of all Christianity only the Orthodox Church gets it right and matches well with the scientific aspects of God's design for hair as stated in this book. If hair grew very long as to reach the belt where the small of the back is, then they recommend, for those uncomfortable with hair that long, nothing more than:

> ... trimming off the hair that falls below the middle of the back. We are not talking about the modern haircut, which is, in fact, the equivalent of the desecration of the head that led to Samson's loss of strength and power.[348]

---

346 Philip Schaff, 96th Canon of the Council of the Trullo, accessed June 4, 2010 http://www.ccel.org/ccel/schaff/npnf214.pdf

347 "Concerning the Tradition of Long Hair and Beards: St. Nikodemos the Hagiorite's Comments on Canon 96 of the Sixth Oecumenical Synod." Orthodox Christian Information Center, accessed May 30, 2010 http://www.orthodoxinfo.com/praxis/clergy_hair.aspx

348 "Concerning the Tradition of Long Hair and Beards: Uncut Hair and Beards of the Clergy," accessed May 30, 2010 http://www.orthodoxinfo.com/praxis/clergy_hair.aspx

This is why Leuring remarks that long hair on a man is a symbol of God's divine strength.[349] And this "glory of God" is to be displayed along with a full beard. This upholds other followers of Christ including the long-haired "brother of our Lord" James called the Just, first Bishop of the church at Jerusalem who also wrote the epistle of James in the New Testament.[350 351 352]

The Long Hair of Early Christianity

James and his followers were all Nazarites.[353] Abbé Constant Fouard informs us that his being called "the Just" was for good reason. James prayed continually upon his knees for all people, went about barefooted, abstained from meat and alcohol, and from birth a razor never touched his long hair![354 355] Imagine uncut hair from childbirth! It must have hung all the way down the back. Because of today's unlAWFUL American culture James would never be hired by most churches, nor would he be hired by the western Christian educational system. In his style of Christianity, he upheld God's laws including long hair. C.M. Kerr tells us about James who:

> loved peace more than faction ... and who perceived that religious communities with different forms of observance might still live and work together in common allegiance to Christ.[356]

Three years after his conversion, Paul went to Jerusalem and saw James, the Lord's brother (Galatians 1:19). Both men were Nazarites – James from the womb, Paul as a temporal Nazarite who cut his hair off occasionally as

---

349 H.L.E. Luering, "Hair," The International Standard Bible Encyclopaedia, ed. James Orr, Vol. 2 (Hendrickson Publishers ed. 2nd Printing March 1996. 4 vols.).
350 Doremus Almy Hays, "James, Epistle of," The International Standard Bible Encyclopaedia, ed. James Orr. Vol. 3 (Hendrickson Publishers ed. 2nd Printing March 1996. 4 vols.).
351 H.E. Jacobs, "Brethren of the Lord," The International Standard Bible Encyclopaedia, ed. James Orr, Vol. 1 (Hendrickson Publishers ed. 2nd Printing March 1996. 4 vols.).
352 C.M. Kerr, "James." The International Standard Bible Encyclopaedia, ed. James Orr, Vol. 3 (Hendrickson Publishers ed. 2nd Printing March 1996. 4 vols.).
353 Eisenman.
354 C.F. Cruse, trans., Eusebius' Ecclesiastical History. Book 2, Chapter 23. Complete and Unabridged, New Updated Edition (Peabody, MA: Hendrickson Publishers, 1998, Fifth Printing – June 2006).
355 Abbe Constant Fouard, Saint Peter and the First Years of Christianity, trans. From 2nd Ed. by George F.X. Griffith (Fort Collins, Colorado: Roman Catholic Books, 1892), 193-195.
356 Kerr.

previously discussed. James, Jude, the brother of James (Jude 1), and Jesus were all raised to be holy with uncut long hair. Apparently, many groups descended from James were of the same long-haired belief.[357] After A.D. 70 many of the long-haired Jewish Christians such as the Nazoreans ended up in Syria, Egypt, and parts of Arabia.[358] In fact Eisenman in his "The New Testament Code" shows emphatically that Nazarite language is used throughout the New Testament. He also demonstrates that Nazoraean is the same as Nazirite (or Nazarite, N-Z-R), the perfect holiness lifestyle due to Divine visitation, which the early believers were encouraged to follow.[359] Three ancient English translations of Acts 24:5 agree: Tyndale – 1534; Cranmer – 1539; and Geneva – 1557 all translate the Greek ναζωραιων, *nazoraion* as Nazarites (also see Chapter 6).

In fact these long-haired Nazarites existed at least into the 4th century of our era. According to John Francis Wilson, we find that Julian the Apostate refused to use the word "Christian" and used "Nazarites" instead as a "term of ridicule."[360] This sounds terribly similar to those in America today who condemn long hair by calling long-haired men names such as "savages," "hippies," or "dreadlocks," who are, when it comes to hair, the new or neo-Nazarites. This is further proof that America, along with much of the so-called civilized world, is in an apostate condition just like Julian. Church historian Eusebius (late 3rd and early 4th centuries) often makes mention of the "venerable and hoary locks" as being "dignified" of even prominent gray or white-haired (hoary) elderly men such as Valens, deacon of the church of Aelia,[361] and a certain Alexander, the 35th bishop of the Jerusalem church. Great honor is associated with such a "crown" as he describes Alexander's long locks:

> ...though crowned with hoary locks of venerable age, he was cast into prison.[362]

Alexander apparently followed in the footsteps of James the Just, the first bishop of the Jerusalem church. The truth is it is no HAIResy to

---

357 Eisenman, 67.

358 Jeffery J. Butz, The Brother of Jesus and the Lost Teachings of Christianity (Rochester, Vermont: Inner Traditions, 2005), 175-176.

359 Eisenman, 34, 67, 68, 616, 622, 649, 671, 673.

360 John Francis Wilson, Caesarea Philippi (Banias, The Lost City of Pan) (London, or New York: I.B. Tauris & Co Ltd, 2004), 100.

361 Eusebius' Ecclesiastical History, The Book of Martyrs, Chapter 11.

362 Eusebius' Ecclesiastical History, Book 6, Chapter 39.

wear long hair as God Himself designed, but rather it is wrong to force male head shearing, especially as it has become an addiction to scissors and razors. In his commentary on Numbers 6, Elmer Smick comments that Paul and James both saw deep spiritual significance in the Nazarite law.[363] He further states that God desired that His people should become a holy nation: "Becoming a Nazarite was a step … toward attaining this ideal." Proof of longer hair in early Christianity is also seen in pictures at the time (Figure 7-7).

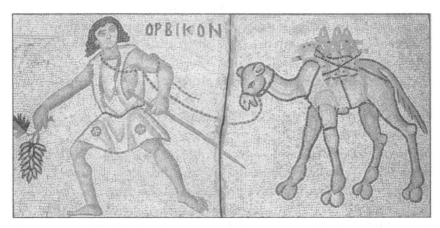

Figure 7-7: Man leading a camel - from a Byzantine church in the Negev. The Roman Byzantine period occurred from A.D. 313 – 636. A somewhat decent head of hair, not really that long but enough length to crown and protect the head and neck. Taken from "Zondervan NIV Atlas of the Bible" by CARL G. RASMUSSEN; CARTA, ISRAEL MAP & PUB CO LTD. Copyright © 1989 by Carl G Rasmussen Maps c 1989 by Carta, Jerusalem. Used by permission of the Zondervan Corporation.

The Gentile followers of the long-hair Nazarite Paul were never forced to fully abide by Old Testament Law. They probably kept their own customs regarding hair, which may be fine. However, the problem is that the modern American Christian education system forces males to be shorn in spite of all the scriptural and historical evidence against it. Or, as Jeffrey Butz relates, as the church gained political power, it became thoroughly Gentile and most of its Jewish roots died.[364] With the exception of the Greek Orthodox Church, Gentile, or better, Roman, customs have invaded too much of the Christian education system.

---

363 Elmer Smick, "Numbers," The Wycliffe Bible Commentary, ed. C.F. Pfeiffer and E.F. Harrison (Chicago: Moody Press, 1990).

364 Butz, 184.

Essentially, many Christian schools have abolished God's laws and created their own manmade anti-male hair laws, a cut against God's intended design in nature. This is the real disgrace. The fact is that the Nazarite James saw his brother's movement as "focused on producing more Nazirites …." For James and those associated with him, Jesus' true identity was his status as a Nazirite.[365] In consideration of all things, the idea to force a man to be shorn has no Scriptural basis. Christian schools must get out of the anti-male hair business, so that families can decide for themselves and develop their own identities per their own unique callings in life. The origin of close-cropped heads lies with pagan idolatry and tyranny (see Chapter 4).

---

365 Butz, 164.

Chapter 8: Killer Cuts

|||||||||||||||||||||||||||||||||||||||||||||||||||||||||||||||||||||||||||||||||||||||||||||||||||||||||||||||||||||||||||||||||||||||||||||||||||||||||||||||||||||||||||||||||||||||

The thief comes only to steal and kill and destroy (John 10:10a; JB).

Thus far we have learned that much baldness is caused by cutting the hair too close (Chapter 3), and pagan idolatry is the origin of this mongrel (Chapter 4). Although many early Christians had long hair, even long white hair, some other early Christians may have worn short hair or limited the hair to a certain length.[366] However, forcing a man to be shorn, as going on today, was never intended by Jesus, the Apostles, and most, if not all, early church leaders, Deacons and Bishops as already demonstrated. The Prophet Jeremiah calls those who cut the corners of the hairline "Crop-Heads," which included men from Egypt (Jeremiah 9:24-26, JB).[367] Recall from Chapter 4 that clipped hair is associated with idolatry, war, and other doom. On the other hand, long hair means peace. Jesus emphasized that the Gospel of God's Kingdom was never to be advanced by force of arms (Matthew 5:9; 26:51-52; Luke 1:78-79; 2:14).

Just like what Baruch witnessed, hair cutting rituals were brought into Christianity but originated in idolatry. Recall that the Romans were already cutting and sacrificing their hair to various false gods. Temples dedicated to their gods stood in all their major cities. Among these are Rome, Athens, Ephesus, Colossæ, Philippi, Thessalonica, and Corinth. Apparently, all their young men of the empire were required to sacrifice their hair to local deities in these cities. This forced hair elimination of men probably continued in their churches as Romans were becoming Christians. In the 2nd century A.D. we see hair a little longer and even beards on Roman men. Perhaps by then the Romans were becoming more influenced by Jesus' example of how hair should be worn? Not really. Their hair was still trimmed above the eyes and only halfway over the ear, a

---

366 David W. Bercot, ed., "Hair," A Dictionary of Early Christian Beliefs (Peabody, MA: Hendrickson Publishers, 1998).

367 The Jerusalem Bible, Readers Edition (New York: Doubleday, 2000).

typical specification in the American Christian education system. These schools follow Roman military standards rather than the example of Jesus. Bringing Roman customs into the Roman church is at the very root cause of the short hair - baldness problem (Figure 8-1).

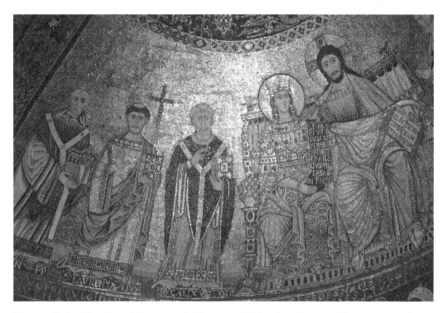

Figure 8-1: Mosaic of Jesus and Tonsured Monks, Rome. This picture shows Roman monks, not only with hair forced above the ears and neck, but even with the intentionally shaved bald spot called a tonsure. Shaving any part of the head is contrary to the teachings of Scripture. This idea was entirely manufactured by the Roman church at the time. The placement of Jesus alongside the monks makes it appear that God requires a shaved head or short hair to serve Him, an abominable lie. Even the 1st century Romans did not do such a thing to their scalps.

D.M. Podolsky informs us that forced hair removal has been going on for centuries and it crept into what is now called the Roman Catholic Church. In the 8th century, the conqueror Charlemagne sported a beard and long hair until he became "Holy Roman Emperor." He then "adopted the Church's [Roman Church] dictates and commanded his subjects to shave"[368] just like Julius Caesar did. Roman Catholic monks were even forced to shave the crown of the head – this artificial hole in the hair of the scalp is called a tonsure (Figure 8-1). Why was this grotesque practice done? Jesus never required any outward form of self-flagellation. On the

368 D.M. Podolsky, Skin: the human fabric (The Human Body) (Tarrytown, New York: Torstar Books, Inc., 1984), 95.

contrary the law for priests states, "They must not wear tonsures, shave the edges of their beards, or gash their bodies" (Leviticus 21:5; JB). For these are sadistic practices.

Why is it that when any organization lusts for power, male hair must be eliminated? The answer is tyranny. This is what the Roman Church, also called the Western Church, wanted, supremacy over the whole church, everywhere, rather than sharing it equally with the other Bishops over Orthodox churches in the other countries of the east. This power play is thought to have begun in the 860s.[369] Close-cropped hair and a shaved face are symbols of tyranny, not freedom, not freedom in the real Jesus Christ. When leaders have a misplaced focus on the hair of their male subjects means they do not know how to work on a man's heart, as one preacher relayed. This is what happened to the Roman Church as it finally split from the rest of the Church in 1054. Igumen Luke puts it rather succinctly:

It is interesting to note that the fashion of cropped or stylized hair and shaved beards found its way into the Roman Catholic and Protestant worlds. So important had this pagan custom become for Roman clergy by the 11th Century that it was listed among the reasons for the Anathema pronounced by Cardinal Humbert on July 15, 1054 against Patriarch Michael in Constantinople which precipitated the Western Church's final falling away from the Orthodox Church: "While wearing beards and long hair you [Eastern Orthodox] reject the bond of brotherhood with the Roman clergy, since they shave and cut their hair.[370]

Word about this event travelled quickly. We see this same negative attitude a few years later with the Roman Saint Wulstan, Bishop of Worcestor, Britain. Sometime after he became bishop (circa A.D. 1062), he pronounced that long hair was "highly immoral, criminal and beastly."[371] This man kept a knife up his sleeve and when those with "shaggy" hair knelt before him, he cut their locks on the spot. This behavior is incomprehensible, especially since he, being a bishop, would have claimed

---

369 Mateja Matejic, Orthodoxy: Courage to be Different, Strength to Remain the Same (Holy Trinity Monastery, 2000).
370 Igumen Luke, "Concerning the Tradition of Long Hair and Beards," reprinted from Orthodox Life, Vol. 46, No. 5, accessed October 1996 and May 24, 2010 http://www.holycross-hermitage.com/pages/Orthodox_Life/longhair.htm, or Orthodox Christian Information Center, http://www.orthodoxinfo.com/praxis/clergy_hair.aspx
371 Podolsky, 96.

to worship Jesus. The Roman Catholic Church well knows that Jesus wore long hair and a full beard, as God Himself created it to be. In effect, so-called "Saint" Wulstan declared that Jesus was a highly immoral criminal! Is this not antichrist? How could such a person become Bishop in the first place? Well, he was part of the Roman Catholic Church after its split from Orthodoxy. It became a rampage of hair hating. Pope Gregory (1073 – 1085) rightfully called "insane," forced bishops and clerics to shave their beards.[372]

To be perfectly clear, forcing a man to cut off his hair or shave is a form of stealing, one of the ten great sins (Exodus 20:15). Hair removal, as bad as it is, is the least of the atrocities committed by the Roman Catholic Church. As they rose to a powerful political force, after their departure in 1054, abominable brutality was launched against their fellow man and continued for about 900 years. The degenerate behavior, war, corruption, drunkenness, gambling, greed, and many other disturbing practices led to the Protestant reformation beginning in 1517 under Martin Luther.[373] Protestant denominations are the offspring of the Roman Catholic Church and did inherent some Roman ideology, including hair removal. It is only in comparatively recent times that the Roman Catholic Church has regained some semblance to early Christianity. It isn't until after World War II, especially after the 1960s, that we finally see some hair for a change, even long hair and beards and a true love for Jesus in certain religious Orders within Roman Catholicism. John Michael Talbot of the Little Portion Hermitage in Arkansas is one such blessing.

Nevertheless, the close-cropping ways of Julius Caesar and the Romans have been exported around the world, especially in the west. As proved earlier, a shaved head or its kin, ultra-short hair, was the mark of a slave or simply death to the individual. When the British became a world power they did the same thing to conquered foe as they harvested slaves in Africa. In "Hair Story," the "shaved head" was done "to erase the slave's culture." A member of a prominent West African family who was kidnapped and forced into slavery said it was the "highest indignity" to have his head and beard shaved as if he was a "prisoner" of war.[374] Like the

---

372 "Concerning the Tradition of Long Hair and Beards: St. Nikodemos the Hagiorite's Comments on Canon 96 of the Sixth Oecumenical Synod." Orthodox Christian Information Center, accessed May 30, 2010 http://www.orthodoxinfo.com/praxis/clergy_hair.aspx

373 Matejic, 26.

374 Ayana D. Byrd and Lori L. Tharps, Hair Story, Untangling the Roots of Black Hair in America (New York: St. Martin's Press, 2001), 10-11.

Gauls, the Ainu people also considered enforced hair cutting as a severe punishment associated with loss of honor.[375] To the Scandinavians it was a shameful disgrace or "a mark of infamy" to cut off the hair.[376] The beliefs of the Scandinavians, Gauls, Ainus and many, many others concur with a plethora of statements in the Old Testament concerning hair such as this one spoken by God Himself (Yahweh or Jah):

> That is why my heart sobs like a flute for Moab, sobs like a flute for the men of Kir-heres: that accumulated treasure all lost! Yes, every head is shorn, every beard cut off, gashes are in the hands of all, sackcloth round all their loins (Jeremiah 48: 36-37; JB).

God's "heart sobs" because "every head is shorn, every beard cut off!" In America this heartless forced hair removal began with the systematic destruction of another race, the Native Americans. The problem began in the later half of the nineteenth century, arguably the most abusive period against the Native Americans. In his book "First People," David C. King informs us that from 1870 to 1900 all remaining Native American tribes were forced onto reservations. During this time period, Richard Henry Pratt founded the Carlisle Indian Industrial School (1879-1918) in Pennsylvania. This federally funded program was an attempt to "civilize" the Native Americans by assimilation through "education." As King puts it:

> ... the goal was to remove the children from their familiar surroundings – separating them from their family, village, food, clothing, customs, and even their language.[377]

The effort was to convince them that their former lives were "savage and repugnant." These were military-type schools and many cropped up all across the country. They forced short haircuts on boys and both boys and girls wore uniforms. Certain Christian missionaries were involved, but to be fair, there were some brave, God-fearing Christians who rose up in defense of the natives. Personally, I recall (although the reference alludes me) one in those days who said something like "I would rather live amongst Christian savages than with savage Christians." Unfortunately, many

---

375 Arthur Rook and Rodney Dawber, eds., Diseases of the Hair and Scalp, 2nd Ed. (London: Blackwell Scientific Publications, 1991), 462.

376 "Hair: Spiritual Theosophical Dictionary on Hair," accessed May 29, 2010 http://www.experiencefestival.com/a/hair/id/200608

377 David C. King, First People (New York: DK Publishing, 2008), 148.

modern Christian schools today have decided to follow militant ways. Did they all somehow forget about the long hair of Jesus, and even the long hair of the white founding fathers of the U.S.A.? When will Christianity ever learn that the message of Jesus is for everyone regardless of their customs, especially in regards to a person's natural outward appearance (read Matthew 5-7)? What about the results of such "education?"

Well, these anti-Christian things happened to the Native Americans. Families were torn apart, many children ran away and "hundreds died of influenza or tuberculosis, and hundreds more succumbed to alcoholism or suicide." Of the rare success stories touted, Jim Thorpe for example, thousands literally perished.[378]

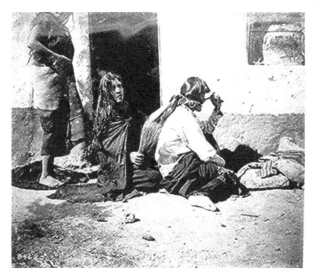

Figure 8-2: Native American "Hopi" Man having his Hair Brushed. He holds his hair in place by a rope, while she brushes his hair. In this way, hair would not be dislodged from the scalp. They knew how to take care of their long hair. The Hopi and other tribes were not savages. The savage idea was by those who deem themselves superior to others. Children were removed from families like this in late 19th century America in a fruitless effort to tame the so-called "savage." Photograph courtesy of the U.S. National Archives and Records Administration.

It was considered a disgrace by many Native American cultures to have their hair cut off short. Instead, they considered it a blessing and took care of it rather than cast it away as a worthless thing (Figures 8-2 and 8-3). It was traumatic for many students to have their hair cut off, which caused

378 King, 148-149.

stress. Michael Cooper informs us that the Sioux cut their hair only as a sign of sadness or shame.[379] Sound familiar? This is how nearly all the ancients and races felt about their long hair. We must remember that many Native American tribes arrived on this continent in the centuries before Christ. Their beliefs appear reminiscent to the Nazarites.

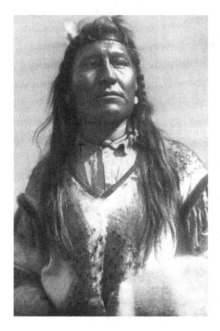

Figure 8-3: Native American called "New Chest," Piegan – Blackfeet Tribe. Long hair is a symbol of health, vitality, and nobility, dedication to the God of nature. He was no "savage." Too bad most moderns cut themselves short.

In 1897 on many reservations, agents were sent to force all males to cut their hair short. The reason given was that their long hair was a sign of "wildness." King quotes the officer in charge of ridding the long hair on the males at the Mescalero Apache Reservation as follows:

> As with Samson of old, the Indians' wildness lay in their long hair …. All energies were bent to compel the adult males to cut their hair and adopt civilized attire …. The Indian office; at my request, issued a preemptory order for all to cut their hair and adopt civilized attire; and in six weeks from the start, every male Indian had been changed into the semblance of a decent man, with the warning that confinement at hard labor awaited any backsliders.[380]

379 Michael L. Cooper, Indian School: Teaching the White Man's Way (New York: Clarion Books, 1999), 5.
380 King, 153.

Remarkably, one of God's own long haired Nazarites, Samson, was used as an example against the Native Americans. What an absurdity of biblical ignorance. There can be little doubt that this plague was instigated by some careless, irresponsible person who was obviously half asleep during Sunday school. The mind fog about Samson aside, what about, "Thou shalt not kill" (Exodus 20:13). For the Native Americans, the individuality of each was removed and they were killed as a people, the cutting of the hair symbolized it and many literally perished: "...in three years nearly one half of the children from the Plains were dead."[381] As said before, the truth is that the Creator exalted his long haired heroes and said to raise your sons that way:

And I raised up of your sons for Prophets, and of your young men for Nazirites. Is it not even thus, O ye children of Israel, saith the Lord? But ye gave the Nazirites wine to drink, and commanded the Prophets, saying, Prophesy not (Amos 2:11-12, The 1599 Geneva Bible).

The parallels of the long haired Nazirites in Amos to the Native Americans are striking. The amount of alcohol given was no small amount as recommended by Paul (1 Timothy 5:23), but this was with the intent to make one drunk. The destruction of the Native Americans was not only the elimination of their long hair, but by persuading them to drink strong alcohol. Both ideas were introduced to them by wicked men.

As eluded earlier, the tribal communal lifestyle of the long-haired Native Americans has ancient connections overseas. The prophet Jeremiah (chapter 35) tells us that the Rechabites were commended by Yahweh (God) for their obedience to the order given by Jonadab, son of Rechab. The orders were never to drink wine, nor to build houses to live in, nor to farm. They were to dwell in tents. Incredible! This is precisely how the Native Americans lived, as they did not farm and moved from place to place in their wigwams, a style of tent. Both the lifestyles of the Rechabites and Native Americans are one and the same. And what was the Lord God's view of them? God honored them and said they would never lack a male descendant to stand in His presence (Jeremiah 35:19). Dr. William Smith informs us that the Rechabite's "Nazarite" way of life "gained for them admission into the house of the Lord."[382] In fact, one of these long

---

381 King, 149.
382 William Smith, ed., "Rechabites," *A Concise Dictionary of the Bible, Comprising its Antiquities, Biography, Geography, and Natural History* (Boston: Little, Brown, and Company, 1865).

haired descendants was there at Jerusalem and tried desperately to stop the martyrdom of James the Just, brother of the Lord, from the cutthroat mob.[383] Smith also mentions that the Nabathaeans and Wahabys tribes were similar in that their customs matched those of Nazarites.[384] The freedom of long hair was once everywhere.

The domino effect of head shearing the Apache began America's move away from freedom. The erasure of the male head symbolizes this loss of freedom and as all feel today, freedom has been on a steady decline since that time. The late 19th century peer pressure to be cut short was systematically placed against all men in American society. By the beginning of the 20th century anyone with "hair even slightly long" was labeled a "poet" or a "musician."[385] Apparently people already forgot about the long hair of the white founding fathers of the United States. This is quite evident even in some writings at the time. In 1913, doctors Charles T. Jackson and Charles Wood McMurtry believed that a man's hair could only grow to a maximum length of six to eight inches.[386] How could they believe that? Did they not have the same access to the historical and archaeological documents that we have today? Did they not even observe the portraits of their own ancestors? Or, were they just somehow blind to the facts of simple observation? Of course, there may not have been any men in London, where they published their book, with long hair at that time. But what about old photographs, portraits, and sculptures plainly visible in the museums of London – did they never see these things? Thus, their remark that a man can only grow hair from six to eight inches is far removed from the simple facts of observation of nature itself.

The rise of modern military in the early part of the twentieth century has been no friend to man's crown. As a former military man said to me: "they [the military] want everyone to be the same: you become State property." "The Oxford Companion to Military History" informs us that one reason the "radical haircuts" are done is to "underline the equality of recruits."[387] But after this initiation rite into the military, why are they not

---

383 Eusebius' *Ecclesiastical History*, Book 2, Chapter 23. trans. C.F. Cruse, Complete and Unabridged, New Updated Edition (Peabody, MA: Hendrickson Publishers, 1998, Fifth Printing – June 2006).

384 William Smith, "Rechabites."

385 Ann Charles and Roger DeAnfrasio, *The History of Hair* (New York: Bonanza Books, 1970), 165.

386 Charles T. Jackson and McMurtry, *A Treatise on Diseases of the Hair* (London: Henry Kimpton, 1913).

387 Richard Holmes, ed., "Hair," *The Oxford Companion to Military History* (New York: Oxford University Press, 2001), 394-395.

allowed to grow their hair back so that it at least protects the head? The ultra-short hair issue of the early twentieth century culminated in World War II (WW II). As a result, the shorn head look became part of the civilian culture. "The 1960s reaction against the short hair made common by WW II" is believed by Holmes to be "in many ways a political as well as a counter-culture phenomenon." This is unfortunate that so many moderns think of male hair in this way. The situation in the American military now appears even worse than WW II. Why must a man be bald to serve?

In his brilliant "The significance of male hair," Raj Singh informs us that the truth of forced hair-cutting is to bestow upon males a "feeling of nothingness." It means you are not a "free person."[388] In "Bald No More," Dr. Morton Walker's research reveals the same idea. He found that removing head hair makes someone a non-person with "no distinct identity." "Specifically, when women are forced to hide their hair under a veil and men are forced to hide their hair by being shorn, these things symbolize a lack of individuality and sexuality.[389] This attitude against human head hair is in opposition to creation, where people in the resurrection are compared to stars, each one being a distinct individual with his or her own glory (1 Corinthians 15:40-41). The intent of the longhaired founding fathers of the United States was freedom for everyone.

Along these same lines of reasoning, one fourteen year-old Protestant boy related the following account. The boy wanted to grow his head hairs longer, but his mother quickly informed him, "long hair is for the privileged." She kept his hair clipped as if he was still an infant, at about one inch in length. I never saw him smile. The message she sent to the poor lad is that you are not privileged, thus he is not free. As documented earlier, a shaved head or really short hair was the mark of a slave. Logically, it follows that by the power of her tongue, she unconsciously condemned the boy to a life of bondage or slavery to other men. And this is what is being taught in America, "the land of the free and home of the brave"? Who will stop the war against the head?

Most people wear longer hair for one main reason, they like it that way. Longer haired men and even women are often persecuted for no reason other than their long hair. Name-calling and snide remarks against those who let their own God-given hair grow are still common in America. Individuals have been called savages, typical slang for Native Americans,

388 Raj Kumar Singh, The significance of male hair – Its presence and removal, The Backlash!, July 1998, 10 (Raj Singh, Valparaiso University, 1997), accessed September 3, 2003 http://www.choisser.com/longhair/rajsingh.html.
389 Morton Walker, Bald No More, (New York: Kensington Publishing Corporation, 1998), 17.

sinners, wild, uncivilized, rebels, hippies, and so forth. Older people with longer hair are often accused of being immature or having a midlife crisis. Here the idea is that long hair is just for the youth, more stupidity. According to Dr. Pickart, "Many women are taught that by age 30, their hair should be no longer than shoulder length." Sometimes women, who have destroyed their hair by over-manipulation, encourage other females with long beautiful hair to cut it off and donate it. In truth, they could care less about charity and are really motivated by jealousy. And who is teaching the rubbish that women should only wear shoulder-length hair? Has anyone realized that it was men who used to wear majestic shoulder-length hair, while women used to wear their hair well past the shoulders, long and healthy hanging down the back all the way to the belt?

The truth is that long hair is "majestic on a mature woman ... it downplays wrinkles and makes her look younger."[390] Long hair does the same for men. As typical, persecution of long hairs always comes from short-haired people, who, by choice, have decided to cut theirs off. Has anyone ever noticed that long hair people never condemn those with short hair? In general some of those with close-cropped heads realize that long hair means freedom. These people do not promote freedom. Remember, any time a society resorts to close-cropping their heads never means anything good (Jeremiah 7:29).

The real reason prisoners' and soldiers' hair is cut short is to remind them that they are not free and cannot do as they wish with their own body.[391] Those in the American military at the present time confirm that this is so. In discussions with some of these men, it is no secret among the enlisted that many will lose their hair due to atrophy of the hair follicle, and over-scrubbing with shampoo, and eventually go bald.

Singh's research demonstrated conclusively that as "to the significance of cutting a man's cranial hair, numerous investigators have agreed on one symbolic meaning: castration".[392]

The Bible teaches the same thing and also compares the cutting of hair with circumcision:

> See, the days are coming – it is Yahweh who speaks – when I am going to punish all who are circumcised only in flesh: Egypt, Judah, the sons of Ammon, Moab, and all the Crop-Heads who live in the

390 Loren Pickart, *Reverse Skin Aging: Using Your Skin's Natural Power* (Bellevue, Washington: Cape San Juan Press, 2005), 117.
391 Singh.
392 Singh, 11.

desert. For all these nations, and the whole House of Israel too, are uncircumcised at heart (Jeremiah 9:24-25[26]; JB).

The "Crop-Heads" are those "that have the corners of their hair cut off" as "The Jerusalem Bible: Koren Publisher's" version (the other Jerusalem Bible) puts it.[393] Obviously, God is not impressed with short haircuts, another form of outward circumcision, which Paul said is not necessary for anything (Galatians 5:6). In fact, Paul in Galatians appears to be restating what the Prophet Jeremiah said many centuries earlier (Jeremiah 9:24-25,26). While teaching on circumcision even Jesus said "Judge not according to the appearance, but judge righteous judgment" (John 7:24). God is all about having your heart circumcised spiritually, not any physical part of the body.

Circumcision of the foreskin itself may be considered healthier. However, circumcision of a man's head hair is quite the opposite. Indeed, it is a very unhealthy thing to do. Forcing a man to have his head circumcised is against nature, God's law for all men generally (Leviticus 19:27), and can even lead to mutilation and death (see next chapter). This may be a secondary reason why Jeremiah condemns head-cropping. Like all the laws, the intent of Leviticus 19:27 was a light for all men of all nations, not just Israelites: for all who are Christians are considered the Israel of God (Galatians 6:15-16). America, loosen your locks and let long hair prevail as Deborah and Barak sang (Judges 5:2, see Chapter 5). On the other hand, forced hair cutting is, as Singh says, "castration."

Let's face the facts. Nearly all men have some facial hair and nearly all have the built-in ability to grow long hair. They just do not show it due to constant cutting, a form of self-mutilation. They war against their own head and expect everyone else to follow. But in truth, a man with long hair and a beard of some sort is the way a man was designed to look. It seems quite odd, if not incredible, that a completely opposite, artificial look (ultra short hair and a shaved face) has been pushed on men off and on since the times of the Romans and other crop-headed societies. In many circles today a man is just not allowed to look like the man God designed him to be. Unfortunately, many church people and employers in America today still force their males, as unnatural as it is, to be as shorn as possible, following customs even worse than 1st century Rome. Many

393 The Jerusalem Bible. Jerusalem: Koren Publishers, 2000. This Bible is just the Old Testament from a different publisher in Jerusalem and must not be confused with the Roman Catholic's "Jerusalem Bible" (JB) quoted above in Jeremiah 9:24-25 and throughout this book.

modern-day Protestants seem to have inherited this ideology from Rome. And this comes from people who claim to believe in creation, that God created all things.

Whether male or female, human head hair grows longer and faster than any other hair of the body – it is a proven, observable scientific fact (see Chapter 2). Did God create hair this way so that men would have it cut off every week or two in the barbershop? Stop and think about how crazy this is for a moment. Back in 1828 Noah Webster informs us that those who frequented barbershops were called barbermongers and fops.[394] Furthermore, did God create the beard so that men would have to shave it off as it re-appears each morning? This is markedly ludicrous. On the contrary, God already told us not to cut the hair or beard unnaturally short (Leviticus 19:27). This, along with the fact that hair is built to last, demonstrates conclusively that long hair is no infraction. Rather, it is intentionally designed to be long by the Great Designer Himself. It was created that way as an ornament of beauty, and to protect your head.

Since the late 19th century those simpletons who forced the Native Americans to be shorn brought a most wicked doom on all our heads. Not only does really short hair symbolize tyranny or a great reduction in freedom, but skin cancer of the white man's head, ears, and neck is what we receive, and this fulfills the saying you will reap what you sow. Or, as long haired Prophet Jeremiah declared:

> The crown is fallen from our head: woe unto us, that we have sinned (Lamentations 5:16; JB).

Unfortunately, hair-hacking Delilah's run many of our Christian schools. The truth is that long hair is majestic, and certain hardhearted, crop-headed individuals should never have been placed in positions of power. The pattern that emerges is quite clear. Just like Julius Caesar, the torch of pagan hair removal now occurs in our modern Christian schools. The typical male hair specification that has been copied and passed around is usually something like this: hair must be above the eyes, no more than halfway over the ear, halfway over the collar; and absolutely no facial hair. They act as though someone with a shorn head is somehow more righteous than a person who allows his long hair to show. What a pretense

---

394 Noah Webster, American Dictionary of the English Language, 1828. Facsimile First Edition (Chesapeake, Virginia: Foundation for American Christian Education, 1995, 13th printing, August 2000).

of religion. This absurdity is against God's Law and it is against nature itself. Furthermore, this is the minimal amount of hair needed to protect the scalp and should not be the maximum allowed. The fear of facial hair is also senseless. Are we afraid of manhood? And the men setting this so-called example are themselves brainwashed as they lead others to destroy their hair and beards, which God created for our benefit. According to Rook and Dawber, the sacrifice of hair, such as seen with monks and Buddhists, is a substitute for human sacrifice![395] Again, we see that hair removal, especially shaving any part of the head, symbolizes death. Does anyone care that they are getting away with killing? Seriously, those who force you wear short hair may be responsible for your death via melanoma (see Chapter 9).

Jesus completely upheld God's Laws in the Old Testament, which the New Testament teaches are suppose to be written on our hearts:

Think not that I am come to destroy the Law, or the Prophets. I am not come to destroy them, but to fulfill them. For truly I say unto you, Till heaven and earth perish, one jot or one tittle of the Law shall not escape, till all things be fulfilled. Whosoever therefore shall break one of these least commandments, and teach men so, he shall be called the least in the kingdom of heaven: but whosoever shall observe and teach them, the same shall be called great in the kingdom of heaven (Matthew 5:17-19, The 1599 Geneva Bible).

To "fulfill" the law means that God's Laws are suppose to be written on our hearts (Hebrews 8:10). The mutilation of one's hair is precisely one of the "least" of the commandments Jesus spoke about. It is against God's Law and natural law. What Jesus said and what many Christian schools do, are diametrically opposed. The truth is that Scripture teaches us that it is a disgrace to intentionally bring baldness to our heads. This means close-cropping and shaving any part of the head. Recall Chapter 3 where you learned that unnaturally short hair accelerates baldness. People who enforce and teach this whether directly or by example will be low in the eternal hierarchy, "the least in the kingdom of heaven."

It appears in American society that the only people who either are free or feel completely free to wear their hair however they wish are women,

---

395 Arthur Rook and Rodney Dawber, eds., Diseases of the Hair and Scalp. 2nd Ed. (London: Blackwell Scientific Publications, 1991), 462.

not including black women. In contrast, most black women and most men, regardless of skin color, are not completely free to wear their own hair how they please. In many places, males are forced to be as shorn as possible. Unnaturally short hair often includes petty rules against masculinity, such as when men are forced to even shave their facial hair. Males who want to wear mature, natural, longer hair are often fired, not hired or not promoted. The interesting thing is that hair has nothing to do with the quality of one's work. In some circles, prejudice seems to be quite high against long-haired males and black people's hair overall. For a detailed listing of court cases against male hair (including Rastafarians, Native Americans, Nazarites, Sikhs, Jews and others), see Raj Singh's, "The significance of male hair." Who would have ever thought that a time would come when a man is not allowed to work unless he has the mark of real short hair? If you cannot work, then you will not earn money. Without money one cannot buy or sell. So they would rather see you dead. Truly, we live in unnatural times.

Another reason to discard the razor is that Gillette is a ringleader in the spy chip business.[396] These radio frequency identification devices, some small as a grain of sand, are being used to track products and transmit private information about you to marketers, criminals, or government agents. Spy chips have already been used on pets and livestock, some people have been tagged, and they are embedded in passports. What if one day our government forces you to be implanted with a chip? Think about that for a moment. Do you really want to support corporations like Gillette? Or, would it be better to beard than succumb?

---

396 Katherine Albrecht and Liz McIntyre, Spy Chips, How Major Corporations and Government Plan to Track Your Every Purchase and Watch Your Every Move (New York: PLUME (a member of Penguin Group), 2006).

Chapter 9: Cutting Corners and the Desecration of the Temple

||||||||||||||||||||||||||||||||||||||||||||||||||||||||||||||||||||||||||||||||||||||||||||||||||||||||||||||||||||||||||||||||||||||||||||||||||||||||||||

I will scatter them to the winds, those Crop-Heads, and bring disaster down on them from every side (Jeremiah 49:32, JB).

The Great Architect of the temple hopes His people maintain full health of the body. But close-cropped hair greatly increases health risk. For one thing, the rays of sunshine are incredibly powerful and can burn the head. Because of the fear of sunburn and its weathering effects, some people avoid the sun completely. But is this wise? Since modern men are taught to remove as much head hair as possible, men have sought alternative artificial means of protection, such as sunscreen. Is this the best thing to do? Modern studies demonstrate that sun avoidance and chemical sunscreens are both unhealthy.

For most people, with the apparent exception of albinos, a certain amount of sunlight is necessary for good health.[397] But overexposure may produce skin damage, wrinkling, and other unwanted effects. If your hair is too short then your ears and posterior neck may become overexposed. The questions are how much sunshine is good for you and what is the best way to protect the head, ears and neck from overexposure?

Sunlight activates a gene called pom-C. According to Dr. Loren Pickart, pom-C helps create melanin that "determines skin color" and "enhances sex drive," the endorphins or "happiness hormones," and leptin, which helps burn fat and keep you thin. As Pickart said, "farmers out in sunlight live longer."[398] The truth is that sunbathing increases longevity because it heals just about every disease including skin

---

397 Loren Pickart, Reverse Skin Aging: Using Your Skin's Natural Power (Bellevue, Washington: Cape San Juan Press, 2005), 137.
398 Loren Pickart, Telephone communication with him at his business, Skin Biology, Inc., Bellevue, Washington, October 28, 2004.

cancer.[399] Dr. Bernarr says that proper sunbathing "heals skin cancer" and "heals wrinkles." The people who get skin cancer and wrinkles from sun exposure are those who have made bad health choices including poor diet, especially polyunsaturated fat, smoking, and who "over consume coffee and tea, which contain toxic caffeine and tannic acid." Then "under the influence of sunlight these toxic foods are brought to the skin."

Therefore, tanning itself is not harmful, but a good thing to do. The production of melanin is good because it creates a powerful protective and anti-oxidant system in the skin.[400] Apparently, melanocytes form a second barrier, beneath the acid mantle of the skin's surface, of protection from the "damaging effects of ultraviolet radiation."[401] The key is to obtain a tan with a minimum of free radical damage to other areas of the skin. During the summer months, clothing can protect the body from over-exposure to the sun, but the head remains unclothed. There are two common things people do to protect their head, ears, and posterior neck from over-exposure to the sun: (1) wear a hat, bandana, or scarf; and (2) sunscreen. As it turns out, many sunscreens are problematic.

Problems with Sunscreen Chemicals

Dr. Pickart informs us that many commonly used chemical sunscreens may be dangerous to your health. He relates the problem: up to 35 percent of sunscreen chemicals applied to the skin can enter your bloodstream![402] Because of this, many sunscreen chemicals are banned in the European community. Chemical sunscreens should not be confused with mechanical sunscreens such as zinc oxide or titanium dioxide, both of which are not known to alter or harm the skin's functions.

According to Pickart, irresponsible cosmetic companies and a few very vocal, publicity-seeking dermatologists have strongly advocated that chemical sunscreens should be heavily applied before any exposure to sunlight, even on young children. These publicity seekers insist that sunscreen use would prevent skin cancer and protect your health. He relates these particular

399 Bernarr, "Sick? Well? ... Sunbathing Helps You and Everyone," accessed July 2, 2010 http://www.healself.org/sun.html
400 Pickart, Reverse Skin Aging: Using Your Skin's Natural Power, 137.
401 Arun Kumar, "Summary of Current Research Programs: Human Skin Smart biological Interface Bio-MEMS / sensor," accessed December 6, 2005 http://www.eng.usf.edu/~arunk/
402 Loren Pickart, "The Chemical Sunscreen Disaster," accessed July 2, 2010 http://www.skinbiology.com/toxicsunscreens.html

dermatologists to those 12,000 plus physicians who advocated cigarette smoking in 1927![403] This is because many scientists involved in cancer studies have come to virtually the opposite conclusion: sunscreen chemicals may increase the incidence of cancer. In Dr. David G. Williams publication "Alternatives," he writes extensively about the prevention of disease. Concerning how chemical sunscreens can cause cancer, he states:

> For years we've been told to stay out of the sun and use sunscreen to avoid skin cancer. But since the invention of sunscreen years ago, skin cancer rates in the U.S. have gone up, not down. Doctors can't explain this. Nor can they explain why the incidence of skin cancer in tropical countries (where the sun's rays are the strongest) is extremely low. The explanation is simple, though: Sunshine isn't bad, it's actually good for you. Besides being our main source of vitamin D (a potent cancer fighter), sunshine causes your body to produce *melanin*, your natural protector against skin cancer.[404]

Overall, sunlight exposure actually decreases human cancer rates and improves health. Garland's research also concluded that sun exposure is the main source of vitamin D. Vitamin D and its metabolites reduce the risk of cancers of the colon, breast, prostate, and others.[405] Likewise, Podolsky informs us that without enough sunshine to set vitamin D in motion, "the body would be unable to properly absorb calcium and phosphorus, the minerals that give bone its rigidity."[406] Thus, moderate sun exposure is needed and highly encouraged.

Heavily-used chemical sunscreens are problematic because they may actually increase cancers by virtue of their free radical generating properties. Another disastrous effect is that sunscreen chemicals also have strong estrogenic actions. This can cause serious problems in sexual development and adult sexual function, and may further increase cancer risks.[407]

---

403 Pickart, "The Chemical Sunscreen Disaster."
404 David G. Williams, "How Sunscreen Can Cause Skin Cancer," Alternatives, New Health Breakthroughs Christians Can Depend On. Special Introductory Issue (sent in mail – no date). http://www.drdavidwilliams.com
405 C.F. Garland "More on preventing skin cancer: sun avoidance will increase cancers overall," BMJ 2003 Nov. 22; 327(7425):1228 PMID: 14630775 30, accessed August 30, 2005 http://www.ncbi.nlm.nih.gov/entrez/query.fcgi?cmd=Retrieve&db=pubmed &dopt=Abstract&list_uids=14630775&query_hl=2.
406 D.M. Podolsky, Skin: the human fabric. (The Human Body) (Tarrytown, New York: Torstar Books, Inc., 1984), 73.
407 Pickart, "The Chemical Sunscreen Disaster."

Ironically, the compounds in sunscreens were never viewed as benign substances.[408] The problem is that these chemicals are widely used to start free radical reactions during chemical synthesis.[409] These substances are mixed with other chemicals, and flashed with an ultraviolet light. The ultraviolet absorbing chemicals then generate large amounts of free radicals that initiated the desired chemical reactions. All the while, the lab technicians making the stuff wisely keep the poisonous brew away from their skin.[410] Free radicals are "atoms or groups of atoms that can cause damage to cells, impairing the immune system and leading to infections and various degenerative diseases."[411] In summary, chemical sunscreens disrupt the natural protective mechanisms of the skin and can cause skin cancer.

Para-Aminobenzoic Acid (PABA) is on the Canadian hot list of bad cosmetic ingredients.[412] PABA can cause allergic eczema and sensitivity to light in people with sensitive skin. Some sunscreens are now PABA free. Another especially harsh chemical in sunscreens is oxybenzone. Oxybenzone is derived from isopropanol, which is highly toxic. In fact, an ingested amount of only one fluid ounce is fatal.[413] Are there any *chemical sunscreens* that are completely safe? Probably not. Ruth Winter says among chemical sunscreens there is a "low concern about the safety" of "octinoxate" and "octisalate." She does say that octinoxate is an excellent UV absorber, but may cause allergic skin rashes in some people. To reduce exposure to chemicals in chemical sunscreens, a lower SPF (sun protectant factor) rating may prove to be better for you, if you feel you must use sunscreen. A lower SPF rating means a lesser amount of chemicals that can potentially harm you.

Let's say your skin burns in one hour due to sun exposure. An SPF 4 sunscreen gives four times the protection to the sun, which means your skin should not burn until four hours, theoretically. Continued application of an SPF 8 sunscreen means you should not burn until eight hours of sun

408 C.F. Garland, F.C. Garland, E.D. Gorham, "Rising trends in melanoma. An hypothesis concerning sunscreen effectiveness," Ann Epidemiol, 1993 Jul; 3(4):451 PMID: 8287144 accessed August 30, 2005 http://www.ncbi.nlm.nih.gov/entrez/query.fcgi?cmd=Retriev e&db=pubmed&dopt=Abstract&list_uids=8287144&query_hl=2.
409 Pickart, "The Chemical Sunscreen Disaster."
410 Pickart, "The Chemical Sunscreen Disaster."
411 Phyllis A. Balch and James F. Balch, Prescription for Nutritional Healing, 3rd ed. (New York: Avery – a member of Penguin Putnam, 2000), 53.
412 Ruth Winter, A Consumer's Dictionary of Cosmetic Ingredients (New York: Three Rivers Press, 2005).
413 Winter.

exposure. Eight hours is essentially all day in the sun. But what if your skin burns in a half hour? Then an SPF 8 sunscreen would offer protection for four hours. This raises another question. Why in the world would anyone need a sunscreen with an SPF 30 or SPF 60? This is like putting chemical icing on your body. The higher the SPF, the more potential there is to introduce your skin to excessive free radicals. In lieu of chemical glaze, why not start tanning little by little in the spring? In this way, your healthy tan skin will reduce sunburn later in the sunnier summer months. Tanned skin increases the amount of time you can spend in the sun before burning.[414] To prevent burning, it is better to acquire sunshine when the sun's angle is slanted, early morning or late afternoon.[415] In lieu of high SPF chemical sunscreens, a very high-quality natural oil called MexitanTM is available (Appendix II).

Hair, the Creator's Natural Sunblock

From a dermatologic standpoint presence of scalp hair certainly does have valuable protective function as to prevention of sun damage and skin cancer.[416]

In lieu of dangerous chemical sunscreens, why not use your own God-given hair (natural head clothing) to protect the scalp, ears and neck. Walker informs us of two main scientific purposes of hair: (1) conservation of body heat, and (2) external protection.[417] Other than personal beauty, hair protects the head, ears and posterior neck from overexposure to the sun in the summer and from cold air during winter. The top of the head or scalp and tops of the ears are particularly prone to damage since these parts face the sun directly. But if you do not grow enough hair, then how is it supposed to protect your head?

Did you know that white men in particular suffer from skin cancer, even the worst kind, malignant melanoma (Figure 9-1)! Ironically, popular locations of skin cancer occur on the ears, the scalp, and back of the neck, and are more common in males because the hair is cut unnaturally short:

414 Podolsky, 76.
415 Bernarr.
416 Paul Subrt, Westside Dermatology Clinic, Katy, TX. This doctor's personal correspondence was given to me while discussing the matter in his office on April 16, 2010.
417 Morton Walker, Bald No More, (New York: Kensington Publishing Corporation, 1998), 70.

...these cancers frequently occur on the sun-exposed areas of the head and neck.[418]

Most tumors arise on the sun-exposed regions of the head and neck.[419]

Scalp cancer is more common in men who have lost their hair.[420]

The incidence of melanoma has been on the rise, with a high incidence occurring in men on the head [and] neck."[421]

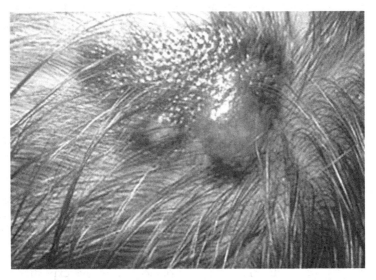

Figure 9-1: Melanoma in the Scalp. Is short hair worth the risk of deadly malignant melanoma? Something like this would not even look good on the Frankenstein monster. Photograph courtesy of John L. Bezzant, M.D.

418 L.A. Goldenberg, "The sun and skin cancer: What you need to know about diagnosis and treatment," Northwest Dent, 2000 Mar-Apr;79(2):19-25. PMID: 11413579 accessed August 31, 2005 http://www.ncbi.nlm.nih.gov/entrez/query.fcgi?CMD=Display&DB=pubmed.

419 Fred J. Stucker, Cherie-Ann O. Nathan, and Timothy S. Lian, "Cutaneous Malignancy," Head and Neck Surgery – Otolaryngology, 3rd Ed., Vol. Two, eds. Byron Bailey et al. (Philadelphia, PA: Lippincott Williams & Wilkins, 2001) 1,223.

420 MayoClinic.com. Scalp Cancer. "What can you tell me about scalp cancer?" accessed April 10, 2004 http://www.ohiohealth.com/healthreference/reference/4080484E-8717-43E2-A3DA4123D17E84D5.htm?category=questions.

421 L.S. Phieffer, E.C. Jones, M.G. Tonneson, D.A. Kriegel, "Melanoma of the scalp: an underdiagnosed malignancy?" Cutis. 2002 May;69(5):362-4. PMID: 12041815 accessed August 31, 2005 http://www.ncbi.nlm.nih.gov/entrez/query.fcgi?CMD=Display&DB=pubmed.

What true statements. The question is, how are these poor men losing their hair in the first place? The manmade causes of hair loss cited in this book may have the answers for many. Short hair accelerates baldness. Some may say, but I have to "look professional" for my job. Aside from what hogwash this is, there are many professionals now with longer hair just like all the true professionals who wore long hair in the past.

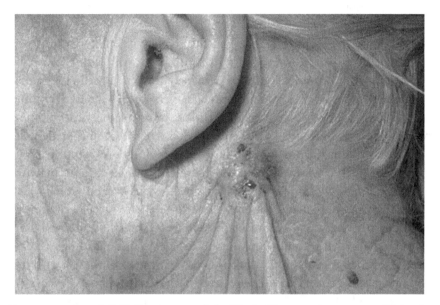

Figure 9-2: Basal Cell Carcinoma of the Neck. Photograph courtesy of John L. Bezzant, M.D. According to Dr. Bezzant, this patient spent her younger years in Chihuahua, Mexico, and was exposed to "a lot of sunlight as a young person." This is what can happen when a female either wears her hair up too much or wears short hair outdoors. Repetitious sunburns lead to skin cancer. Bezzant says that this "basal cell carcinoma originated within the epidermis and extended through the skin fat, and attached to the underlying muscle."

In yet another example, a male tennis player got malignant melanoma of the scalp. The French doctors concluded that "hair protects only partially the skin from ultraviolet damages."[422] But this comment by A.L. Fraiture is only *partially* true. No doubt, this male tennis player wears his hair ultra-short. If his hair was long enough and thick enough, he would probably be cancer-free. Rook and Dawber agree. They understand quite well that

---

422 A.L. Fraiture, F. Henry, C. Pierard-Franchimont and G.E. Pierard, "Image of the month. A hidden melanoma hidden in a tennis player." Rev Med Liege, 2001 Nov;56(11):737-8 PMID: 11789384 accessed August 31, 2005 http://www.ncbi.nlm.nih.gov/entrez/query. fcgi?CMD=Display&DB=pubmed.

tumors are rarely found in the scalp of those who retain a good protective cover of hair.[423] What if men would just simply wear longer hair, the way many males did throughout the centuries? After all hair does protect the ears, scalp, and back of the neck. This is child's play. In "ABC's of the Human Body," Alma Guinness informs us that one of the chief purposes of head hair is to screen out harmful ultraviolet rays from the sun![424] Even women are not exempt from sunburn if they leave their hair up too long while outdoors (Figure 9-2).

Many do not seem to realize that skin cancer is "the most common form of cancer" and overexposure to sunlight is its "leading cause."[425] There are several types of skin cancer, including basal cell carcinoma, squamous cell carcinoma, and melanoma, which are all related to "chronic sun exposure," especially in men.[426] Actinic kerotoses is the most common premalignant lesion with a 20 percent potential to become malignant. Keratoacanthoma begins as a smooth round nodule exhibiting rapid growth. The center of this growth becomes filled with keratinous material and looks like a "volcano."[427] Squamous cell lesions can be virulent and can metastasize to regional nodes. When this happens in the head or neck area, death is certain. Because of the unpredictability of all these skin cancers, removal is recommended, even surgical excision leading to scars. Even after the cancer is surgically removed, recurrence of these horrifying and mutilating cancers on the nose, ears, neck, scalp, and other places on the face is quite possible.[428] Melanoma is the leading cause of death from malignancies of the skin, accounting for 2 percent of all cancer deaths in the United States.[429] The median age of malignant melanoma is 55 years, but some as young as 12 years are diagnosed with this deadly cancer. Most of these could have been avoided by a healthy head of hair of adequate length to protect the head.

According to "The Complete Book of Cancer Prevention," fair-skinned people are at the highest risk in developing skin cancer. In 1989,

423 Arthur Rook and Rodney Dawber, eds., Diseases of the Hair and Scalp, 2nd Ed. (London: Blackwell Scientific Publications, 1991), 541.
424 Alma E. Guinness, ed., ABC's of the Human Body (New York: The Readers Digest Association, 1987), 150.
425 Podolsky, 75.
426 Stucker, et al, 1,226.
427 Stucker, et al, 1,227.
428 Stucker, et al, 1,228.
429 Jeffery Myers and Andrew Nemechek, "Malignant Melanoma," Head and Neck Surgery – Otolaryngology, 3rd Ed., Vol. Two, eds. Byron Bailey et al. (Philadelphia, PA: Lippincott Williams & Wilkins, 2001).

Prevention's editors estimated about 422,000 cases each year. For every 100,000 people, only three to four blacks, but more than 230 whites will acquire sun-induced skin cancer. There is an "increased sensitivity of individuals with blonde and red hair to sunburn and skin cancer."[430] Another researcher says the same thing in another way: the "pigmentary phenotype characterized by red hair, fair complexion, inability to tan and tendency to freckle is an independent risk factor for all skin cancers, including melanoma."[431] Also, the fairer the skin the earlier the onset of horny skin growths, warts, and the like, under the same exposure to the sun as darker individuals.[432]

Most of the cancer hits the same places of the body the sun does, such as the "tops of the ears and scalp," especially in balding men. In 1991, just two years later, John Feltman and his colleagues increased the amount of skin cancer cases to more than 500,000 per year, and further stated that one out of every seven Americans will get skin cancer.[433] This figure is feared to be increasing to one out of five.[434] They go on to tell us that the sun causes 90 percent of all skin cancers. In 1999, an astonishing 1,000,000 new cases of skin cancer were diagnosed in the United States.[435] But remember, this is overexposure to the sun. Twenty percent of all Americans will get skin cancer. Is it wise to cut the hair so short that it offers no protection?

If you get malignant melanoma on the neck, what do you think your options are? Well, first of all the tumor must be removed from your neck via dissection.[436] Unless you think removing body parts is fun, perhaps

430 S. Takeuchi, W. Zhang, K. Wakamatsu, S. Ito, V.J. Hearing, K.H. Kraemer, D.E. Brash, "Melanin acts as a potent UVB photosensitizer to cause an atypical mode of cell death in murine skin," Proc Natl Acad Sci U S A., 2004 Oct 19;101(42):15076-81. PMID: 15477596 accessed April 16, 2006 http://www.ncbi.nlm.nih.gov/entrez/query.fcgi?CMD=Display&DB=pubmed.
431 F. Rouzaud, A.L. Kadekaro, Z.A. Abdel-Malek, V.J. Hearing, "MCIR and the response of melanocytes to ultraviolet radiation," Mutat Res., 2005 Apr 1;571(1-2):133-52. Epub 2005 Jan 26. PMID: 15748644 accessed April 16, 2006 http://www.ncbi.nlm.nih.gov/entrez/query.fcgi?CMD=Display&DB=pubmed.
432 Rook and Dawber, 546.
433 John Feltman, ed., Prevention's Giant Book of Health Facts (Emmaus, PA: Rodale Press, 1991), 478.
434 "What is Skin Cancer?" "Skin Cancer Rates Rising," accessed July 2, 2010 http://www.skincarephysicians.com/skincancernet/whatis.html.
435 Goldenberg.
436 S.R. Fisher, T.B. Cole, H.F. Seigler, "Application of posterior neck dissection in treating malignant melanoma of the posterior scalp," Laryngoscope. 1983 Jun;93(6):760-5. PMID: 6855400, accessed April 10, 2004 http://www.ncbi.nlm.nih.gov/entrez/query.fcgi?CMD=Display&DB=pubmed.

you should go to a skin cancer hospital and see for yourself. After they remove the tumor then who knows. Perhaps you will need chemotherapy or radiation if they think the cancer has spread to other areas. Hair is not a waste product. So why treat it as such, that your skin must combat the sun all by itself? The same thing could be said of the ears (Figure 9-3). Men of fair skin have cancers like this removed all the time. Is very short hair worth the health risk? If we personify the body parts as Paul did in 1 Corinthians 12:18-26, then *how can the eye or ear say to the hair, I have no need of you?* Hair over the ear would have protected these men from this abuse.

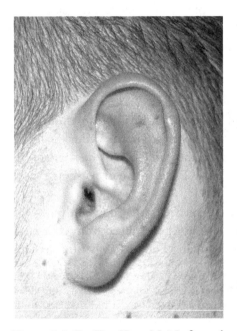 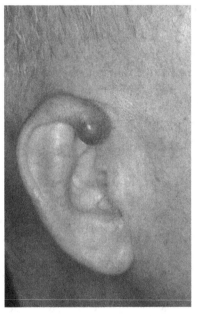

Figure 9-3: Do You Hear Me? Left: sunburned red inflamed ear of a 19- year-old man. This young man spends much time outdoors in the sun. Premature weathering and skin damage are already apparent. The ears become red because blood rushes to the area in an effort to heal the damage. Photograph by the author, 2009. Right: malignant melanoma cancer of the ear in an old man. Dissection is the probable method of treatment. Is unnaturally short hair so important that you would rather have your ears cut off? Photograph: courtesy of DermAtlas; http://dermatlas.org.

Please recall that the first rule of science is simple observation. Have you ever noticed a fair-skinned white man with short hair who has been over-exposed to the sun? If so, then you would have observed inflamed red ears and a red neck parched considerably in the posterior. The ears and neck turn red due to increased blood flow, the skin's way to speed "healing."[437] In some men, this redness seems to glow most of the year, an indicator that the healing process is not given a chance to end. On closer observation, you can even see the damaged skin of the ears and neck from repetitious sunburns. Glowing red ears especially stand out on a man with fair skin. This can be readily observed on even young males today. Repetitive abuse causes the normally smooth skin of the ears to become rough, weathered and almost scaly, possibly those horny skin growths, in appearance. Freckles and other skin damage abound. Thus, cutting the hair so short that it remains above the ears is a very bad idea, an idea with no basis in wisdom at all.

By simple observation, it is quite evident that shaving the corners of the hairline of the posterior neck is an equally disastrous idea. Anyone who is observer of nature can plainly see that the corners of the hairline drop quite low. This natural neck hairline occurs near or at the height of the chin. In some men it occurs even lower than chin level, and this is where the hair begins to grow. The hair begins to grow there because it is seeking a certain programmed length, a length that should be allowed to grow to the bottom of the neck at least (Figures 9-4, 9-5, 9-9). But those who shave it often show an entire array of damaged and irritated skin. This includes pimples, warts, sun-parching, pock marks (scars from shaving pimples?), infections such as barber's rash, and pseudofolliculitis barbae (see Dinulos and Graham). Hair that is allowed to grow to cover the neck is most wise. The hair is designed to protect you. Besides, the low level of the hairline proves that head hair is designed to cover and protect the neck. Since this is true, and to make hair look balanced, the ears should either be partially or wholly covered. Shaving the neck and intentionally tapering the hair so none of it falls over the ears could potentially threaten your health (Figures 9-3, 9-7, 9-8).

This brings us to another point. It seems that male hairstyles in the late 1960s and 1970s were right on target with most of our other longer-haired ancestors throughout history. Hair has many important purposes. We must face the observable facts. How many balding rock stars, Rastafarians, or Sikhs do you see? An honest person would admit that most of them do not thin or bald much. Why? Longer hair is healthier and short hair leads to scalp atrophy, skin cancer, and other problems. We must get rid of ultra-short, unnatural, male hair policies. Thankfully, many schools do believe in nature and freedom (Figure 9-5).

---

437 Podolsky, 76.

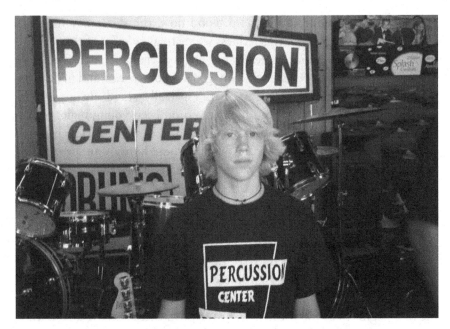

Figure 9-4: Young male 14 years of age with hair of adequate length. This is this person's natural hair unaltered by any means. Note the natural way the hair curls to form an umbrella effect, which offers much shade for the head and neck. The head, ears, and neck are thus protected from over-exposure to the sun. Hair on the forehead even offers additional shade to the face. In all wisdom, preacher Billy Graham said on one of his nationally televised sermons that there must be a compromise with regards to male hair length. If there must be a compromise, then it is the author's opinion that this should be that length is acceptable, and nothing less. If one wishes to wear their hair shorter, then this is their personal choice (and risk), and should not be forced on others. No one should risk another person's neck. Besides, hair of this length is still in the realm of short hair, scientifically. Photograph by the author, August 2005.

Even in the Scriptures, *all* the males were told by God Himself:[438]

Ye shall not round the corners of your head, neither shalt thou mar the corners of thy beard (Leviticus 19:27).

Modern Orthodox Jews, called Hasids, interpret Leviticus 19:27 to mean that the two corners in front of the ears (i.e., sideburns or sidelocks (called *peyot*)), and beard must not be cut at all.[439] They cut the rest of the

---

438 Leviticus 19:2 explains that these hair laws were for all men, laypeople. Clergy had similar rules, but those are described in Leviticus 21.

439 H.L.E. Luering, "Hair," The International Standard Bible Encyclopaedia, ed. James Orr, Vol. 2 (Hendrickson Publishers ed. 2nd Printing March 1996. 4 vols.).

head hair really short (Figure 9-6). The problem is that this hairstyle is of rather recent origin. The Lubavitcher Headquarters, Brooklyn, NY informs us that this hairstyle originates from a Hasidic custom that began with the teachings of Rabbi Israel Ben Eliezer, also known as the "Besht," in 18th century Eastern Europe.[440] Do the "corners" just mean sideburns or the temple region as they allege? No, this view is rather odd, one-dimensional, and based on a misinterpretation of Leviticus 19:27. Unfortunately, notations in some protestant study bibles have furthered this error.

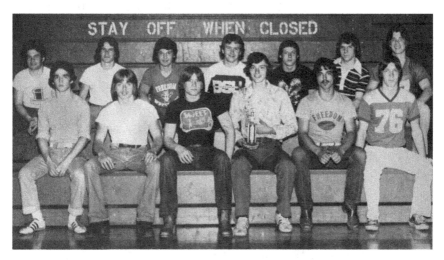

Figure 9-5: Hair length of students, Freedom High School, Pennsylvania 1977.
No one has long hair in this picture, based upon scientific measurement. The length is in short to medium range (see Figure 2-6). But at least the hair is long enough to protect the head, ears and neck. "Freedom" is a good name for this school for at least they were free to wear their own hair in this natural way. Based on the hairstyles of the founding fathers of the United States, certainly they would have agreed.

One article called "The Pharisees" says "Some Hasids grow their peyot [sidelocks] long and almost *crew cut* the rest of their head, not realizing that it's a primitive and pagan gesture." [441] "Why do religious Jews grow long sidelocks ..." says, "in ancient times it was a pagan custom to shave the sideburns."[442] The writer of "The Pharisees" says it was pagan to accentuate the sidelocks by cutting the rest of the head hair short. The other writer

440 Lubavitcher Headquarters, Brooklyn, N.Y. accessed March 20, 2009 http://philtar.ucsm. ac.uk/encyclopedia/judaism/hasidim.html.
441 "The Pharisees," accessed February 16, 2006 http://www.nabion.org/html/the_pharisees. html.
442 "Why do religious Jews grow long sidelocks ("peyos")?" accessed February 16, 2006 http://www.askmoses.com/qa_detail.html?h=256&o=2413.

says it was pagan to shave off the sides of the head. Both are probably true since both are unnatural. The ancient contemporaries of the Hebrews were the Hittites. According to Pickart's "Hair Biology, Hair Care, and Loss," it was the Hittites who shaved off their beards and patches of hair near their temples, but wore the remainder of their hair long.[443] The original intent of Leviticus 19:27 may have been an effort to prevent the removal of the sidelocks and beard, or parts thereof, since most of the interference seems to have been with the hair on those parts in ancient times. So the relatively new idea that all the head hair is to be cut off short except for the sidelocks and beard is unfounded.

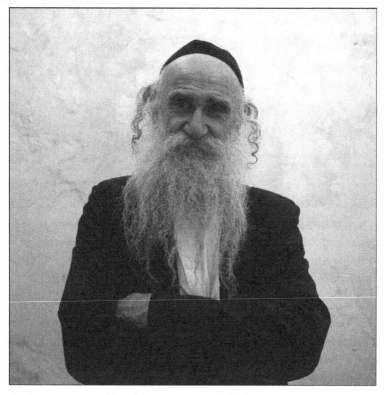

Figure 9-6: Orthodox Jew with Long Sidelocks and Long Beard. Notice how this man may be balding on top, which is not at all like most of his longer haired ancestors who lived in the centuries before Christ.

Rounding any corners of the natural hairline is unnatural. It truly does desecrate the temple, meaning your body. God wishes that men would

443 Loren Pickart, Hair Biology, Hair Care, and Loss, accessed November 6, 2010 http://www.skinbiology.com/hairbiology,care&loss.html.

wear their hair naturally as He created it without mutilating any part of it. Like any ethical contractor, the Master Builder does not cut corners, otherwise the temple could fall. In fact, just a few verses prior to Leviticus 19:27 the Lord says thou shalt love thy neighbor as thyself (Leviticus 19:18). Through God's love, many of His basic laws are actually for the betterment of your health.

When the natural hairline is traced around the circumference of the head, a three dimensional consideration, one would find that there are several "corners." As far as the sides of the head are concerned, there are at least four prominent corners of the hairline. Two corners occur before the ears and the two behind the ears. Dr. William Smith recognizes this in his "A Concise Dictionary of the Bible" and says it was forbidden for the "locks along the forehead and temples and behind the ears" to be removed.[444] Bickel and Jantz, while answering the question "Are tattoos wrong?" in their book, say the same thing, that the meaning of Leviticus 19:27 is "you shouldn't cut your hair or clip off the edges of your beard."[445] John Graybill emphasizes this point in his writing on Jeremiah,[446] where it literally reads:

And I will scatter them to all winds, those who cut the corners [of their hair]. And I will bring their calamity from all sides of it, says Jehovah. And Hazor shall be a dwelling for jackals, a ruin forever (Jeremiah 49:32b-33; "The Interlinear Bible").

Certainly, the basic rule is not to cut any of the hair unnaturally short. Jeremiah's cutting of the "corners of the hair" relates to disaster from "all sides." This passage makes it clear that the "corners" occur on "all sides" of the head, not just sidelocks. And the sad truth is those who cut their natural hairline bring disaster upon themselves, "ruin" in the forms of weathered skin, burns, and skin cancer. God created all the corners around the circumference of the head, none of them should ever be removed. The common practice of rounding these corners, especially by shaving them off,

---

444 William Smith, ed., "Hair," A Concise Dictionary of the Bible, Comprising its Antiquities, Biography, Geography, and Natural History (Boston: Little, Brown, and Company, 1865).

445 B. Bickel, and S. Jantz, Bible Answers to Life's Big Questions (Eugene, Oregon: Harvest House Publishers, 2006), 133. While answering the question "Are tattoos wrong?" they relate that Leviticus 19:27 means that neither the hair nor the beard was to be cut.

446 John Graybill, "Jeremiah," The Wycliffe Bible Commentary, eds. C.F. Pfeiffer, and E.F. Harrison (Chicago: Moody Press, 1990). The better translation of Jeremiah 49:32 is "who cut the corners (of their hair)."

is not a well thought out idea, it brings about "ruin." Or did you not know that some of God's laws are actually for your health? In his commentary on Jeremiah 9:26, Graybill also remarks that those who cut the corners of their hair is a heathen practice. As stated earlier, "The Jerusalem Bible's" translation of "Crop-Heads" says that certain Arab groups did this. Why are most modern American men the worst, by literally cutting and shaving all the natural corners of the hairline?

Leviticus 19:27 really means that none the head hair was to be cut, or rounded off, short. None of the corners were to be removed. The ancient Israelites knew what the passage meant. They wore all the scalp hair fairly long, as discussed and proved earlier, not just long sideburns or sidelocks. Some men wore long beards (Psalm 133:2), but others apparently kept beards trimmed (2 Samuel 19:25). The only difference between the instructions given in Leviticus 19:27 and Numbers 6 is that the former was allowed to trim, or dress, the hair only after a full length was achieved. The latter was not permitted to touch the hair at all with a blade, the Nazarite vow. In either case, all the ancient Israelites wore all the head hair long, not just the sideburns. The long hair symbolized their respect and protection, not only for the sake of their own heads, but for others as well:

> ... thou shalt not wholly reap the corners of thy field ... thou shalt leave them for the poor and the stranger [e.g., travelers through their land] (Leviticus 19:9-10).

Even here we see God's heart where the corners of the fields of crops were never to be harvested so the poor and sojourners would not starve. Fields have more than two corners, do they not? Furthermore, it demonstrates that those who do cut corners of their hair may be cheapskates. Most salesmen today are crop-heads, servants of money rather than God. Those who sell razorblades do not even realize all the damage they have caused. If they do not even care about their own head health, do you really think they care about you? Rather, is it not an addiction to the razor?

A wise person might ask, is short hair worth the potential health risk? If one out of every five people get skin cancer, then it is most advisable to protect the head with hair long enough to do an adequate job, hair long enough to shade the head, ears, and neck. Hair trimmed around the ears and above the collar is not only unnatural, but it unnecessarily exposes areas of the head to ultraviolet rays, which can lead to skin cancer. The common modern practice of rounding these corners, shaving them off, is the first step towards eliminating natural neck protection. I have observed some men who appear to have shaved their natural neckline to an absurd height of nearly half-way up the backside of their skull. Exposure of the tops of ears and neck is a potential health risk that is just too high. The odds are a one in five (1/5) chance of getting skin cancer if you wear your hair too short. The odds are greater with those who have blonde and red hair. Be wise and protect your head. This is the reason the corners of the natural hairline grow on the neck (Figures 9-7, 9-8, 9-9).

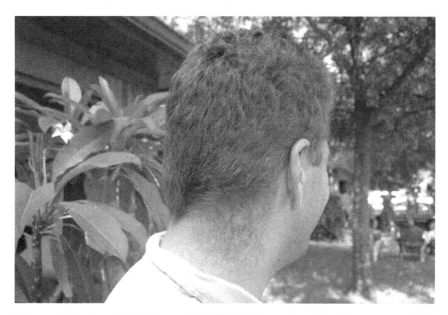

Figure 9-7: Natural Hairline of the Neck. Notice how low the corners of the natural hairline grow on this man's neck. This low altitude, even to the base of the neck or bottom of his natural collar, proves that, by design, men are supposed to wear their hair longer than the modernistic practice of super- close cropping. The hairs are designed to grow out and protect the neck. An exposed neck leads to severe sunburns. If the neck hairs are unsightly, it is only because the hair from above is meant to cover the corners. The structure of the hairline is to direct longer hair towards the shoulders so that they too can be protected. All individuals have corners similar to the man shown here. The basic design proves that men are intended to wear shoulder length hair at the very least. Note also the infectious barber's rash caused by razor burn in the beard area, which is also very evident in those who shave the corners of the neck. Photograph by the author.

The power of the sun is often displayed on those who wear longer hair as was observed in Jesus' hair (Chapter 6). Damaged hair is better than damaged skin. Sun-bleached or highlighted hair is damaged, weathered hair. These natural highlights represent a process of decay. However, they do add beauty to the individual as testified by those who get their hair artificially highlighted at a salon. Sun-bleached hair is analogous to beautiful autumn leaves, which also represents decay. So even though sun damaged hair (natural highlights) increases beauty, sun damaged bare skin decreases beauty. Thus, weathered hair is better than weathered skin, because weathered skin leads to wrinkles, premature aging, skin problems, and even cancers. So then, why is hair is built to last? The obvious answer is because hair is designed to take much more of a beating than bare skin. Protect your head, ears and neck from abuse with your own hair. Otherwise you can get skin cancer, even melanoma, as the young man has in Figure 9-8. Protect your hair with a temporary cover, if needed.

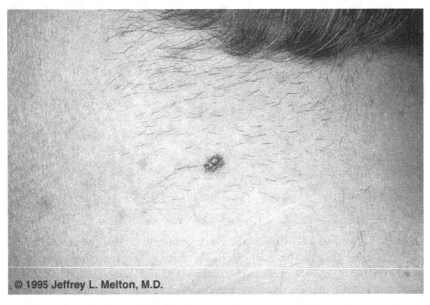

© 1995 Jeffrey L. Melton, M.D.

Figure 9-8: Melanoma of the Neck. Note the position of this malignant cancer, it is right in the midst where the natural hairline (left corner of the posterior neck) has been removed by shaving, probably repeatedly during each haircut! Could it be that damaged skin caused by frequent shaving, along with sunburn, caused this cancer? This no doubt is the situation. Photograph courtesy of Jeffrey L. Melton, M.D. (drmelton.com).

Hair grown to the base of the neck protects the neck from sunburn in the summer, and protects the neck from cold air during the winter, and even protects the neck from insects. One of the worst ideas ever is shaving off the hairs of the natural neckline, a form of rounding off the corners. The manmade sister-idea to this dogma is that a man's hair should be "above the collar," a manmade piece of clothing. The truth is that hairs emerge lower than the top of a manmade shirt collar. When allowed to grow, the hairs have a natural umbrella effect and behold, no more sun-burnt red necks occur.

Hair draped over the neck even protects from insect bites. Furthermore, the oil on the hair secreted by the sebaceous gland (sebum) keeps the neck and other skin parts well oiled. In this way, premature wrinkling is inhibited. Consider an automobile with a leather interior. Leather is cow skin. If leather is not kept well-oiled, it fades, wrinkles, and cracks apart. It weathers. Not only is hair designed to take the weather instead of bare skin, it also spreads the oil extruded by the follicles about the head, ears and neck keeping the skin moist and pliable. This is how longer hair keeps you from looking old and weathered with scorched, dry, crusty ears and a wrinkled, leathery neck. It seems quite apparent that the Creator knew what he was doing when He designed our bodies. In fact, the Prophet Ezekiel (29:18) seems to indicate that when head hair is removed the shoulders are left unprotected as well:

Their heads have all gone bald, their shoulders are chafed … ("The Jerusalem Bible")

Every head was made bald, and every shoulder was made bare … ("The 1599 Geneva Bible")

Bare shoulders or chafed shoulders are mentioned after the removal of the head hair in this prophecy against Tyre. Ezekiel always relates the removal of long head hair with impending doom (Ezekiel 5:1-13). The importance of human head hair cannot be overstated. Long hair is designed to protect the head and shoulders. The following personal testimonies will help drive the point even further.

There are many interesting encounters people have with insects, even deadly encounters.[447] For example, while mowing his mother-in-law's lawn a man related how he was attacked by a swarm of bees that bit his head and neck. The problem is that he has no head hair. He shaves his entire head bare. Since there was no barrier the flying swarm attacked his head

---

447 A. Kunitomi, Y. Konaka and M. Yagita, "Hypersensitivity to mosquito bites as a potential sign of mantle cell lymphoma," Intern Med. 2005 Oct;44(10):1097-9. PMID: 16293926 accessed June 26, 2006 http://www.ncbi.nlm.nih.gov/entrez/query. fcgi?CMD=Display&DB=pubmed.

and neck directly. Not only does head hair protect, it also provides sensory perception. When insects land on your hair, you can feel them. By feeling their presence before being bitten is far better than after the fact. This is especially true of the head and neck. Poisons injected into the head and neck potentially have quick access to the victim's brain.

One day in January 2006, I personally witnessed the following event. While working at a construction site south of Houston, Texas, on this beautiful sunny day, one of the workers, Jason, ran up to his boss, Ron. Jason insisted on immediate attention from Ron while I stood there and listened. Jason proceeded with something like, "I was just stung on the back of my neck by a bee and you must take me now to get Benadryl [a popular antihistamine] for I am highly allergic to these stings and could die." They left the site.

When they returned Jason had already taken six pills. Later, after he recovered, I explained to him the purpose of hair and how it is designed to cover the neck for its protection. Jason said "yeah, the insect probably would have just got entangled in the hair and not stung me." I concurred. Later another thought occurred to me – could it be that certain insects are attracted to shiny, sweaty, red necks?

About a week earlier, at this same construction site, the superintendent Marvin, about 65 years old, jokingly said, "when you going to get that hair cut boy?" So I asked Marvin, "what is the purpose of hair?" Marvin responded, "it's for looks." I said, "yes that is true, but what else is it for? What is it for scientifically?" He said, "I don't know, what?" I explained, "head hair is for the protection of the head, back of the neck and ears from overexposure to the sun. It can keep you from getting skin cancer in these areas." Immediately, Marvin exclaimed "I have been overexposed," and proceeded to show me the tops of both of his ears where skin cancer was "burned off." He had the same problem on his arms, so now he wears a long-sleeved shirt year-round to protect his arms from overexposure to the sun.

During our conversation I noticed that Marvin's head hairs were just beginning to touch the tops of his ears. Ironically, and in spite of the awesome knowledge he was just given, he got his hair cut about a week later. Apparently, it is ingrained in his mind that his hair must be kept above his ears and above his shirt collar regardless of common sense. Such mentality is commonplace in America and other so-called "civilized" nations today. Apparently, it is okay to wear a long-sleeved shirt to protect the entire arm, but not okay to wear his own God-given hair long enough to protect his head, ears and neck. The irrational, nonsensical beliefs of modern people are devastating. By the way, and by simple observation, hard hats, now worn on most construction sites, do not protect the ears and posterior neck from overexposure to the sun. Why do many men run to the barber when the hair barely touches the ears (Figure 9-9)? Are they gluttons for punishment in the form of more cancer?

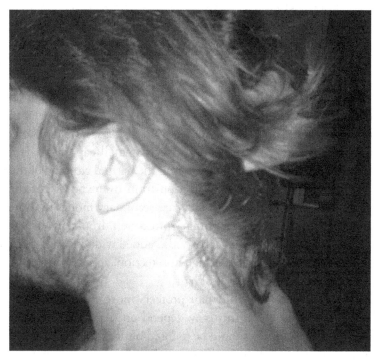

Figure 9-9: Hairs How to Protect Your Neck. The corners of the head including the neckline are not shaved off. Thus, the hair grows and protects both the ears and the neck from overexposure to the elements, such as too much sun, from insects, and other ills. If you really want to prevent skin cancer to head and neck region, this is the way to do it. Photograph by the author, 2005.

The too much sun problem cannot be resolved by most sunscreens for there is now ample evidence that these chemicals cause more cancer than they prevent. To cause cancer means that some of these chemicals apparently induce DNA damage, just like too much ultraviolet light, which "gives rise to skin cancer."[448] Once DNA is damaged, skin cancer may follow. It would be quite wise to start tanning little by little, day by

---

448 Rouzaud, et al.

day, beginning in the spring. Use a milder sunscreen with a lower SPF as discussed earlier.

What about Hats?

What about wearing a hat? The only type of hats that may protect the tops of the ears and posterior neck are either cowboy hats or sombreros. But many of these are not always adequate protection – it depends upon the sun's angle. Another problem is that big hats are not very practical in modern society most of the time. Why should a person drag a big hat around all day if their own hair (natural protection) can do the job? If the hair is thick enough and long enough, an artificial covering will rarely be needed. Hair lays flat over the ears and neck. Because of this fact, the sun's angle does not matter. If your hair is long enough but you feel a need for secondary protection, like when the sun is directly overhead, then a small cap or bandana will suffice during those couple of hours. Hair is the natural clothing of the head and thus the primary mode of protection from overexposure to the sun. Hair never blows off in the wind. Hats are secondary modes of protection and should never be considered primary protection. Ironically, the modern Hasids, beginning in the 18th century, also added wide-rimmed black hats as part of their dress.[449] The hat is man's protection, apparently worn in lieu of God's natural protective cover of hair.

Some may argue that while hair protects most of the head region, it does not protect the nose. This may depend on how far one's own nose sticks out. Nevertheless, it should be pointed out that the nose secretes the highest amount of sebum, the oil produced by the sebaceous gland within the hair follicle, than any other place on the face.[450] This is why the nose has a greasier feel than elsewhere on the face. According to Desmond Tobin, moderate amounts of sunshine or ultraviolet rays (UV) increase the levels of sebum, which improves "barrier performance."[451] Apparently, the sebum helps to screen out UV rays. Thus, the nose is already designed to protect itself to a certain extent. Washing the face with detergents or soaps before doing outdoor activities is probably not a good idea. Plus, is it wise to face the sun while working outdoors? Before the invention of sunglasses,

449 Lubavitcher Headquarters, Brooklyn, N.Y.
450 T. Igarashi, K. Nishino, S.K. Nayar, "The Appearance of Human Skin," Technical Report: CUCS-024-05 (New York: Department of Computer Science, Columbia University, June 2005), 26.
451 Desmond J. Tobin, "Biochemistry of human skin – our brain on the outside," Chemical Society Reviews, 2006, 35, 56.

who would have even dreamed to face the sun? Our eyes are designed to look away from the sun, not at it, not for any long amount of time. When we simply turn our heads away from the sun, our noses turn with it.

The truth is that many men wear their hair so short that you rarely see them without a hat. In America, the hat is usually a baseball cap, which seems to be worn in place of the hair. These men become very attached to the hat. In essence, it becomes their hair. Typical male summer-wear in America is a short-sleeved T-shirt and baseball cap. A baseball cap offers protection to the face, nose, and top of the scalp from over-exposure to the sun, but does nothing for the ears or neck. For those who like baseball caps, hair over the ears and neck along with this cap would provide much protection. But keep in mind, your God-given hair is the primary natural protector of the head.

If you have sparse coverage (thinning hair) then a hat is a good idea, especially when the sun is directly overhead. Thinning hair is a sign that your scalp is already damaged. Overexposure to the sun will damage it more. But if you wear some type of hat or cover, make certain that it circulates the air through the hair. With the exception of construction hard hats, most other hats and caps do provide some ventilation. Generally, most experts agree that baseball caps and cowboy hats do not cause baldness.[452] On the other hand, the plastic lining in some hard hats can irritate the scalp by rubbing. If you wear hard hats, make sure to wear a cotton cushion or bandana between your scalp hair and the hard hat's lining. Continual rubbing action of the hard hat's plastic lining can cause scalp irritation leading to hair loss. You want to minimize scalp irritation as much as possible. About a century ago doctors said an unventilated stiff hat should be avoided because it traps too much heat.[453] In general, any type of hat or helmet that causes any sort of scalp irritation or stress can cause hair loss and must be avoided.

Other problems by wearing hats all the time are lack of air circulation and lack of adequate sunshine, before overexposure, for both are needed for good hair growth.[454] Wind blowing through the hair is an excellent way to stimulate the scalp. When hair remains perfectly still, hair follicles are not stimulated. The special sensory nerve endings, mechanoreceptors that surround each follicle remain silent. But when hair moves, "a burst of nerve

---

452 Walker, Bald No More.

453 Charles T. Jackson and McMurtry, A Treatise on Diseases of the Hair (London: Henry Kimpton, 1913), 55.

454 Jackson and McMurtry, 55.

impulses is initiated."[455] Movement of hair, particularly long heavier hair, stimulates the neuromuscular system of the scalp. This is best achieved during normal outdoor activities when the hair can move and bounce. The constant wearing of hats and hair spray prevent normal and natural movement of the hair. Thus, the function of the neuromuscular system of the scalp is reduced to a weakened condition.

Many modern men wear their hair too short, unnaturally short. Think about it. If you have enough overlapping hairs, how can the sun beam through to the scalp? How can insects get through for a bite? The thicker and taller the forest, the less sunshine reaches the ground because the rays are diffused. This is a good thing for the forested ecosystem. Tall trees keep the ground from being parched. This analogy works the same way for scalp health. By design, scalp hair is the natural clothing of the head and posterior neck and thus the natural protector of the skin surface from overexposure to the elements, and from pestilence. Or as Jerry Bergman related, hair protects against mosquitoes and biting flies, sunburn, and skin cancer.[456]

This is why the clergy in Orthodox Church, and rock stars for that matter, set the best example for all men the importance of natural long hair and beards:

"... a beard and uncut hair are ... no more or less important to a Priest than feathers are to a bird."[457]

What better way to protect the head and neck than with one's own hair. It is the only way to fly. As already discussed, healthy skin leads to healthy hair. Longer hair, adequate sunshine, but not overexposure, a good diet, and physical activity, preferably outdoors, all contribute to healthy skin and healthy hair. For Jesus' sake, protect your head and neck with your own hair!

---

455 Richard S. Snell, Clinical Neuroanatomy for Medical Students, 3rd Ed. (Boston: Little, Brown and Company 1992), 123-124; 417-419.

456 Jerry Bergman, "Why Mammal Body Hair is an Evolutionary Enigma," Creation Research Society Quarterly, v. 40, March 2004, p. 240-243.

457 "Concerning the Tradition of Long Hair and Beards." "Uncut Hair and Beards of the Clergy." Orthodox Christian Information Center, accessed May 30, 2010 http://www.orthodoxinfo.com/praxis/clergy_hair.aspx.

Chapter 10: Hair of Fame

But the very hairs of your head are all numbered (Matthew 10:30).

What good is it to say all our hairs are numbered, if the Creator wishes us to reduce these numbers and bring baldness on our heads? This is no good at all and contrary to the importance of our hair as stated throughout Scripture. Down through all the ages when men have worn longer hair, baldness was extremely rare. Furthermore, when these men wore longer hair throughout life, they still had hair, even when old. Race (i.e., skin and hair type) is not a factor. The proof of this can be seen in just about any sculpture, portrait or photograph prior to the early 20th century. Even when shorter hair was in style at certain times in the past, it was still worn long enough to at least protect the head and prevent baldness.

For example, the Italian explorer Christopher Columbus (Figure 10-1) and Protestant reformer Martin Luther (Figure 10-2) both had modest amounts of hair. Although in the realm of short hair scientifically, it was still long enough to protect the ears and neck. And, as far as we know, neither went bald except for the intentional tonsured scalp of Luther in his former life as a Roman Catholic monk.

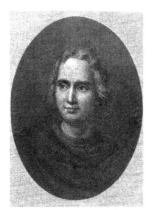

Figure 10-1: Christopher Columbus, 1451 - 1506.

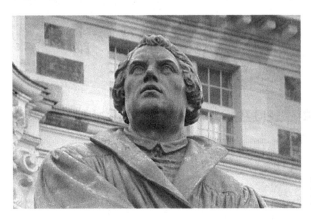

Figure 10-2: Martin Luther, 1483 - 1546.

Remarkably, as great as these men were, both would have trouble being hired in many places today even with modest amounts of hair. The situation would even be worse for those great men of the past who truly did wear long hair. Nevertheless, they are the ones who had the healthiest scalps of all. The following images represent some of these longer haired men of history over the past 500 years up to the present time. Since they have worn their God-given hair longer, their scalps became strong and healthy. By doing so they gained a crown of long hair for life, the hair of Samson.

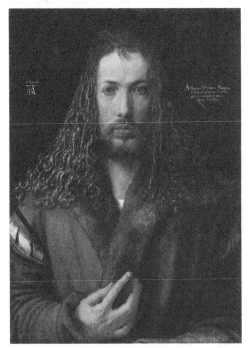

Figure 10-3: Albrecht Durer, 1471 – 1528. Durer, a German artist, painted his self-portrait when he was 28 years old. He wore his hair in "reverent imitation of Christ" says art historian Erwin Panofsky.[1]

---

1   D.M. Podolsky, Skin: the human fabric (The Human Body) (Tarrytown, New York: Torstar Books, Inc., 1984), 80.

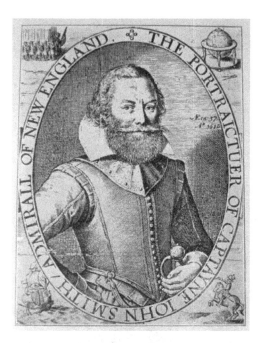

Figure 10-4: Captain John Smith, 1580 – 1631. This Public Domain image is from his map of New England in 1616 when Smith was 36 years old, with no hint of any receding hairline.

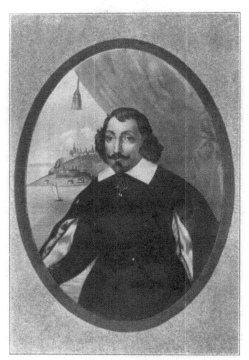

CHAMPLAIN
Fondateur de Québec

Figure 10-5: Samuel de Champlain, 1580 – 1635. This French explorer and founder of Quebec City is yet another example of a healthy head of hair. U.S. Library of Congress, Prints and Photographs Division.

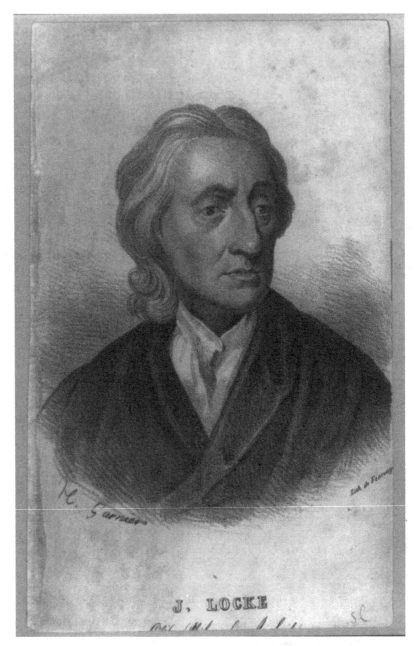

Figure 10-6: John Locke, 1632 – 1704.

Locke's contributions to political philosophy are reflected in the American Declaration of Independence. He is shown here in his 60s with a full head of hair with no receding hairline. U.S. Library of Congress, Prints and Photographs Division.

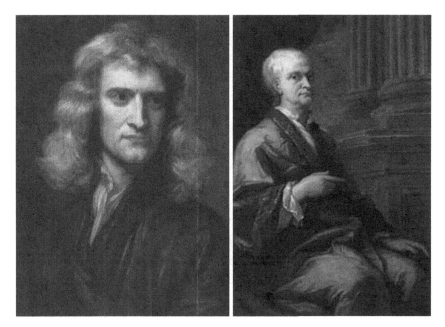

Figure 10-7: Sir Isaac Newton, 1643 to 1727.

Left: Newton at the age of 46 with hair about 12 to 14 inches in length. Painting by Godfrey Kneller, 1689.

Right: Newton at the age of 69 with a full head of white hair, although his hair is shorter in his old age. The neuro-muscular system of Newton's scalp was trained to be strong and healthy in his younger days. Wear hair long when young and have a full head of hair when old. Portrait by Sir James Thornhill, 1712.

The father of the Methodists, John Wesley, had a full head of shoulder-length hair throughout his life with no apparent receding hairline (Figure 10-8). He preached at a time when the Church of England fell into "lifeless formalism."[458] Wesley was not allowed to preach in the churches so he went to the common folk in the fields, mining camps, and street corners. Since Wesley sincerely cared, he became one of "earth's greatest." As seen in Figure 10-8, Wesley still had a full head of long white hair with no receding hairline, even when he was quite old.

---

458 Henry M. Halley, Halley's Bible Handbook, 24th Ed. (Grand Rapids, Michigan: Regency Reference Library, 1965), 797.

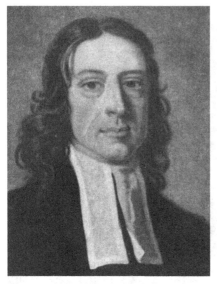

Figure 10-8: John Wesley, 1703 – 1791.

Left image: Some claim Wesley was 48 years old when this oil painting was done. But according to Jennifer L. Woodruff Tait of Drew University, they have pretty conclusive evidence that the original painting was done in 1742, which would make him 39 years old at the time. Courtesy of Drew University and the General Board of Global Ministries of the United Methodist Church. Right image is public domain.

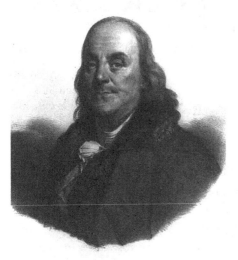

Figure 10-9: Benjamin Franklin, 1705 – 1790. U.S. Library of Congress, Prints and Photographs Division.

Benjamin Franklin, one of the great long haired founding fathers of the United States, could be cited as one having a "predisposition" (e.g., recall the sensitive skin issue) for baldness, but why did he not go bald? Yes, he did have a receding hairline. However, he was far from bald. Surely, if Franklin was a product of the excessive hair-cutting of the 20th century, he probably would have become quite bald in his older years. Short hair along with strong detergents in shampoos and the consumption of unnatural foods would have caused him to lose most of his hair probably by age 50.

Lucky for him he lived during the 18th century when longer hair was the way. In 1779 when Franklin was 74 years old, his portrait shows somewhat of a receding hairline, but nevertheless he still had quite a full head of hair even on top, at this grandfatherly age (Figure 10-9).

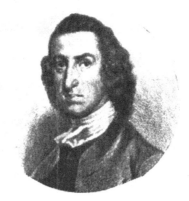

Figure 10-10: William Livingston, 1723 to 1790.

Founding Father of, and a signer of, the Constitution of the United States, and Governor of New Jersey from 1776 to 1790. He is probably in his early 50s when this portrait was done, showing a full head of shoulder-length hair and no receding hairline.

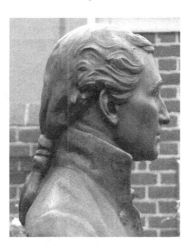

Figure 10-11: James Monroe, 1758 to 1831.

Monroe was the fifth president of the United States. Since he grew up as a long hair ponytail, James Monroe had a healthy head of hair for life, even when old. But in America today he would be banned from employment by most crop-headed corporations. Are we really sure America is still a land of freedom? Photograph by the author, July 2008, at the James Monroe Museum, Fredericksburg, VA.

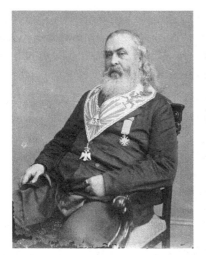
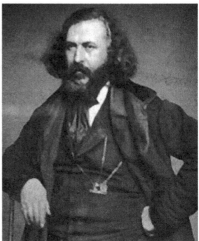

Figure 10-12: Albert Pike, 1809 to 1891. Albert Pike was no barbermonger and felt that nature reveals the mighty wisdom of God. The design in nature is long hair for both sexes, or at least shoulder-length hair for men. The photograph to the right is Pike in his younger days. As an old man he still has a full head of long hair as designed by the Creator. Even his hairline along the forehead is the same in both photographs: no recession at all. Pike certainly represents how white men are designed to look. U.S. Library of Congress, Prints and Photographs Division; Brady-Handy Photograph Collection.

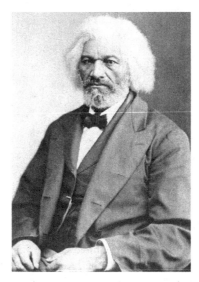

Figure 10-13: Frederick Douglas 1818 – 1895.

Frederick Douglas believed in the equality of all people, whether they were blacks, women, immigrants, or Native Americans. The United States Declaration of

Independence says the same, that "all men are created equal." The rights in this great document include "Life, Liberty and the pursuit of happiness." Long hair represents all of these ideals. His lectures filled Protestant churches in Great Britain. Once a slave, in 1872 Douglas became the first African American nominated as a vice presidential candidate. This photograph was taken in 1894, when Douglas was 76 years old and he still has a full head of majestic hair with no receding hairline. No doubt he grew his hair and beard because he was a free man. Long hair is the symbol of true freedom, life, and liberty. A shorn head represents none of these things, especially if done by rule, written or unwritten, or force. He represents how many black men are designed to look. U.S. Library of Congress, Prints and Photographs Division.

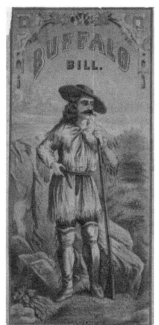 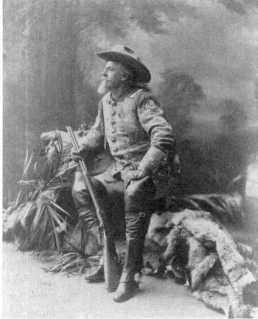

Figure 10-14: William "Buffalo Bill" Cody 1846 – 1917.

Left: Buffalo Bill at 24 years of age - Monsch Bros, Cincinnati, Ohio, 1870.

Right: photograph from 1903 when Cody was 57 years old. How do you have a full head of hair for life? Wear it long. Both images are from the U.S. Library of Congress, Prints and Photographs Division.

It is wonderful to know that not all white men succumb to scissors and razor. Buffalo Bill was a friend to Native Americans and his family suffered much persecution for their stance against slavery. He was a believer in freedom. Long hair symbolizes freedom.

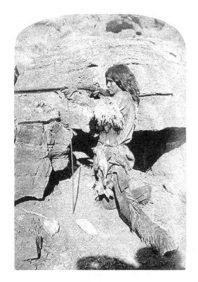

Figure 10-15: Young Native American – Uainuint Paiute, Southwest Utah. This young Native American's natural hair length is determined by his genetic code, by God's design. The length appears to be about 14 inches or so. Wear your hair like this and chances are you will not lose your hair even when an old man. Photograph by John K. Hillers in 1873, United States National Archives.

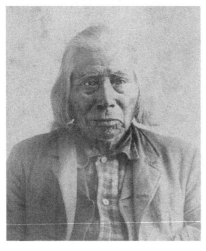

Figure 10-16: Chief of the Spokanes. Photograph taken in the year 1892. This Native American chief looks to be around 90 years old and he still has a full head of white hair with no receding hairline. The only difference is that his white hair is straight, while Frederick Douglas' had tight curls. Each crown type is based on their own genetic code designed by God. He lived at a time to watch his people, including their naturalistic ways, give way to the modern artificiality of the industrial revolution. Courtesy of James J. Hill Papers, James J. Hill Library, Saint Paul, MN.

The Native Americans endured much persecution. By the late 19th to early 20th centuries they were deemed long-haired savages by many of a so-called civilized bent, the barbermongers. Many Native Americans have succumbed to the unnatural ways of modern society and are now shorn and assimilated into the present culture. Likewise, the long-haired Ainus of Japan have also suffered centuries of oppression, racism, and forced assimilation policies.[459] Their mix of European and Asian traits is unique in Asia. The shame is that modern socialization has caused recent generations to even deny their very Ainu heritage.

---

459 Andy Thomason, "The Ainu of Japan: The History, Culture, and Discrimination Against this Aboriginal Group," Suite101.com July 2, 1999, accessed March 28, 2009 http://www.suite101.com/article.cfm/fourth_world/22057.

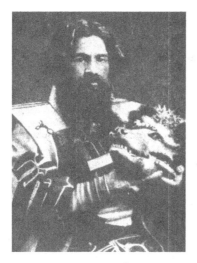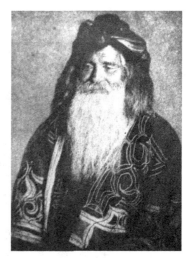

Figure 10-17: Ainu Men of Japan.

The young man on the left is perhaps in his early 30s. The old man on the right is probably mid 70s. For them, like many people, it was a dishonor to be forced to shear their heads of thick wavy hair. Long, healthy, natural hair when young equates to long healthy hair when old. Photographs taken late 19th to early 20th century: both from "The Secret Museum of Mankind."

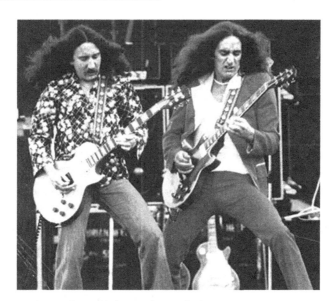

Figure 10-18: Legendary Rock Band: Uriah Heep.

Mick Box (left) and Ken Hensley (right) of Uriah Heep, playing at a concert, mid-1970s set an excellent example of how hair should be worn. Courtesy of Mick Box – see www.uriah-heep.com for more about this awe-inspiring band.

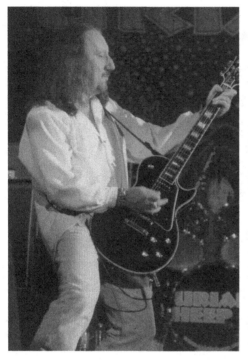

Figure 10-19: Mick Box of Uriah Heep.

Mick Box about 60 years old (year 2007?) and he still has a full head of hair with little, if any, recession. Incidentally, Ken Hensley also has a full head of hair with no receding hairline. Since long hair increases stimulation to the brain, it brings about a hair more creativity in music. Ken Hensley had the longest hair of all and is an extremely gifted songwriter. Courtesy of Mick Box, www.uriah-heep.com.

The forgoing illustrations show three obvious differences in skin and hair types. Native American, called red but actually mid-brown, black or African American, and white or European American. A man's so-called race, along with his personal skin and hair type, apparently does not influence natural hair length. It does demonstrate simply that longer hair leads to less fallout, and a thicker healthier scalp for life, as designed. If you wear your hair as designed, natural and longer, then chances of going bald are reduced as long as you make changes with regards to the other manmade causes of hair loss cited in this book. The longer hair also demonstrates the great variety and brings about a unique identity of each individual.

Many other portraits and photographs of long haired men of all races could be shown as proof, the evidence for the healthiness of longer hair. Their portraits are easily found in history books or on the Internet. You can check them out for yourself. The observational evidence mandates that if longer hair is worn at least to the base of the neck or tops of the shoulders, then chances of going bald are greatly reduced. Furthermore, those that do so generally have healthy heads of hair even when advanced in age.

Benefits of Longer Hair Summarized

How long should I wear my hair you ask? If you want a healthy scalp health, then the longer the better. Modern females are allowed to wear their hair any way they please, including very long hair if they want. But many men of the modern western world have butchered their heads far worse than any group in history, even the first century Romans. Why opt for the ultra-short butchered hair of the tyrants instead of the natural hair styles of freedom, for example the Native Americans, Founding Fathers of the U.S.A., humble Christian leaders such as John Wesley, James Ussher, Frederick Douglas, and many, many others? I realize the facade of corporate America pressures you to be shorn. However, just because practically everyone is doing it does not make it right. If you are a male, there are several lines of common sense greatly needed in our overly materialistic modernistic society. The following list indicates logical reasoning, rules of thumb if you will, for male hair length.

1. Exposing the thin-skinned scalp is not a good idea. If you can see the skin of your scalp, assuming you still have hair, then the hair is cut far too short. The scalp is abused. Examples of ultra-short hair styles that lead to potential health problems include any close-cropped cut including crew cuts, flat tops, high-and-tight cuts, spiked hair, or any style that forces hair to remain above the ears and collar.
2. Since the hair of the scalp is designed to be longer than body hair, then it should be worn longer than body hair for your health. Body hair grows slow and stays relatively short, and yet at certain places, these body hairs reach three inches in length.
3. In contrast, scalp hair grows fast and grows long, by design. For this reason alone, every single hair that grows on the head should be allowed to grow longer than the longest body hair. And naturally scalp hair would grow much longer if it was not cut so frequently. I know some men who cut their hair too short and too frequently, every week or two. This is abusive and traumatizes the scalp. It promotes hair loss via atrophy of the hair follicles' neuromuscular system. It also wastes valuable time and money.
4. A hair five inches in length weighs five times more than a hair one inch in length. Recall that the extra weight causes the hair follicle to become larger leading to a healthier scalp. You must strengthen the muscles of your scalp.

Unfortunately, most people consider scalp hair as a matter of "style" only. This seems to be a major concern of females who always want to present the styles of the times. But human hair serves many vital purposes besides following prevailing fashions. These purposes include (1) preservation of heat; (2) protection; (3) stimulation; and (4) personal beauty. Most seem to understand the beauty part only, especially young people. The other purposes are quite enlightening. For example it has been long known that the purpose of eyebrows and eyelashes, other than being just a decoration, is to protect the eyes.[460] [461] Likewise, underarm hair and pubic hair reduce friction (prevents bare skin from rubbing and acts as a cushion) and increase sensitivity in these areas.[462] [463] Head hair forms a thick elastic cushion and is considered an "admirable defense" to the skull against blows and falls.[464] Jackson and McMurtry also considered hair as an adornment, saying "natural hair is known to soften and render less conspicuous hard facial features or blemishes." Besides manly beauty, even mustaches and beards have purpose. Since men were designed to work outdoors, the mustache is considered a respirator and the beard protects the larynx from cold weather.[465]

Consider Tables 10-1 and 10-2:

Table 10-1: Purposes of Various Human Hair Types

Hair Type	Purpose 1	Purpose 2
Eyebrows	Personal Beauty	First line of defense to keep sweat out of the eyes
Eyelashes	Personal Beauty	Acts as a broom to sweep away dust
Body Hair	Personal Beauty	Sex appeal including the increase in sensitivity (makes touching feel good); some hair acts as a cushion: for example auxiliary hair does so by keeping the skin from rubbing as the arm swings.
Mustache	Personal Beauty	Respirator.
Beard	Personal Beauty	Protects the larynx.

Note: All body hair is designed to grow slowly and is programmed to reach a certain length. The length of body hair is rather short, but can be more than inches in length, such as pubic hair.

460 Charles T. Jackson and McMurtry, A Treatise on Diseases of the Hair (London: Henry Kimpton, 1913), 48-49.
461 Truman J. Moon, Biology for Beginners, (New York: Holt, Rinehart and Winston, Publishers, 1981), 421.
462 Jackson and McMurtry.
463 D.M. Podolsky, Skin: the human fabric (The Human Body) (Tarrytown, New York: Torstar Books, Inc., 1984), 82.
464 Jackson and McMurtry.
465 Jackson and McMurtry.

On the other hand, scalp hair, by design, grows fast and grows long. The importance and purposes of scalp hair are indicated in Table 10-2.

Table 10-2: Benefits of Mankind's LONG HAIR of the Head

Benefits of LONGER HAIR Summarized	
Appearance	Adds personal beauty and nobility to both males and females – it is your God-given personal crown.
	Gives males a stronger appearance; facial hair also adds strength.
	Gives breadth to the head. This may be important for those with narrow heads, which, oftentimes looks merely like an extension of the person's neck, when the sides are close cut.
	Hides veins, nooks, crannies, knobs, bumps, flat spots, blemishes, scars, birthing sutures of the skull, and other unsightly features.
	Keeps the neck, ears, and head in youthful, unweathered condition – reduces aging (prevents wrinkling and hides wrinkles).
	Makes a person more visible: a unique identity.
Health Reasons	Protects the head, ears, and neck from the ultraviolet rays of the hot sun reducing the chances of skin cancer to these areas of the head.
	Hair acts as your first layer of clothing by conserving heat and thereby protects the head, ears, and neck from cold air during the winter. I recall my short-haired friends in the 1980s – while their ears were freezing, mine were fine.
	The extra weight of longer hair keeps the scalp healthier - causes the follicle to become larger leading to thicker skin, which is very important especially on top. The chances of scalp atrophy of the follicles are reduced.
	Cushions the head, for example, if struck on the head, hair serves to cushion the blow.
	Protects the scalp from exposure to strong shampoo chemicals and other air-borne pollutants and chemicals.
	Protects the head, posterior neck and ears from the stings and bites of insects.
	Makes the scalp more pliable, thus when struck, the skin will not split open as easy.
	Anoints the head, ears and neck with oil (sebum), which is distributed by the hair. This keeps the skin in youthful health.
	Increases sensitivity or touch so you can feel when something is about to happen, for example, before you bump your head.

Scalp hair is designed to grow long and fast and is an emblem of female and male beauty. But greater than the appearance issues are the health and protection issues. The evidence is everywhere to be found. We have already learned that, when long and thick enough, head hair protects the scalp, ears, and neck from cold, overexposure to the sun (eliminates sunburn and prevents skin cancer), insect bites, and other things. The cushioning effect of longer hair is another significant truth. All fighters (e.g., boxing; karate) and other athletes should consider this: if struck on the head, hair serves to cushion the blow.[466] The present-day shaved head idea is not very well thought out. Constant shaving is highly destructive and without the weight of longer hair, there is no way to prevent the scalp from becoming even thinner and more brittle. Let them hit hair rather than bare naked skin.

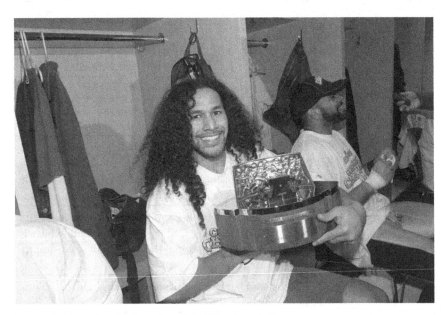

Figure 10-20: Troy Polamalu of the Pittsburgh Steelers.

Polamalu is holding the AFC championship trophy – AFC Championship Game – Pittsburgh Steelers vs. Denver Broncos – January 22, 2006. As Lycurgus the Spartan said, long hair makes a handsome man even better looking. At 24 years old in this photo, Polamalu is well on his way to a healthy head of hair for life. He is a humble man and God gave him a great crown.

Long-haired Troy Polamalu, safety for the Pittsburgh Steelers, is an excellent case in point. When Polamalu wore short hair, he had repetitious

466 Alma E. Guinness, ed., ABC's of the Human Body (New York: The Readers Digest Association, 1987), 150.

concussions. Then as a junior at the University of Southern California (USC), he let his hair grow and "the repeated concussions that he had suffered stopped."[467] He has not cut it since, like the Nazarites of old. In all wisdom, there are several long haired players in the National Football League (NFL), who no doubt have similar testimonies. Seriously, why have your brain joggled if you can protect it with the additional cushion provided by your own long hair?

Polamalu is also quoted as saying: "my fiancée's mother (Katina Holmes) told me that every great warrior throughout all of world history has had long hair, starting with the Samurais, the Greeks, the American Indians, the Chinese....You name it. They've all had long hair. I don't know why it's so different now to have long hair."[468] Well, if the reader has read the previous chapters, then you already know where difference comes from. To recap, the problem stems from the hair-hating modern military that shears the head practically bald, and those same types of people who are novices with their poor handling of Scripture along with a complete lack of understanding with regards to the import of created things.

The truth is all people are created by God Himself to grow long hair. As far as I know, He does not make mistakes. Longer hair adds life to the scalp, appearance and is an indicator of internal health. Longer hair is the way we are designed. With the exception of those with rare diseases, all people have longer hair, but many just do not show it.

467 Jerry DiPaola, "Polamalu has emerged as one of NFL's top safeties," Tribune-Review, January 21, 2005, accessed March 21, 2006 http://www.pittsburghlive.com/x/tribune-review/sports/steelerslive/s_295403.html
468 DiPaola.

Chapter 11: Scalp Trauma, Chemicals and Related Insults

||||||||||||||||||||||||||||||||||||||||||||||||||||||||||||||||||||||||||||||||||||||||||||||||||||||||||||||||||||||||||||||||||||||||||||||||||||||||||||||

...their root is dried up, they shall bear no fruit (Hosea 9:16).

Thus far we have learned the dangers of constant daily head shaving, excessive hair cutting, and cropping of hair too close. The name 'Butch' has always been a shorter form of 'butcher'. These practices lead to baldness, skin cancer and other ills all against God's will for your life. Mankind is the crown of creation and yet the crown of hair is being destroyed by self-inflicted trespasses, perhaps at the instigation of other ignorant people. Now we will look a little closer at so called hair-care products.

Trichology is the holistic scientific study of the hair and scalp. Very few people are trained in this unique field of study. But if their training was well done, they should know two basic things: (1) chemicals can damage the hair and scalp; and (2) natural methods can heal the scalp. There are differences between trichologists. One says to wash your hair as often as you want.[469] In this chapter you will learn that is a mistake, especially with the wrong products. On the other hand, trichologist Riquette Hofstein says to gather all "your hair care products" and throw them away because they all cause "hair damage and loss."[470] This includes gels, hair spray, relaxers, dyes, mousses, and conditioners, even the expensive ones purchased at the salon. You may think she is just being extreme by telling you to throw those things away, but nevertheless she is right. Dr. Loren Pickart puts it this way:

---

469 David H. Kingsley, The Hair-Loss Cure, A Self-Help Guide (Bloomington, IN: iUniverse, 2009), 11.

470 Riquette Hofstein, Grow Hair Fast – 7 Steps to a New Head of Hair in 90 Days (Naperville, Illinois: Sourcebooks, Inc. 2004), 33.

The effect of the hair-care industry on hair health has been overwhelmingly negative in the opinion of many people, including Russian Physician George Michael.[471]

Dr. Michael observed that Russian women in their 60s had well pigmented waist-length hair, but the New York City women who frequented salons could barely grow hair six inches in length. Artificial processes damage natural hair and the scalp. These include permanents, chemicals to straighten the hair, methods to alter the color, excessive heat (hair irons, too much blow-drying), excessive hair cutting, over-shampooing, and use of other products that build up on the hair and scalp.[472][473] Split ends, dull color, brittle hair, and thinning hair result from many of these manipulations. Split ends are easy proof of damaged hair. When split ends form, a person has no choice but to trim the damaged ends. If you continue to damage your hair and hair follicles, then the ends will have to be trimmed more often. Over time you will be forced to wear your hair shorter and shorter. Because of atrophy the hairs thin as the follicle withers. Who knows, if you are lucky you may not go bald. But chances are better than not that you will be unable to produce long healthy hair.

Bleaching and permanents are potentially "very damaging" and hair straightening chemicals can cause permanent scars on your scalp.[474] All these processes cause the hair to become fragile and extremely weathered. In "Diseases of the Hair and Scalp," hairspray and hair setting lotions irreversibly weaken hair. In short, all these unnatural processes cause the opposite effect of what you have hoped. If hairsprays, hair setting lotions, bleaching, and other hair alteration chemicals cause irreversibly weak, damaged, fragile, and highly weathered hair, then think of how these same things act upon your scalp where the hair is made. Recall that Riquette Hofstein says all these things cause hair loss. Presumably, these hair care products have the same affect on the scalp and hair follicles over time. Ultimately, if you persist in doing these things then your scalp and hair will age prematurely. This is not what you want is it?

---

471 Loren Pickart, Reverse Skin Aging: Using Your Skin's Natural Power. (Bellevue, Washington: Cape San Juan Press, 2005), 101.

472 Hofstein, 21; 33-35.

473 Pickart, Reverse Skin Aging: Using Your Skin's Natural Power, 101-104.

474 Arthur Rook and Rodney Dawber, eds., Diseases of the Hair and Scalp, 2nd Ed. (London: Blackwell Scientific Publications, 1991), 474-479.

Another abusive situation occurs in the black community. Recall that the hair follicle of blacks is set at an acute angle to the skin surface. Hair extruded from these types of follicles is flattened and tightly coiled.[475] Many black women use incredibly strong artificial chemicals to straighten their otherwise naturally coiled hair. The process of producing straight hair with chemicals, oils and heat causes hair fracture, scalp scarring, and either temporary or permanent hair loss.[476] In "Hair Story," some black ministers related that to straighten the hair like a "white" person was the "work of the devil!"[477] These preachers may not have been too out of line. For we all know the devil's work involves destruction. Scars and hair loss caused by harsh chemicals is surely destructive.

But it should be pointed out that it was the blacks who originally concocted methods to straighten their hair because the whites did not consider their bushy hair as "real hair."[478] The pressure some African Americans feel about their hair in a society controlled by whites is related by Cheryl Browne. In "Dreads" she points out that "you don't have to have straight hair to be beautiful."[479] In fact, in the late 1960s the popular slogan "black is beautiful" was coined to promote the goodness of African American hair. Therefore, the blacks grew out their hair in a natural afro. They were right, so what happened? If black is beautiful, then why do so many modern black women straighten their hair and why do so many black men either shave it off completely, or crop it too close so that all the lumpy features of the skull are seen? Is it because they have been convinced by our plastic society that their hair truly is unwanted? Ademole Mandella said it best: "God made only good hair."[480] Dreadlocks are beautiful.

The bottom line is to wear your hair naturally without chemical alteration. If you have straight hair, wear it straight. If wavy, wear it wavy. If curly, keep it curly. If your hair naturally locks, then grow dreadlocks or Nubian locks. Likewise, wear your hair's natural color. Minor highlights may be okay on the ends but keep dyes off the scalp. If you do these things you will have a healthier crown.

---

475 B.L. Johnson, R.L. Moy, and G.M. White, Ethnic Skin, Medical and Surgical (St. Louis, MO: Mosby, Inc., 1998).

476 Johnson, Moy, and White, 4.

477 Ayana D. Byrd, Lori L. Tharps, Hair Story, Untangling the Roots of Black Hair in America (New York: St. Martin's Press, 2001), 39.

478 Byrd and Tharps, 14-17.

479 Francesco Mastalia and Alfonse Pagano, Dreads, (New York: Artisan 1999), 61.

480 Ademole Mandella, Authentic Hair (New York: Cosmic Nubian Enterprises, 2002).

The Shampoo Problem

As a reminder, sebum is the oily substance secreted from the oil gland beneath the skin's surface (Figure 2-1). Sweat is the salty, watery solution produced by sweat glands, which have their own separate microscopic openings to the skin surface. Please note that sweat pores are a distinct structure from the hair follicle. Sweat is part of the body's cooling system.[481] The function of the follicle is to produce hair and make the oil called sebum.

As sebum and sweat migrate and mix on the skin surface, a protective layer is formed called the acid mantle. This acid mantle has a pH range from about 4.0 to 5.5. The acid mantle is designed to protect the skin, which ultimately protects you from weathering effects, bacteria, and fungi. Dr. Arun Kumar puts it quite well, saying "If the acid mantle is disrupted or loses its acidity, the skin becomes more prone to damage and infection. The loss of acid mantle is one of the side-effects of washing the skin with soaps or detergents of moderate or high strength."[482] [483]

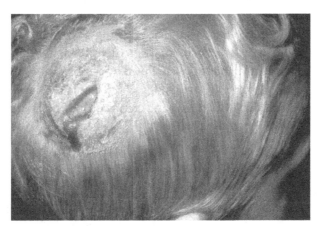

Figure 11-1: Severe Fungal Infection of the Scalp. Did this poor soul's head lose its acid mantle due to excessive shampooing? The acid mantle protects against fungi. It is vital to treat such conditions with an oral antifungal and an oral or ingestible steroid to quickly reduce the inflammation and thereby preserve the hair follicles, and prevent permanent hair loss. Sometimes six months of oral antifungal therapy is required to eradicate it. Photograph courtesy of John L. Bezzant, M.D.

481 D.M. Podolsky, Skin: the human fabric (The Human Body) (Tarrytown, New York: Torstar Books, Inc., 1984), 67.

482 Arun Kumar, "Summary of Current Research Programs: Human Skin Smart biological Interface Bio-MEMS / sensor," accessed December 6, 2005 http://www.eng.usf.edu/~arunk/.

483 "Sebum, Sweat, Skin pH and Acid Mantle," accessed September 25, 2005 http://www.smartskincare.com/skinbiology/sebum.html.

Other than extreme inflammation and scarring, a fungal infection of the scalp can cause permanent hair loss if not corrected. According to Dr. John Bezzant, it can take up to six months of oral antifungal therapy to eradicate the fungi (Figure 11-1). As already suggested, the most probable culprits are detergents of moderate to high strength. Most shampoos are indeed detergents of this magnitude. According to Ruth Winter, shampoos are of recent origin.[484] Original products were made of coconut oil and castile soap. In 1930, liquid shampoos were introduced, followed by the cream type, and then the liquid cream shampoos. She says that shampoos are among the most frequently cited in complaints to the FDA for eye irritation, fuzzy hair, split hair, tangled hair, and scalp irritation.

Sodium Lauryl Sulfate (SLS) and Other Brutal Chemicals

For many years now it has been well known that a dangerous chemical lurks in most shampoos. The chemical is called sodium lauryl sulfate. The technical name is *sulfuric acid monododecyl ester sodium salt* as indicated on the material safety data sheet. The warning of its dangers was given quite frankly in the "Alert-Cosmetic Ingredient Review 1983," the same year Elder's final report about the chemical was published in the "Journal of the American College of Toxicology."[485] [486] Lauryl sulfates have been linked to eye and DNA damage and nitrosamines, a carcinogen that could lead to cancer, and hair loss![487] The reason SLS causes hair loss

---

484 Ruth Winter, A Consumer's Dictionary of Cosmetic Ingredients (New York: Three Rivers Press, 2005).

485 "Alert-Cosmetic Ingredient Review 1983," accessed September 27, 2005 http://www. healthy-communications.com/slsalert.html. Indicates that deposits of detergents on the scalp damage hair follicles. Elaborates about how SLS, etc. is used in engine degreasers, garage floor cleaners, etc.

486 Robert L. Elder, ed., "Final Report on the Safety Assessment of Sodium Lauryl Sulfate and Ammonium Lauryl Sulfate" (Safety Assessment of Cosmetic Ingredients). Journal of the American College of Toxicology, vol. 2 no. 7 (1983): 127-128. This study tested animals. Concentrations of 10 percent to 30 percent Sodium Lauryl Sulfate caused "skin corrosion and severe irritation" and "Solutions of 2 percent, 10 percent, and 20 percent Ammonium Lauryl Sulfate were highly irritating and dangerous" (p. 127). Also says concentrations should not exceed 1 percent for prolonged use. If you use these shampoos then you should use a very small amount, be brief by rinsing it out quickly and thoroughly! Avoid shampoos that have high volumes of these ingredients.

487 Linda Chae, "Are Foam and Bubbles Worth Bad Health? (The Truth about Sodium Lauryl Sulfate)," accessed September 24, 2005 http://www.lindachae.com/Truth_about_ sls.htm. The report summarizes the health hazards of SLS including DNA damage, eye damage, skin penetration, hair loss, and how it can produce carcinogens.

is because it is a proven skin irritant. But the present position of the Cosmetic Ingredient Review is that information about sodium lauryl sulfate circulating the Internet is a myth. Their seven member expert panel has this to say:

The Cosmetic Ingredient Review (CIR) has fully assessed the safety of this ingredient [SLS] and found it to be safe.[488]

However, this statement does not concur with everything else they say about SLS. In fact it actually contradicts Robert Elder's 1983 report which the CIR cites. Here it is:

Sodium Lauryl Sulfate and Ammonium Lauryl Sulfate are irritants in patch testing at concentrations of 2 percent and greater and that irritation increases with ingredient concentration. In some cosmetic formulations, however that irritant property is attenuated. The longer these ingredients stay in contact with the skin, the greater the likelihood of irritation, *which may or may not be evident to the user* [this means that you not feel it as it damages your tiny hair follicles].

Although Sodium Lauryl Sulfate is not carcinogenic in experimental animals, it has been shown that it causes *severe epidermal changes* to the area of the skin of mice to which it was applied. This study indicates a need for tumor-enhancing activity assays.

Auto radiographic studies of rat skin treated with radio-labeled Sodium Lauryl Sulfate found *heavy deposition of the detergent* on the skin surface and *in the hair follicles; damage to the hair follicle could result from such deposition.* Further, it has been reported that 1 percent and 5 percent Sodium Lauryl Sulfate produced significant number of comedones when applied to the pinna of albino rabbits. These two problems – *possible hair loss* and comedone formation – along with proven irritancy should be considered in the formulation of cosmetic products.

Sodium Lauryl Sulfate and Ammonium Lauryl Sulfate appear to pose less potential hazard when in products designed for brief, discontinuous use, following which they are *thoroughly rinsed* from

---

488 Cosmetic Ingredient Review, SLS, accessed July 10, 2010 http://www.cir-safety.org/ alerts.shtml http://www.cir-safety.org/staff_files/alerts.pdf

the surface of the skin....for prolonged contact with the skin, concentration should not exceed 1 percent (emphasis mine).

As you can plainly see there is a need for concern. Severe skin damage and heavy deposition in the follicles leading to damage and hair loss is possible, and you most likely will not even feel it happening! This is why in so many words Elder recommends low amounts of SLS to be placed in formulations. Not only that, but brief, discontinuous use is necessary along with thorough rinsing. How do you know microscopically if you have thoroughly rinsed? Also, instructions on shampoo bottles tell you to use it everyday (continuous use) and state to wash-rinse-repeat. This does not sound like brief, discontinuous use. Plus, as you will soon learn, there are very high volumes of SLS in many shampoos, many times higher than the recommended 1 percent.

Ruth Winter's "A Consumer's Dictionary of Cosmetic Ingredients" defines thousands of cosmetic ingredients from a safety standpoint. This book should be on everyone's shelf because it is vital that you know what you are putting on your skin, hair and scalp: "The real key to safety is your own knowledge." The following list shows the most common detergents utilized in most shampoos. These detergents are made from lauryl alcohol (1 dodecanol), a colorless, crystalline compound produced from coconut oil. Sodium Lauryl Sulfate appears to be the worst. Another sinister chemical, methylisothiazoline, often called MIT for short, has a neurotoxic effect on cells.

Sodium Lauryl Sulfate (SLS) – a detergent, wetting ingredient, and emulsifier widely used in bubble baths, emollient creams, cream depilatories, hand lotions, cold permanent waves, soapless shampoos, and toothpastes. It is prepared by sulfation of lauryl alcohol followed by neutralization with sodium carbonate. It emulsifies fats. It also causes drying of the skin, is associated with eczema, and is a skin irritant.

Sodium Laureth Sulfate – the sodium salt of sulfated ethoxylated lauryl alcohol, widely used in baby and other nonirritating shampoos. It has caused eye and skin irritation in animals and some humans. The irritant effects are similar to those produced by other detergents and is affected by concentration. Dr. Loren Pickart and Thymuskin® representatives have both said that it is much more mild than sodium lauryl sulfate.[489]

---

489 Telephone conversations on October 28, 2004 with Dr. Loren Pickart, Skin Biology, Inc., Bellevue, WA and with an unnamed person at Biotechne, Cleveland, GA the importer for Thymuskin hair loss treatment and shampoo both consider sodium laureth sulfate to be a mild detergent.

Ammonium Lauryl Sulfate – the ammonium salt of lauryl sulfate. It is a mild anionic surfactant cleanser widely used at mildly acidic pH values. Thoroughly rinse from skin – for prolonged contact with the skin concentrations should not exceed 1 percent.

Ammonium Laureth Sulfate – a compound that breaks up and holds oils and soil so they can be easily removed from the skin.

Sodium Myreth Sulfate – a shampoo containing 7 percent of this ingredient induced mild to moderate eye irritation in some animal studies. Some natural shampoos contain this ingredient in low concentrations.

Methylisothiazolinone (MIT) – a biocide that has neurotoxic effect on cells: this means it causes nerve damage.

According to a University of Pittsburgh study led by Dr. Elias Aizenman, methylisothiazolinone "inhibits the development of particular neuron structures that are essential for transmitting signals between cells."[490] This important study was presented at Cell Biology 2004, the 44th annual meeting of the American Society for Cell Biology. In 2005, Mike Adams, the "Health Ranger," displays his outrage in his online article "Popular shampoos contain toxic chemicals linked to nerve damage."[491] Remember if MIT or SLS destroys your nerves surrounding the follicle, then hair loss will result. Dead or severely damaged nerves cannot activate further cell production in the hair follicle!

What can be easily deduced is this: Do not use shampoos with sodium lauryl sulfate or methylisothiazolinone, they are hazardous to your scalp and health. If you use a shampoo with the more mild detergents (sodium laureth sulfate, ammonium lauryl sulfate, ammonium laureth sulfate) then use as little shampoo, by volume, as possible. Concentration of the detergent matters as much as the amount of shampoo used. If you use these types of shampoos, then you must find out how much (percent volume) of the detergent is in the shampoo, and dilute it with water if necessary.

---

490 "Common ingredient in some shampoos (methylisothiazolinone) stunts developing neurons of rats," December 6, 2004, The Medical News from News-Medical.Net – Latest Medical News and Research from Around the World, accessed July 5, 2010 http://www.news-medical.net/news/2004/12/06/6699.aspx.
491 Mike Adams, "Popular shampoos contain toxic chemicals linked to nerve damage," accessed September 13, 2009 http://www.naturalnews.com/003210.html.

According to several sources, sodium lauryl sulfate penetrates the skin[492] [493] [494] [495] and "high levels of skin penetration may occur at even low concentration."[496] In fact, sodium lauryl sulfate is used to purposely irritate the skin in scientific studies.[497] [498] Skin barrier damage, even with highly diluted SLS (0.1 percent or 0.3 percent) significantly increases the penetration rate of other chemicals, such as pesticides.[499] In this study it should also be noted the damage to the skin produced by SLS "remained unchanged for an experimental period of 48 hours." That is two full days of skin damage caused by one application of SLS! Are you sure you still want to shampoo everyday? Remember, it takes about 30 days for your skin to replace itself.

Another study involved warm airflow after a 0.5 percent SLS solution was applied to the skin.[500] The study was done to mimic the aftereffects of SLS in dry climatic conditions and local heat sources. Twenty volunteers were exposed to airflow at two different temperatures, approximately 75o F and 109o F. Warm airflow alone, at either temperature, did not

492 Elder.

493 David M. Homer, "Biolife Cleansing Guide: Understanding How Your Body Cleanses & Purifies Itself, Inner," accessed October 4, 2003 http://www.innerlifewellness.com/articles/internalcleansing1.html. Explains how skin replaces itself every 28 days as the cells migrate upward towards the skin surface. The skin is the largest organ of the body – it expels toxins, especially through exercise. The bad news is that the skin is also the largest organ to ingest toxins from the environment through cosmetics like shampoos. Quote "Be mindful of things you put on your skin".

494 David Steinman,"Sodium Lauryl Sulfate in Shampoos: The Real Story," accessed September 12, 2003 http://www.aubrey-organics.com/about/articles/shampoo.cfm. On this website, scroll down and hit the link: "10 Synthetic Cosmetic Ingredients" you should avoid. Lists most of the problems associated with SLS including skin inflammation and severe epidermal changes. The site also lists popular shampoos that contain this ingredient.

495 "Material Safety Data Sheet on Sodium Lauryl Sulfate," accessed September 12, 2003 http://www.healthy-communications.com/msdssodiumlaurylsulfate.html. SLS is absorbed by the skin and could cause skin irritation or allergic reaction.

496 Elder.

497 J.W. Fluhr, J. Praessler, A. Akengin, S.M. Fuchs, P. Kleesz, R. Grieshaber, P. Elsner, "Air flow at different temperatures increases sodium lauryl sulphate-induced barrier disruption and irritation in vivo," Br J Dermatol. 2005 Jun;152(6):1228-34. PMID: 15948986 accessed September 25, 2005 http://www.ncbi.nlm.nih.gov/entrez/query.fcgi?CMD=Display&DB=pubmed.

498 J.B. Nielsen, "Percutaneous penetration through slightly damaged skin." Arch Dermatol Res. 2005 Jun;296(12):560-7. PMID: 15834614 [PubMed – in process] accessed September 26, 2005 http://www.ncbi.nlm.nih.gov/entrez/query.fcgi?CMD=Display&DB=pubmed.

499 Nielsen.

500 Fluhr et al.

lead to water loss of the skin. However, the addition of sodium lauryl sulfate was a different matter entirely. First, the 0.5 percent solution of SLS was applied to the skin, which caused its normal "barrier function" to become impaired. Second, the addition of warm airflow caused even more damage to occur well beyond the irritation already produced by SLS alone. What this means is if you wash with medium to strong detergents and live in a dry climate, then the effects of SLS are even worse. Who knows, you may even wrinkle like a prune with this sort of abuse. Normally the skin provides a good impermeable barrier as long as your natural oil or sebum is not stripped away. Therefore, a desert climate does not damage and wrinkle the skin. However, a dry climate in conjunction with soaps or products with SLS may wrinkle your skin, the prune effect.

The article "Hidden hazards in body care products..." in the July/August 1994 issue of "Spectrum, The Wholistic News Magazine," reported the toxic effects of sodium lauryl and laureth sulfates, and indicated that greater than 90 percent of shampoos contain these type ingredients.[501] These ingredients are used mainly because they are cheap and make the foam. Ingredients listed on the bottle appear in order of abundance. Water is the main ingredient by volume. However, usually one of these brutal surfactants is listed as the second item, just after water! This means the concentrations are much higher than safe. These ingredients are proven not to be "safe" in formulations designed for continuous use.... concentrations should not exceed 1 percent.[502] [503] I suppose if something had two or three percent that would not be bad – you could dilute it with water. The problem is that "The Alert-Cosmetic Ingredient Review 1983" reports that many shampoos have an astonishing 10-20 percent of the chemical or at least ten times more than "safe"! Some shampoos contain even 50 percent SLS.[504] Are you beginning to get the picture?

---

501 "Hidden hazards in body care products Sodium lauryl sulfate, a known toxin, lurks in most shampoos." (reprinted from Spectrum, The Wholistic News Magazine, July/August 1994 Issue, p. 37), accessed September 27, 2005 http://www.altmednetwork. net/articles/sodium_lauryl_sulphate.html and/or http://miracleii-4u.com/hazards. htm. This report gives the horrible conclusion: SLS penetrates and damages the skin, hair follicles deteriorate, the hair growth cycle is impaired and the hair loss phase is prolonged from the normal three months up to 24 months – the sad result – thinning hair.
502 "Alert-Cosmetic Ingredient Review 1983."
503 Elder.
504 Winter.

In 2004, skin irritant studies utilized a 20 percent solution of SLS, which is more indicative of actual amounts in many shampoos.[505] [506] The study conducted by H.R. Smith and colleagues demonstrated that individuals vary in response to the "pro-inflammatory" irritation effects caused by SLS. But of course individuals vary – this is common sense. Skin is an organ of the body. Like other organs, some have a sensitive heart. Another may have sensitive lungs, or sensitive kidneys, etc. For example, a few people who smoke may never have any lung problems, thus their lungs are apparently not very sensitive to tobacco smoke. So the sensitivity of each organ, including the skin, varies between individuals with regards to how much abuse each organ can take. Only the healthiest scalp can stand up to the daily abuse of SLS based shampoos on their head.

Elder's research indicates that SLS has a "degenerative effect on the cell membranes because of its protein denaturing properties."[507] Shampoos like these strip the hair and scalp of its natural oils and destroy beneficial bacterial that are essential to a healthy scalp.[508] Most shampoos cause allergic contact dermatitis because they contain biocides.[509] Once the good bacteria are gone, harmful germs cause allergic reactions and hair loss. In fact, millions of microorganisms live on the scalp in an "interdependent network of delicately balanced communities."[510] Tobin agrees and says any "chemical substances foreign to the biological system" can damage the skin.[511] Once the micro-biological "balance" is disturbed, normal skin bacteria can no longer combat intruding types of harmful bacteria. Skin is designed to combat intruders in two main ways: (1) daily skin loss; and (2) by forming it's own acid. The acid mantle of the skin forms when the natural resident skin bacteria break down sebum into fatty acids. Normal skin acidity deters harmful microorganisms.

---

505 H.R. Smith, G.E. Orchard, E. Calonje, D.A. Basketter, and J.P. McFadden, "Irritant threshold and histological response of epidermis to irritant application," Contact Dermatitis, 2004 Nov-Dec;51(5-6):227-230. PMID: 15606645 accessed September 25, 2005 http://www.ncbi.nlm.nih.gov/entrez/query.fcgi?CMD=Display&DB=pubmed.

506 H. Zhai, R. Fautz, A. Fuchs, S. Bhandarker, and H.I. Maibach, "Human scalp irritation compared to the arm and back," Contact Dermatitis. 2004 Oct;51(4):196-200. PMID: 15500669 accessed September 25, 2005 http://www.ncbi.nlm.nih.gov/entrez/query.fcgi?CMD=Display&DB=pubmed.

507 Elder.

508 Pickart, Reverse Skin Aging: Using Your Skin's Natural Power, 114-115.

509 Rook and Dawber, 468.

510 Podolsky, 52.

511 Desmond J. Tobin, "Biochemistry of human skin – our brain on the outside," Chemical Society Reviews, 2006, **35**, 52-67.

Hair and the thin-skinned scalp are not designed for any harsh treatment. This includes too many antibiotics, man-made chemicals, and most soaps and shampoos. It is one thing to be clean, but be reasonable. Squeaky-clean may be good for your automobile, but it is not good for you. The truth is that you do not need foam to be clean. Do not fall for pretty, colorful bottles and tiny amounts of so-called good ingredients. These are marketing tactics to persuade you to buy. Marketers care more about money than they do about your scalp health. Besides, most people selling you these products are completely ignorant of the sad facts provided in this book.

Recall that hair follicles reside in the skin and damage to follicles results from Sodium Lauryl Sulfate. According to the report "Cancer Causing Chemicals in Personal Care Products," SLS is so corrosive that it is utilized in garage floor cleaners, engine degreasers, and car-wash soaps.[512] SLS cleans by corrosion. It is regulated as a pesticide. SLS penetrates and damages the skin barrier, so the hair follicles deteriorate. When hair follicles deteriorate, this is very bad news. "This impairs the hair growth cycle and prolongs the hair loss phase from the normal three months up to 24 months!!! The result – thinning hair."[513]

Short hair is especially problematic. This is because too many concentrated suds reach the scalp rather than just the hair. Long hair naturally prevents an overabundance of suds from reaching the scalp. Think about it. Suds can actually cause your hair follicles to deteriorate and prolong the hair loss phase for up to two years! This is an incredible amount of damage to this tiny complex structure, the factory called the hair follicle.

Specifically, it is even possible that products with high amounts of detergent damage the genetic code of the DNA of the hair follicle. In their study, "Analysis of DNA in hair fibers," Heywood, Skinner and Cornwell found that surfactant, detergents such as sodium lauryl sulfate, erase DNA from human hair shafts.[514] DNA resides in the cuticle, the outer portion of the hair shaft. They found that levels of DNA were "higher at the root-end compared to the tip-end of hair." This makes sense because the hair is younger at the root-end, and older at the tip-end. They concluded that

---

512 "Cancer Causing Chemicals in Personal Care Products," accessed September 26, 2005 http://www.healthy-communications.com/5cancercausingchemicals.html.

513 "Hidden hazards in body care products Sodium lauryl sulfate, a known toxin, lurks in most shampoos," (reprinted from Spectrum, The Wholistic News Magazine, July/August 1994 Issue), 37.

514 D.M. Heywood, R. Skinner, P.A. Cornwell, "Analysis of DNA in hair fibers." J Cosmet Sci., 2003 Jan-Feb;54(1):21-7. PMID: 12644856 [PubMed] accessed May 11, 2009 http://www.ncbi.nlm.nih.gov/entrez/query.fcgi?CMD=Display&DB=pubmed.

DNA was "lost" with surfactant washing. This "loss" accelerated with "prolonged or an increasing number of washes." Their study demonstrates how effective detergents are. After you shed an old hair, the hole leading down into the follicle is open. At his time detergents can enter the follicle directly. Proven skin irritants, like sodium lauryl sulfate, do much damage. If such harsh surfactants or detergents can completely erase the remnant DNA from the cuticle of the hair shaft, then would it not be likely that these chemicals can enter the follicle and cause the so-called "decreased gene expression"?[515] Therefore, if your DNA becomes damage by parts being erased, then how can the follicle make hair? As this occurs, the roots of your hair whither away and a fruitless scalp is the result, with thinning hair and baldness. Your head will now have the landscape of the desert.

Doctors in 1913 stated, "the most fertile single source of spreading diseases of the hair and scalp is the hair-dressing establishment."[516] Hairdressers are exposed to several irritants and allergens.[517] The problems encountered are irritant contact dermatitis, DNA damage, allergic inflammatory disease, and tumor necrosis factor alpha. Some of the products they touch with their hands end up on your scalp. Get the picture? Apparently, Riquette Hofstein is right, that your hair care products all cause hair loss and should be discarded.[518] To be fair, some salons use better products than others, but it is up to you to find out what exactly is being placed on your scalp.

Major Hair Care Recommendations

1. Long hair expert Dr. George Michael insists that hair must be treated like fine silk![519] You would not use harsh detergents in hot water to clean a silk shirt would you?

515 T. Midorikawa, T. Chikazawa, T. Yoshino, K. Takada, S. Arase, "Different gene expression profile observed in dermal papilla cells related to androgenic alopecia by DNA macroarray analysis," J Dermatol Sci. 2004 Oct;36(1):25-32. PMID: 15488702 accessed April 16, 2006 http://www.ncbi.nlm.nih.gov/entrez/query.fcgi?CMD=Display&DB=pubmed.

516 Charles T. Jackson and McMurtry, A Treatise on Diseases of the Hair (London: Henry Kimpton, 1913), 57.

517 D. Cavallo, C.L. Ursini, A. Setini, C. Chianese, A. Cristaudo, and S. Iavicoli, "DNA damage and TNFalpha cytokine production in hairdressers with contact dermatitis," Contact Dermatitis. 2005 Sep;53(3):125-9. PMID: 16128749, accessed May 31, 2006 http://www.ncbi.nlm.nih.gov/entrez/query.fcgi?CMD=Display&DB=pubmed.

518 Hofstein.

519 Jennifer Bahney, "A Visit with Dr. George Michael," accessed October 4, 2003 http://www.bbahneycomm.com/longhairlovers/gmvisit.html.

2. Find a mild shampoo over the Internet or at the local health food store. Do not use shampoos with harsh corrosive detergents, especially sodium lauryl sulfate. In fact, you may wish to avoid foaming-type shampoos altogether. If the shampoo contains detergent, make sure that it is way down on the list of ingredients, not one of the first shown. Use just a small amount of shampoo. Pour it in your palms and gently wash your hair. Start shampooing on the back of the neck where the skin is thick, and work your way towards the sides where the skin is still thick. Wash the top of the sensitive, thin-skinned scalp last. In this way the shampoo will be even more diluted, and surprisingly, it still cleans. According to Dr. Loren Pickart: "If it [any shampoo] foams you've used too much."[520] It really does not take much shampoo to clean your hair.

3. Do not shampoo every day.[521] One to three times maximum per week is plenty, even with the mildest of shampoos. In the early 20th century it was recommended not to wash hair more than once or twice per week even with cold water because this practice "removes too much natural scalp oil."[522] Back then shampoo was only recommended once or twice a month unless exposed to high concentrations of dust. Jackson and McMurtry also suggested that men who over-wash the scalp may be a reason why they go bald.

4. Never shampoo twice as instructed on the bottle. You know the typical slogan: *lather – rinse - repeat.* These instructions are there so you buy shampoo more often.[523]

5. Do not let too many suds reach the scalp. Rinse quickly and thorough. When you are sure that all suds are gone, rinse another 30 seconds more, even with "mild" shampoos. In this way, all chemicals sitting on your crown can be rinsed away.

6. On days when you do not shampoo, try just gently brushing the hair, or rinse the hair with water only, if needed.

7. Exercise patience! Recall that your skin won't replace itself for a month or longer. Likewise, recall the Spectrum article: your hair loss phase may have been greatly prolonged from the normal three months up to 24 months! So it may take several months, even a

---

520 Pickart, telephone communication on October 3, 2003.
521 Bahney.
522 Jackson and McMurtry, 52.
523 Pickart, Reverse Skin Aging: Using Your Skin's Natural Power, 115.

year or two, to observe a difference. For those who are not that patient, read on.

The truth is that "our longer-haired ancestors went months between hair washing and had healthy hair."[524] Shampoo on top of short hair adds insult to injury.

Brushing hair every day, dredlocks or Nubian locks not included, keeps the scalp healthy and improves blood circulation that feeds the hair follicle, and it distributes the skin's natural oil down the length of the hair shaft.[525] A wooden boar's hairbrush is best.[526] The gentle "pulling" during brushing mimics the effects of the weight of longer hair. So the tugging effect during brushing stimulates the proper function of the tiny *erector pili* muscles to squeeze the sebaceous glands, which lubricates the hair.[527]

Chlorine

Shampoo is not the only problem in the shower. Another simple thing you should do is get a chlorine filter for your showerhead. Why, you ask? Chlorine destroys protein in our bodies and "cause[s] adverse effects on skin and hair."[528] Chlorine softens the hair's protective outer shell, its scaly cuticle. In fact, "under an electron microscope, the cuticle can be seen to have melted or worn away."[529] According to Alma Guinness, it only takes 10 hours of chlorine exposure to damage the hair. If chlorine can "melt" hair, think about the damage it can cause to the hair follicle itself. Taking long, hot showers is a health risk. The problem is that chloroform and chlorine by-products form in a hot steamy shower. The heat causes these toxic gases to vaporize. The poisonous gases are then inhaled and absorbed through your skin.[530] [531] [532] Not only is chlorine toxic to the body, other chemicals may lurk in your tap water. Neurotoxicity from dibromoacetic acid in

524 Pickart, telephone communication on October 3, 2003.
525 Pickart, Reverse Skin Aging: Using Your Skin's Natural Power, 117.
526 Hofstein, 45.
527 Hofstein, 46.
528 D.V. Riddle, "Evaluation of the Sprite RSF shower filter for chlorine removal characteristics," Kemysts Laboratory, June 1997.
529 Alma E. Guinness, ed., ABC's of the Human Body (New York: The Readers Digest Association, 1987), 155.
530 John Archer, "The Water you drink: How safe is it?" Pure Water Press, 1996.
531 H.W. Kuo, T.F. Chiang, I.I. Lo, et al. "Estimates of cancer risks from chloroform and trichloroethene from tap water," Environmental Health Perspect, January 1996, v. 104, n. 1, 48-51.
532 Riddle.

drinking water is linked to hair loss.[533] Again, anything that damages the tiny nerves attached to hair follicles leads to hair loss.

Besides chlorine's drastic effect on hair and the skin, where the hair is made, there are even worse health problems. According to Riddle, "Scientific studies have linked chlorine and chlorination by-products to cancer of the bladder, liver, stomach, rectum, and colon, as well as heart disease, arteriosclerosis (hardening of the arteries), anemia, high blood pressure, and allergic reactions."[534] So it seems that chlorine in public supply water, tap water, poses greater dangers than those things (e.g. bacteria) it was used to eliminate. This reminds me of the chemical sunscreen problem. I suppose one could form an alliance and storm city hall with torches and pitchforks but there might be a less time-consuming way to combat this problem. An inexpensive way to remove chlorine from your water supply is to purchase a chlorine filter for the showerhead (see Appendix II).

A chlorine filter purchased from Morrocco Method International comes (at least ours did) with a sheet of scientific quotes from 42 different sources documenting the problems of chlorine. The same showerhead filter can be purchased at other local hardware stores as well. The chlorine filter itself fits inside the showerhead and lasts about six months. Also, keep in mind that a chlorine filter only removes chlorine from the water supply, nothing else. My wife and I both noticed a big difference even in our first shower. The gaseous shower odor from toxic chloroform was eliminated. And our skin, where the hair is made, is no longer dry and brittle. Remember, healthy skin leads to healthy hair. By the way, do not drink tap water. Instead, do yourself a favor and get a water treatment system for your drinking water and icemaker.

High Heat

After you wash your hair there is another thing you need to consider. Temperatures more than 120o F, damage hair follicles.[535] If hair follicles become damaged, the hair-making process is hindered. One day I observed my daughter pressing the hand-held electric hair dryer against the top of her scalp. I shrieked in horror. My shriek startled her quite a bit. Then

---

533 V.C. Moses, P.M. Phillips, A.B. Levine, K.L. McDaniel, R.C. Sills, B.S. Jortner, M.T. Butt, "Neurotoxicity produced by dibromoacetic acid in drinking water of rats." Toxicol Sci., 2004 May;79(1):112-22. PMID: 14976349 [PubMed] accessed August 20, 2006 http://www.ncbi.nlm.nih.gov/entrez/query.fcgi?CMD=Display&DB=pubmed.

534 Riddle.

535 Pickart, Telephone communication on October 3, 2003.

she heard my instructions to never do that again because the hot air will destroy your hair follicles, therefore hair loss is inevitable.

The hot air as it exits our hand-held hair dryer has a temperature of about 145o F! This temperature, being 25o higher than the tolerance level, is much too high for the scalp. The lesson learned is to hold the hair dryer as far from the scalp as possible. The better way would be to let the hair dry naturally. One should also be careful with hot oil hair/scalp treatments. Make certain that the temperature is less than 120o F. Excessive heat from blow dryers and hot oil treatments can "literally boil the follicles."[536]

Recall earlier the problem with sodium lauryl sulfate-based shampoos: warm airflow damages the skin even more when combined with SLS.[537] This is adding insult (warm or hot air flow) to injury (inflamed scalp caused by SLS based or similar shampoos). The bottom line is this: if you destroy the roots, you will have no forest.

---

536 Pickart, Telephone communication on October 3, 2003.
537 Fluhr et al.

Chapter 12: Stress Related Hair Loss

But God shall wound the head of his enemies, and the hairy scalp of such an one as goeth on still in his trespasses (Psalm 68:21, KJV).

What Nerve

Stress and hair loss form a vicious circle – hair loss causes stress and stress causes hair loss.[538] It is well known that hair loss causes stress. Also, just having the hair cut causes stress for many. Thirdly, stress in the form of mental or spiritual anguish causes hair loss. Job loss, divorce, death, abortion, and other life-changing events cause stress.[539]

The loss of head hair causes mainly anxiety, depression, and loss of self-confidence.[540] One study found that more than 76 percent of patients think hair loss is caused by stress, and more than half of the 80 people (38 males and 42 females) questioned also believe that hair loss has had major consequences on their lives.[541] Even though most patients think that their hair loss is, or was, caused by stress, this may not be necessarily so. Recall the other causes cited in this book. Nevertheless, it is a proven scientific fact that stress is certainly a cause of hair loss in some people.

538 I.M. Hadshiew, K. Foitzik, P.C. Arck, and R. Paus, "Burden of hair loss: stress and the underestimated psychosocial impact of telogen effluvium and androgenetic alopecia," J Invest Dermatol, 2004 Sep;123(3):455-7. PMID: 15304082, accessed September 27, 2005 http://www.ncbi.nlm.nih.gov/entrez/query.fcgi?CMD=Display&DB=pubmed.

539 Riquette Hofstein, Grow Hair Fast – 7 Steps to a New Head of Hair in 90 Days (Naperville, Illinois: Sourcebooks, Inc. 2004), 18.

540 F. Poot, "Psychological consequences of chronic hair diseases," Rev Med Brux, 2004 Sep;25(4):A286-8. PMID: 15516058, accessed September 27, 2005 http://www.ncbi.nlm.nih.gov/entrez/query.fcgi?CMD=Display&DB=pubmed.

541 A. Firooz, M.R. Firoozabadi, B. Ghazisaidi, and Y. Dowlati, "Concepts of patients with alopecia areata about their disease," BMC Dermatol, 2005 Jan 12;5(1):1. PMID: 15644147 [PubMed – in process] accessed September 27, 2005 http://www.ncbi.nlm.nih.gov/entrez/query.fcgi?CMD=Display&DB=pubmed.

In 2004 it was substantiated that stress profoundly inhibits hair growth and causes "hair-damaging pro-inflammatory effects."[542] In January 2006, Peters and colleagues reported that stress-induced hair loss or "hair growth inhibition" can now "serve as a highly instructive model for exploring the brain-skin connection."[543] Apparently processes in the scalp and hair follicle become severely damaged and inflamed. Who has not experienced a tight, inflamed neck during stress? Mental processes occur in the brain. When stressed the nerves and muscles closest to the brain seem to be affected more by tightness and inflammation than distal parts of the body. Thus the nerve collar that surrounds the *erector pili* muscle in each hair follicle must behave in a similar way. Recall in Chapter 2 that stress can cause subluxations of the neck and spine. This places pressures on the nerves and can lead to hair loss. Most likely, this type of stress leads to balding in the vertex region of the scalp (Figure 12-1). As seen in Figure 12-1, the *greater occipital* branch supplies the vertex. The *greater occipital* is a division of the second cervical nerve, which exits through the second cervical vertebra (C2) of the neck.[544] If the C2 vertebra is misaligned, then this could directly affect the nerve supply to the vertex region of the scalp and result in hair loss of that area. Proper curvature of the neck and spine must be maintained for ultimate health of the body.

The follicles of the crown of the scalp are supplied by a different set of nerves, the *supra orbital* branch, than the vertex (Figure 12-1). One day I experienced the effects of stress-induced hair loss of the crown first hand. It was an intense struggle between a young husband and his wife. The problems with this relationship began prior to marriage. They had a child out of wedlock. The man was bothered by this so he wanted to marry the woman and have a normal family home. But the woman never looked upon marriage as a positive thing. Eventually she agreed for the baby's sake. After they were married, the arguments between the two escalated to an intense severity. One day the male sought my help for he needed consoling. While ministering to him, he explained that his wife was given advice by her church friends to divorce him. This miserable advice is apparently from the same

---

542 Hadshiew et al.

543 E.M. Peters, P.C. Arck, and R. Paus, "Hair growth inhibition by psychoemotional stress: a mouse model for neural mechanisms in hair growth control," Exp. Dermatol, 2006 Jan;15(1):1-13, accessed August 15, 2006 http://www.ncbi.nlm.nih.gov/entrez/query. fcgi?CMD=Display&DB=pubmed.

544 Henry Gray, Anatomy, Descriptive and Surgical, 1901 Edition, The Unabridged Running Press Edition of the American Classic: Gray's Anatomy, eds. T. Pickering Pick and Robert Howden (Philadelphia: Running Press, 1974), 51, 760.

types of church people who have infected certain "Christian" schools who force males to cut their hair, a form of divorce. Obviously, they have never studied all the Scripture passages referred to in this book, nor have they read that being cut off or divorced is loathsome to God. Personally, I never witnessed their tempestuous battles. But while there, his wife, whom I never met before, came home. All three of us sat there in the living room.

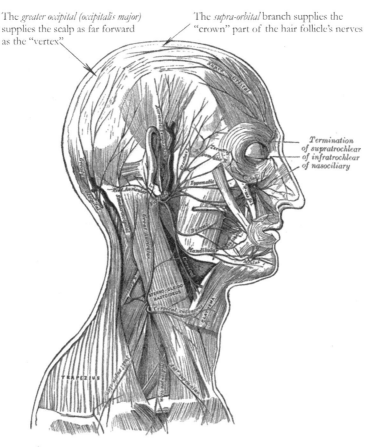

The *greater occipital (occipitalis major)* supplies the scalp as far forward as the "vertex".

The *supra-orbital* branch supplies the "crown" part of the hair follicle's nerves

Termination of supratrochlear of infratrochlear of nasociliary

Figure 12-1: Nerves of the Scalp, Face, and Side of the Neck. The *supra-orbital* branch supplies the skin of your crown. A nerve is attached to the muscle of each hair follicle. Stress hinders nerve supply. As nerves deaden so do the follicles. Short hair does little to stimulate these nerve endings. Long hair provides the extra weight to build larger follicle muscles and help stimulate these nerves all the way to their origin in the brain reducing stress. The *greater occipital* branch supplies hair roots as far forward as the vertex. Vertex balding is more related to internal health conditions and subluxations of the neck and back (see Chapter 3). Therefore, it is vital for overall health to maintain the proper curvature of your neck and back so that nerve supply to any organ is not marred.

During our discussion, the woman informed me of the terribly volatile situation. Then as proof, she ran her hand through the crown of her scalp and produced a handful of hair. Others have told similar stories. As Tobin well knows, nerves of the scalp pass directly to the surface of the brain. Thus hair loss in the crown portion of the scalp can be caused by stress in the brain itself (Figure 12-1). This is obviously the case here considering this woman's mental anguish.

As we learned, the nervous system's communication system is a two-way street. These nerves are shown to pass from the crown down the forehead through the eye sockets and directly into the brain (Figure 12-1). This means that hair from the crown of the head is part of a person's sensory perception. When stressed the brain sends out negative impulses through the nerves of the *supra-orbital* branch directly to the hair follicles of the crown. Apparently, communication signals to the follicles are shut down so that the follicle stops making hair. Again, as Tobin put it: hair is not just a source of neuro-transmitters but also a "target."[545] This is why longer hair is so important. You need it not only to exercise scalp muscles, but to stimulate the brain. Stimulation is the antithesis of stress. The weight of long hair combined with motion sends positive impulses to the brain. This could help fight negative impulses sent out to the follicles for their demise. Ironically, concerning the woman with marital issues, her hair was rather short, only about six inches, and she was overweight, indicating possible poor nutrition leading to follicle starvation. By adding insult to injury, stress also impedes vital nutrients and vitamins needed to maintain proper hair growth. It is, in fact, a drain on the immune system. A good vitamin B complex combats stress (see Chapter 13). But a proper amount of sleep, rest and relaxation are highly needed as well.

Barbermonger

For some people a haircut may be a wonderful thing. However, for many people just having the hair cut produces stress, especially if cut excessively (Figure 12-2). When forced to cut the hair, a person can feel violated or less attractive. Unfortunately, those lovers of haircuts, the crop-heads, do not understand this. One male related that when he was a boy his father used the "dog-clippers" on him as if he was an animal. Another guy recalled that while a young boy and just when his hair started to "look good" he

---

545 Desmond J. Tobin, "Biochemistry of human skin – our brain on the outside," *Chemical Society Reviews*, 2006, 35, p. 52-67.

was taken to the barber he and his friends called Kelly the Butcher and the hair was sheared off. Another youth related, "I love my hair and others do too … every time it just starts looking good, they [private schools] make me cut it off."

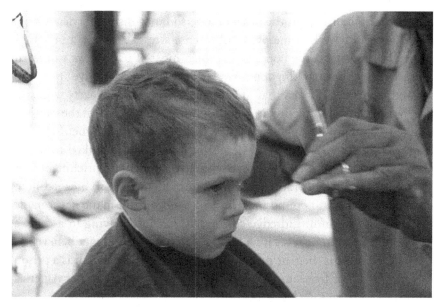

Figure 12-2: Beginnings of a Stress-Filled Life. What a happy smiling face this is – NOT. Notice the frown on this young lad. Many young males do not like haircuts, and rightly so – knowing what we have learned about baldness and skin cancers of the scalp, ears, and neck. This poor soul's hair is cut so short that all his natural protection from the sun's rays is gone. When innocence is lost, their stress is passed on to others. No doubt, this lad will grow up and force others to be shorn as he was. Unbeknownst to crop-heads is how they might inadvertently cause the mutilation or death of another person via skin cancer.

Stress caused by hair cutting is not rare, as some may suppose. Personally, I remember my job search back in 1994. One position I considered was that of air traffic controller. It is probably one of the better jobs in the federal government. The people are highly paid professionals. To help determine if this was something I wanted to do, I took a tour of the Federal Aviation and Administration (FAA) facility at one of the largest U.S. airports. One of the first things the tour guide told me was that "dress code" was essentially up to the individual. Whether someone wore a business suit, or jeans, either was acceptable. If another was comfortable with a beard, that was perfectly fine. If another man wore his hair down his back, that was okay too. Why? Without even asking he informed me that the FAA "must not cause any additional stress on the job for they literally have lives in their hands!" As one who travels by air, it is a relief knowing that such wisdom exists somewhere in this world. The dream is to have such freedom, the elimination of unnatural anti-male hair rules, in all other places of work. Real professionalism is in the heart of a person, not his hair style.

Our cities have become places of intense stress. They are a prison of sorts. To understand the bondage in which most of us live, we can learn much from the animal kingdom. A veterinary study of "captive" primates showed forms of hair loss that are absent in their counterparts who still live in the "wild" or "free-living" conditions.[546] The hair loss of the captives resulted "from grooming or plucking behaviours directed at themselves or at other individuals." This "over-grooming" behaviour is linked to stress, and is "controllable to some extent with environmental enrichment." In "Wild at Heart," John Eldredge compares modern man to a caged lion. He related that a 500 pound male lion with a beautiful mane never made eye contact with him. Eldredge concluded that "after living in a cage, a lion no longer even believes it's a lion ... and a man no longer believes he is a man."[547] This is the true picture of modern urban society. It is a prison under a facade of freedom. The long-haired founding fathers of America wished us to be free. What happened?

America has grown to be a very stressful society. In some regard, modern America resembles first century Rome. Rome, like America, began with long hair. After a while, when a society loses heart, they revert to head shearing. This disintegration of the hair is related to stress or tyranny over their subjects. The Romans cut the hair short and often had it plucked out. According to Scripture, plucking out the hair was a form of punishment (Nehemiah 13:25; Isaiah 50:6). The passage in Isaiah 50:6 reads, "I gave my back to the smiters, and my cheeks to them that plucked off the hair." This is a prophecy that foretold the brutal treatment Jesus would receive at the hands of the Romans prior to His crucifixion.[548] This compares quite nicely with the veterinary study of "captive" primates in the foregoing paragraph who plucked themselves and each other. The civilized Romans

---

546 P. Honess, J. Gimpel, S. Wolfensohn and G. Mason, "Alopecia scoring: the quantitative assessment of hair loss in captive macaques," Altern Lab Anim., 2005 Jun;33(3):193-206. PMID: 16180975 [PubMed – in process] accessed September 27, 2005 http://www.ncbi. nlm.nih.gov/entrez/query.fcgi?CMD=Display&DB=pubmed.

547 John Eldredge, Wild at Heart (Nashville, Tennessee: Thomas Nelson Publishers, 2001), 41.

548 William Neil, Pocket Bible Commentary (Edison, New Jersey: Castle, 1997, Hodder & Stoughton, 1962), 254.

became known as the beard pluckers. They directed their over-grooming and plucking behaviors upon themselves and to others, just like much of corporate America does at the present time.

A Roman-type world is a stress-filled society. Stress and short hair are probably the two principal reasons why many Roman men went bald, and why modern American men, and other so-called civilized societies, bald. As a reminder, short hair causes two problems: (1) it can lead to atrophy of the scalp muscles and reduce the size of the hair follicles; and (2) it exposes the thin skinned scalp to the sun's ultraviolet rays, overexposure of which leads to various sorts of skin damage discussed earlier. The wearing of a tight-fitting helmet was of no help, especially if it rubbed against the top of the scalp. Short hair would not offer much cushion between the scalp and the helmet. The rubbing action could have irritated and inflamed the scalp, causing hair loss.

In truth, the Romans were not more civilized, they merely deemed themselves superior to other peoples, and thus became arrogant and uppity. How many are held captive and treated like slaves in the modern world? I fear too many. Story after story has come to the author's attention in America. Some of these have to do with male hair restrictions and other so-called dress code violations. In many ways, America seems to resemble ancient Rome. In terms of head shearing, America is even worse than 1st century Rome. And this is what is being taught in America's so-called Christian education system, which is in truth, pseudo-Christianity.

Hair Phobias

Why do some people have a fear of hair? And what can we say about people that cut, shave or pluck out their hair constantly? Tricho-, from the Greek, *thrix* (hair), is a prefix relating to hair. Trichophobia is the morbid dread of hair, and is a psychological disorder. Therefore, people with this mental problem need help. Certain psychological disorders like this can arise if one is actually taught (self-taught or forced in the education system - stress) to hate or dread their own hair. The hair loss disaster for others occurs when trichophobic people are placed in top positions of corporations. Trichotillomania and trichotemnomania are two other psychological disorders people suffer from (Figures 12-3, 12-4).

Trichotillomania is the obsessive-compulsive habit of plucking out the hair (Figure 12-3). According to Raikes, nearly 11 million Americans have this hair-plucking disorder. Presumably, it may be caused by stress possibly from bad childhood experiences.

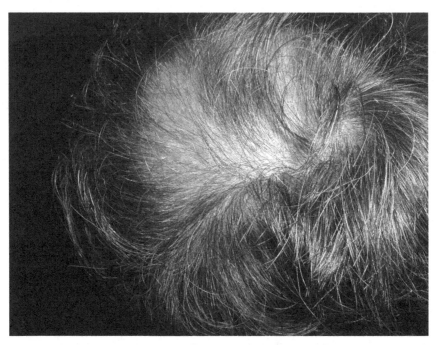

Figure 12-3: Tonsure-Style Bald Spot in the Vertex of the Head. In this case, this bald spot is not natural. This man suffers from an obsessive habit of plucking his hair out, a form of *trichotillomania*.

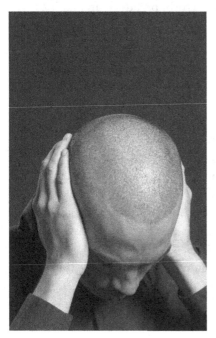

Figure 12-4: Shaved Head and Hair-Cut Madness: Trichotemnomania. Of all the ways of self destruction, shaving off a completely good, thick head of hair is probably the most nonsensical of them all. What, or who, is compelling so many to do such a thing to their heads? Have we forgotten that it was the neo-Nazi skinheads who seem to have started this? Remember cutting off the hair, especially like this, is an act of partial suicide. Constant shaving will damage the head in one form or another. Various skin eruptions from infection, rash, scars, and cancer are the result. Surely, doing this in an obsessive way is a form of trichotemnomania or "hair cut madness." Who will teach this generation the importance of hair before they all destroy themselves and others?

Trichotemnomania is the obsessive-compulsive habit of cutting or shaving the hair (Figure 12-4). Trichotemnomania is similar to trichotillomania except it obviously is not as painful, since it involves shaving and cutting rather than pulling or plucking out the hair. R. Happle's simple definition of trichotemnomania is simply "hair cut madness" derived from the Greek *thrix* (hair), *temnein* (to cut), and *mania* (madness).[549] Are people who cut or shave (a form of plucking) their hair excessively suffering from some borderline version of this psychological disorder? If not psychological, then is it simply the result of a stress-filled society? The truth is that cutting off the hair and casting it away may be a sign that the Lord has rejected that nation as a whole (Jeremiah 7:29; Ezekiel 29:18; compare also Psalm 68:21). If this is true, then could it be that an abundance of baldheads collectively symbolizes the barrenness a nation, a spiritual desert?

549 R. Happle, "Trichotemnomania: obsessive-compulsive habit of cutting or shaving the hair," J Am Acad Dermatol, 2005 Jan;52(1):157-9. PMID: 15627101 accessed September 27, 2005 http://www.ncbi.nlm.nih.gov/entrez/query.fcgi?CMD=Display&DB=pubmed.

Chapter 13: Hairs to Your Health

||||||||||||||||||||||||||||||||||||||||||||||||||||||||||||||||||||||||||||||||||||||||||||||||||||||||||||||||||||||||||||||||||||||||||

Wherefore I pray you to take some meat: for this is for your health: for there shall not an hair fall from the head of any of you (Acts 27:34).

In this chapter we will discuss ways to rejuvenate the scalp, stop hair loss, and re-grow your hair without harsh drugs or surgery. There are a few natural holistic ways to do this. This assumes, of course, that any underlying causes of your hair loss, pharmaceuticals, chlorine, thyroid, stress, poor nutrition, harsh shampoos, fungal infection, and so forth, have been addressed. Age does not matter, but you must still have vellus hairs (i.e., peach fuzz). However, the *length of time* that you have been bald does matter. If you have been thinning or have been bald for 15 years or less there is hope, even if you are 70 years old.[550] But the sooner you address the hair-thinning problem the better. If you have been bald for more than 15 years then your chances of hair re-growth diminish greatly.

In fact, two of the scientists, Loren Pickart and Morton Walker, are both promoting certain products in this section. Both men are quite bald, so why listen to them? After all, how could they recommend products for us, if those same products do not work for them? Good questions. The reason is that both men are older now and have been balding for so long, well past the 15-year mark. Their follicles have no hope for regeneration. These products were not discovered and made available until fairly recent times. For example, Dr. Morton Walker began to bald when he was 28 years old back in the 1950s. In 1995, he was 68 years old. After 40 years of balding there is no hope.[551] By this time the follicles are waxed over and quite dead.

---

550 Telephone discussion with U.S. Thymuskin representative of Biotechne, Cleveland, GA on January 25, 2006.

551 Morton Walker, Bald No More, (New York: Kensington Publishing Corporation, 1998), 23.

Hofstein puts it this way: if you still feel "peach fuzz" (i.e., the tiny vellus hairs), then there is hope.[552] The peach fuzz is a sign that the follicles are not dead, but just dormant. If you still have a full head of hair, the best method is prevention. The following is a brief list of what everyone needs to do to prevent hair loss:

1. Eat healthfully.
2. Drink plenty of water, at least 64 ounces every day.
3. Exercise regularly.
4. Get adequate sunshine, but not overexposure.
5. Get plenty of sleep every night.
6. Reduce stress (e.g., vacations, chiropractic care, massage, yoga, etc.).
7. Install a chlorine filter in the showerhead.
8. Reduce or eliminate, if possible, pharmaceutical and over-the-counter drugs.
9. Change your thinking how to treat your scalp regarding hair length, using the right shampoos, brushing/combing to distribute sebum (natural scalp oil) down the hair shaft, proper shampooing methods, and reduce chemicals such as chlorine, dyes, colors, straighteners, gels, hair spray and others.

Nutrition and Exercise

Test your servants for ten days; let us be given vegetables to eat and water to drink…. At the end of ten days it was seen that they were better in appearance … than all the youths who ate the king's rich food (Daniel 1:12,15 – RSV).

As discovered thus far, many things can contribute to thinning hair. Any one or any combination of the manmade causes already mentioned in this book can contribute to hair loss. Other than shampooing less and getting rid of harmful shampoos, the other things that you can control are proper exercise and nutrition. For optimal health, exercise is not optional. So get up off the couch and do some good old-fashioned physical exercise. Good vigorous exercise leads to better blood circulation. Better circulation brings vital nutrients to starving cells. Along with your new exercise program, assuming you do not have one, begin to eat foods that your body wants.

552 Riquette Hofstein, Grow Hair Fast – 7 Steps to a New Head of Hair in 90 Days (Naperville, Illinois: Sourcebooks, Inc. 2004), 5-6.

It has been well established that "nutritional deficiencies" play a large role in hair loss. In fact, hair and skin care expert Riquette Hofstein says, "the condition of the hair is a direct manifestation of a person's health."[553] Poor blood circulation, poor diet, and vitamin deficiencies help promote hair loss. According to Dr. Morton Walker, non-nutritious "fast food" is a "major source of hair loss for both sexes." He says the chemical additives, excess fats, and free radicals in these foods also cause cancer, heart disease, and other forms of slow death. As an example, Walker relates that many Japanese men used to have thick hair. This is when they ate a traditional Japanese diet of soy foods, a natural DHT blocker. But since they adopted the fattier diet of the latter half of the 20th century, they now lose their hair. Dr. Walker's advice: eat more soy and seafood and less fat.[554]

A diet high in fruits and vegetables and low in starch can help your hair. Fruits and vegetables contain flavonoids, "many of which are antioxidants that may provide protection for the hair follicles and encourage hair growth."[555] An intake of essential nutrients, protein, carbohydrates, a normal amount of fats, and minerals is also necessary for healthy hair. According to Walker, carbohydrates and fats should never be eliminated from the diet.[556] Carbohydrates provide energy that helps the body use protein and improve cell growth in hair follicles. A normal amount of fat is needed as well. Do you remember the sebum produced from the oil gland located adjacent to each hair follicle? Well, sebum is an oil fat, which is designed to keep the follicles lubricated. Therefore, fats are very important for these sebaceous oil glands.

It is interesting that man's original diet consisted of things produced by plants only (Genesis 1:29; 3:18-19). Animals considered "clean," meaning healthy for human consumption, were added after the Great Flood and spelled out in Leviticus 11 and Deuteronomy 14:3-20. Many mammals, birds and fish, as long as the fish have fins and scales, are part of the menu. Kosher or clean animal foods include beef, lamb, goats, deer, gazelle, and among birds are ducks, geese, chicken, and turkey. Several testimonies exist how people have been healed of various diseases using The Maker's Diet.[557]

553 Hofstein, 20.
554 Morton Walker, Bald No More, 131-132.
555 Phyllis A. Balch and James F. Balch, Prescription for Nutritional Healing, 3rd ed. (New York: Avery – a member of Penguin Putnam, 2000), 401-403.
556 Morton Walker, Bald No More, 132.
557 Jordan Rubin, The Maker's Diet (Lake Mary, FL: Siloam Press; Reprint edition, April 30, 2005).

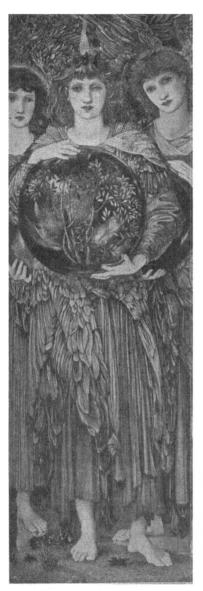

Figure 13-1: Creation of Plants. And out of the ground made the Lord God to grow every tree that is pleasant to the sight, and good for food (Genesis 2:9a). This is reminder to eat your fruits and vegetables for ultimate hair health. Painting was done sometime prior to 1908 from "The Bible and Its Story."

Contrary to the Creator's diet are scavengers, predators and bottom feeders. This is because they can become toxic with poisons and parasites due to the dead and putrid matter they ingest.[558] The typical modern diet consists of an abundance of these things, shellfish and pork as examples. It is commonly argued that as long as these unclean animals are fully cooked then there should be no problem with their consumption. And

---

558 Charles J. Brim, Medicine in the Bible (New York: Froben Press, 1936).

domesticated pork, fed a strict diet in developed countries, are healthier than wild pigs. But if it is true that the Maker's diet heals as Rubin says, then this could mean that unclean (unhealthy) foods may pollute the body over time. After all, even if you fully cook pork, the dead bodies of the worms still remain in the swine's flesh. This does not sound good. Is the consumption of these animals fully understood by science? Should you eat these things or do they add to the baldness problem?

The Prophet Isaiah condemned those who "eat swine's flesh, and broth of abominable things" (Isaiah 65:4, KJV). Swine, the property of Gentile herdsman, are mentioned in the account where Jesus cast the Legion of demons out of a man and into the bodies of 2,000 pigs, which ran down the hill and into the sea where they drowned themselves. This happened in the Gadarene region (Mark 5:1-13). Remarkably, "Strabo in the sixteenth book saith that in Gadaris there is a standing pool of very naughty water, which if beasts taste of, they shed their hair, nails, or hooves and horns."[559] Apparently, you are what you eat! Presumably, the region was infested with parasites.

Furthermore, you must know your ABCs. Vitamins A, B, and C are vital for hair and scalp health. Deficiencies can be disastrous for hair and your looks. Too little vitamin A in the diet is a cause of hair loss. Initially, a lack of vitamin A leads to dry and dull hair. Eventually, the "hair follicle's root lets go so that the hair bulb dies off or forms a cyst around itself."[560] To summarize Walker, vitamin A deficiency causes the outer layer of the scalp's skin layer to actually grow over the mouth of each hair follicle near the sebaceous oil gland. This "overgrowth" obstructs the follicle's opening, impedes the manufacture of hair, and causes improper sebum flow. Then the keratin cells that make hair form "plugs" within the follicles. As this happens, hair will not emerge from the follicle and the sebaceous gland withers. The terrible result from scant vitamin A: "Hair loss must be the result of such blockage."

Graying of hair is even blamed on vitamin deficiencies.[561] A good vitamin B complex must include para-Aminobenzoic acid (PABA), inositol, niacin (B3), and biotin. PABA reverses premature graying and niacin turns gray hair back to its normal color over time.[562] Biotin in the

---

559 Commentary notes of "Mark 5:13" in The 1599 Geneva Bible (White Hall, West Virginia: Tolle Lege Press, 2006).

560 Morton Walker, Bald No More, 133.

561 Alma E. Guinness, ed., ABC's of the Human Body (New York: The Readers Digest Association, 1987), 154.

562 Morton Walker, Bald No More, 133.

diet is needed for "healthy hair and skin."[563] Biotin binds testosterone in hair follicles instead of permitting the testosterone to bind with protein receptors that turn it into DHT.[564] Biotin supplementation also "resulted in gradual regrowth of healthy hair."[565] Phyllis and James Balch indicate that sources of biotin include "brewer's yeast, brown rice, bulger, green peas, lentils, oats, soybeans, sunflower seeds, and walnuts." Vitamin C (ascorbic acid) improves blood flow to the scalp, and is great for skin, hair, and nails.[566] Vitamins B and C also combat stress, which as learned earlier is a cause of hair loss. Protein is also vital for proper hair growth. Protein-calorie malnutrition causes the following problems with hair[567]:

1. Change in color and texture.
2. Loss of natural curl.
3. Brittleness.
4. Thinning hair due to hair fallout.
5. Thinning hair due to a reduction in hair diameter.
6. Growth rate retards.
7. Increases the number of hairs in the telogen (hair loss) phase.
8. Atrophy of the bulb.
9. Loss of the outer root sheath.
10. Frequent loss of the inner root sheath.

Interestingly, "protein deprivation" causes degeneration of the nerve fibers.[568] As stated earlier, nerves supply the power to hair follicles – without this power hair cannot be made. This lack of protein even expresses itself in the hair roots "before changes in blood values occurred."[569] This is direct proof that the overall health of the body can be seen in the quality

---

563 Balch and Balch.
564 Morton Walker, Bald No More, 134.
565 S.M. Innis and D.B. Allardyce, "Possible biotin deficiency in adults receiving long-term total parenteral nutrition," Am J Clin Nutr., 1983 Feb;37(2):185-7. PMID: 6401910 [PubMed] accessed July 11, 2006 http://www.ncbi.nlm.nih.gov/entrez/query.fcgi?CMD=Display&DB=pubmed.
566 Morton Walker, Bald No More, 134.
567 Vlado Valković, Human Hair. Vol. 1: Fundamentals and Methods for Measurement of Elemental Composition (Boca Raton, Florida: CRC Press, Inc., 1988), 24.
568 A. Oldfors, "Nerve fibre degeneration of the central and peripheral nervous systems in severe protein deprivation in rats," Acta Neuropathol, 1981;54(2):121-127. accessed August 15, 2006 http://www.ncbi.nlm.nih.gov/entrez/query.fcgi?CMD=Display&DB=pubmed.
569 Valković, 24.

of one's hair. Pickart informs us that hair is composed of 35 percent sulfur containing amino acids. Methyl sulfonyl methane has "long been used to improve the hair coats of racehorses and are increasingly being used to improve hair health in humans."[570]

Minerals in the diet such as zinc and copper are vital for healthy hair. Zinc deficiency is linked to hair loss.[571] Copper is good for skin and hair. In fact "a lack of sufficient dietary copper can cause hair to lose its color."[572] However, since zinc and copper compete with each other, these supplements should not be taken together. For Pickart relates that excessive zinc can drive out "the copper needed to synthesize hair pigments and turn hair gray." Therefore, if you supplement with zinc in the morning, then take copper in the evening. The bottom line is a poor diet produces ugly hair and ultimate hair loss. Even the Apostle Paul did not want to see the Romans go bald, so he instructs them to eat something since they hungered after 14 days of fasting (Acts 27:33-37).

Although there are many conveniences to modern society, there are also as many problems as there are benefits. Our heads, or better, the hairs of our heads are paying a big price – the price of over-cutting, over-shampooing, fast food restaurants, chemically induced foods, etc., all leading to loss of hair. Besides a proper diet, and the modern problem of not always being able to eat right, vitamins and herbs should be highly considered to supplement the diet (Table 13-1).

Prostate problems could lead to DHT, which adds its negative effects to already damaged hair follicles. Do you get up frequently during the night to urinate? Chances are better than not that you may have a swollen prostate, and even a slightly swollen prostate may cause problems. For prostate health, the herb Saw Palmetto is often used. It is a good herb, but for something stronger you wish to consider other natural products from your local health food or vitamin store. How do you tell if you might have prostate problems? If you wake up a few times every night to urinate, then you may have prostate problems. To verify that this is so, you may want to schedule an appointment with an urologist.

---

570 Loren Pickart, "Improving Hair Growth with Skin Remodeling Copper Peptides," Cosmetics and Medicine (Russia) (July 2004), accessed February 13, 2005 http://www.skinbiology.com/2004RussiaHairRemodeling.html

571 J.S. Prendiville, L.N. Manfredi, "Skin signs of nutritional disorders," Semin Dermatol, 1992 Mar;11(1):88-97. PMID: 1550720 [PubMed] accessed July 11, 2006 http://www.ncbi.nlm.nih.gov/entrez/query.fcgi?CMD=Display&DB=pubmed.

572 Loren Pickart, Reverse Skin Aging: Using Your Skin's Natural Power. (Bellevue, Washington: Cape San Juan Press, 2005), 113.

Table 13-1: Important Supplements for Hair Health

SUPPLEMENT	SUGGESTED AMOUNT	COMMENTS
"Ultra Hair" from *Nature's Plus*. This includes vitamins A, B, C and others.	As directed on label	Contains the necessary nutrients to stimulate hair growth. If your condition is not too bad, this product may be all you need.
Essential Fatty Acids: flaxseed oil, primrose oil, salmon oil are sources	As directed on label	Improves hair texture and prevents dry, brittle hair.
Vitamin B Complex	B3 (Niacin) 50 mg 3x a day	B vitamins are excellent for the health and growth of hair. Fights stress.
	B5 (Pantothenic Acid) 50 mg 3x a day	
	B6 (Pyridoxine) 50 mg 3x a day	
	Inositol	
	Biotin	
	PABA 50 mg 2x a day	
Vitamin C with Bioflavonoids	3,000 mg – 4,000	Aids in improving scalp circulation. Helps with antioxident action in hair follicles. Fights stress.
Vitamin E	Start with 400 IU daily & slowly increase to 800 – 1000 IU	Improves circulation to the scalp

Amounts of B3, B5, and B6 after Phyllis A. Balch and James F. Balch, Prescription for Nutritional Healing, 3rd ed. (New York: Avery – a member of Penguin Putnam, 2000), p. 401-403. All other nutrition supplements in Table 13-1 are also from this work unless noted otherwise. Please note that individual B vitamins in a Vitamin B Complex will vary somewhat from brand to brand: The amounts of PABA are based on Morton Walker, Bald No More, (New York: Kensington Publishing Corporation, 1998), p. 133. When using Vitamin C, start with 1,000 mg per day and increase by 1,000 mg each day until you reach 3,000 – 4,000 mg. Balch and Balch set an upper limit of 10,000 mg per day. Amounts of Vitamin C greater than 4,000 mg per day may be too much and prove to be fruitless.

Before beginning any vitamin regiment, be certain to consult with your physician.

Topical Products

Remember longer hair is healthier. How much baldness would there be if people simply grew their hair naturally long with minimal trimming, the way it was designed to be worn? In truth, thinning hair would be far lesser of a problem. For this reason, some selling products and services to combat baldness may dismiss the idea that longer hair is healthier. It could affect them financially because they would sell less, particularly those who sell drugs. The good news is that in 1989 the U.S. Food and Drug Administration accepted that hair growth could be positively increased by non-drug cosmetic applications to the scalp.[573] As a result, a plethora of heavily advertised products hit the market with little, if any, results. In short, they do not work. On the other hand, several good methods/suggestions/products have arisen to address hair loss from a natural holistic approach, and they actually work for many, especially if the hair loss is due to an abused scalp that led to one's seborrheic dermatitis or related skin/follicle damage. At the same time, some of these products also minimize the hormonal ravages caused by DHT and the immune system.

First I will discuss how I avoided hair loss. Then Dr. Loren Pickart's copper peptides (and emu oil), Super Hair Energizer, Thymuskin®, and the Riquette Hofstein methods will be discussed. These companies manufacture and/or sell good products including topical solutions, shampoos without sodium lauryl sulfate, and/or vital nutrients. The other thing honorable about these particular companies is that none of them spend millions of dollars on marketing through expensive advertising. Their success is measured and backed by powerful testimonies and word of mouth. The benefit to the reader, or user of their products, is a quality product for lower cost rather than hype. No matter which of these products/methods you try it is important that you commit for up to two years. It could take anywhere from a few months up to two years to see a difference. Patience is a virtue. More detail on the time factor will be discussed in each of these five methods.

How I Did and How You Can Avoid Hair Loss

Just by shampooing less often and with a good, natural, high-quality shampoo can stop hair loss in 30 days. The sooner you act to stop hair loss the better. The author of this book's testimony is as follows:

---

573 Morton Walker, How to Stop Baldness and Regrow Hair (Stamford, CT: Freelance Communications, 1995), 8.

In 2003, I became aware of the shampoo problem, those that contain too much sodium lauryl sulfate. Immediately I stopped using sodium lauryl sulfate type shampoos. In fact, I did not shampoo with anything for a week. I then started to use some of the shampoos listed in Appendix II. I reduced shampooing, even with these good shampoos, to twice per week. The days varied each week depending on circumstances. At this time I was 43 years old and I still had a full head of hair that began to thin and recede slightly. My scalp was beginning to feel brittle and tight, and it even started to have pain on the crown area. Apparent inflammation was the probable cause. I felt like I was on the verge of hair loss. During the first 30 days of my new regiment, my scalp flaked horribly with large pieces of skin peeling off my scalp, some even more than an eighth of an inch long. Later I learned from Riquette Hofstein that these dry flakes were not dandruff. She says dandruff shampoos are bunk: "The only cause of flaking is having a dry scalp."[574] Ironically, 30 days of flaking is roughly the time it takes for the skin to replace itself. After these 30 days I realized that the reason my scalp flaked so badly was that my skin was severely damaged (seborrheic dermatitis) due to the harsh detergent-based shampoos I was using daily. My personal immunity to sodium lauryl sulfate detergent was diminishing rapidly as it was destroying the oil (sebum) system of the scalp. I believe this because my scalp was becoming tight with some pain – it just did not feel pliable. But I caught my hair loss in time.

I related this to several of my friends. Those who have heeded this advice have stopped their hair loss. Several shampoo only once per week now with a good quality shampoo (see Appendix II) and their hair and scalp even feel better. Others, who switched to good natural shampoos and shampoo less often, have also related that their so called "dandruff problem" disappeared, their hair either feels better, appears thicker, or has more bounce. If you go this route there are certain criteria for selecting a shampoo.

The pH value of shampoo is very important. Pure water (and apparently milk) has a pH of 7 and is considered neutral. Vinegar and lemon juice are acidic, laundry detergents and ammonia are basic (or alkaline). Chemicals that are very basic or very acidic are reactive and can cause severe burns. An important point to consider is that the pH Scale is logarithmic. In other words a pH of 6 is ten times more acidic than water, and a pH of 8 is ten times more basic than water. A pH of 11 (ammonia) is 10,000 times more basic or alkaline than water (Figure 13-2). Rule number one is that

574 Hofstein, 35.

a shampoo must be pH balanced. Dr. Zoe Diana Draelos informs us that pH balanced means that the shampoo must have a pH around 5.5 to 7.0.[575] Values in this range will have little altercation of the skin's normal acid level or the skin's natural pH.

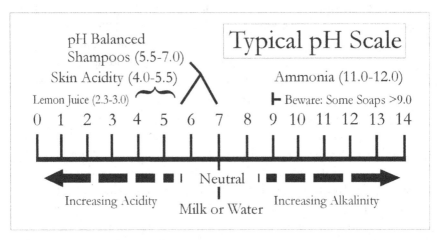

pH Balanced Shampoos (5.5-7.0)
Skin Acidity (4.0-5.5)
Lemon Juice (2.3-3.0)

Typical pH Scale

Ammonia (11.0-12.0)
Beware: Some Soaps >9.0

0 1 2 3 4 5 6 7 8 9 10 11 12 13 14

Increasing Acidity
Neutral
Milk or Water
Increasing Alkalinity

Figure 13-2: Typical pH Scale

The Task: find out which shampoos have no (or very little) detergent and have a reasonable pH for cleaning. High pH shampoos are too alkaline and should not be used for they make your hair look great for only a few weeks. Eventually, the hair will become dry and brittle.[576] Water alone can clean because it is from ten to more than 100 times more basic than the acid mantle of the skin. Obviously, water takes longer to clean than strong detergents. And it does not have those great smelling fragrances. But be very careful of shampoos with a pH much greater than 7.0.

Also note that even many health food/vitamin stores still sell shampoos with lauryl sulfates – you must read the ingredients before buying. If the shampoo does have a lauryl sulfate in it, make sure that it is way down the list of ingredients. This is because ingredients are listed in order of abundance. The first ingredients listed are indeed the most abundant by volume. If you are uncertain about the pH of a particular shampoo or need to find out how much (by percent volume) laurly sulfate (or other detergent) is in the product, then please call the manufacturer before

575 Zoe Diane Draelos, M.D., "Moisterizing mechanism, MVEs; ph-balanced cleansers," accessed January 30, 2006 http://www.dermatologytimes.com/dermatologytimes/article/articleDetail.jsp?id=183469.
576 Pickart, Reverse Skin Aging: Using Your Skin's Natural Power, 114.

buying it. Be aware that some "natural" shampoos may have a pH that is too high for comfort. Preserving natural hair and skin oil is the key to a healthy scalp. The acid mantle or natural acidity of then scalp should not be disturbed. Dr. Pickart recommends that shampoos have a pH between 4.5 and 6.0 because in this way the natural scalp oil or sebum is preserved to protect the scalp from foreign bacteria.[577] Grow longer hair to keep the follicle larger, your scalp thicker and more pliable, and well oiled (i.e., enough oil to keep the scalp's connective tissue pliable). For a list of good quality shampoos see Appendix II.

Some believe there should be absolutely no detergent in shampoo at all. Recall that Sodium *Laureth* Sulfate is a mild detergent, much more mild than Sodium *Lauryl* Sulfate. Also, Pickart (Chapter 11) does say that if any product foams, then you have used too much. Recall the main problem with detergents (i.e., the sulfates) is that the quantity is much too high in most store-bought shampoos. Shampoos with a little detergent will not foam that much. Pickart also believes that a pH of 6.3 is just slightly more basic (or alkaline) than the skin's natural acid mantle is best. Thus far, the author of this writing has tried Folligen, Giovanni, Ginesis, Nature's gate "Organics," Shi Kai, Jason's Aloe Vera 84% Shampoo, and Super Hair Energizer (to be discussed in more detail later).

All these products work very well. Alternating between shampoos is probably a good idea, unless you are using a specialty product such as Super Hair Energizer to regrow hair. There probably are many more mild shampoos on the market. The questions are: (1) is the pH close to neutral or slightly acidic (mimic the skin's acid mantle), and (2) what type of and how much detergent is in the product? Remember to use very little shampoo. If it foams a lot, then that is a sign that you have used too much shampoo by volume. If this occurs, reduce the quantity next time you shampoo until only little to no foaming occurs.

Dr. Loren Pickart's Copper Peptides and Emu Oil

If you want healthy hair then you must have healthy skin. To speed up the process of scalp rejuvenation then you may want to consider Folligen®, a copper-peptide product, and emu oil. Dr. Loren Pickart discovered that skin remodeling copper peptides (SRCPs) increase the size of the hair follicles.[578] His product is called Folligen®, and is considered the best copper

---

577 Pickart, Reverse Skin Aging: Using Your Skin's Natural Power, 114.
578 Pickart, Reverse Skin Aging: Using Your Skin's Natural Power, 159.

peptide product on the market. After all, Dr. Pickart is the discoverer and inventor. The enlarged hair follicle then grows coarser hair (i.e., larger diameter) and also produces stem cells to rebuild the scalp.

Another beneficial product was discovered thousands of years ago by the Australian Aborigines: emu oil. "The fatty acid composition of human skin oil and emu oil is similar."[579] On his website, Pickart quotes Dr. Michael Holick of the Boston University Medical Center, who reported a clinical study in which emu oil accelerated skin regeneration and stimulated hair growth: "The hair follicles were more robust, the skin thickness was remarkably increased…Also, we discovered in the same test that over 80 percent of hair follicles that had been 'asleep' were awakened, and began growing hair."[580]

To get started, discard your store bought hair care products before taking the next step towards healing the scalp. After that, and if you decide to try Folligen and emu oil, start with Folligen first for skin repair. Folligen Solution Therapy Spray is very inexpensive. Later you may want to add emu oil, a rather expensive product, if needed. For hair regrowth, many of Skin Biology's customers have reported that the combination of Folligen (copper peptides) and emu oil often produce great "reductions in hair loss and increased hair growth."[581]

Copper is even good for blocking the negative effects of DHT. As stated earlier DHT, the male hormone problem, can add its negative effects to the scalp and accelerate hair loss. The enzyme system that converts testosterone into DHT occurs in two enzyme forms. The Type 1 form is located in various places of the skin and is the type that is the primary one that damages hair follicles. Copper ion in the skin is more effective in inhibiting the Type 1 form and is applied locally to the scalp with Folligen. The application of copper-peptides inhibits DHT production in the scalp.[582]

Pickart goes on to instruct us that the Type 2 form is located mainly in the seminal vesicles, prostate and in the inner root sheath of the hair follicle. Propecia® (Finasteride), which has a higher affinity for the Type 2 form, is best suited for controlling prostate enlargement. It must be administered by pills, which spread the drug throughout the body.

579 Pickart, Reverse Skin Aging: Using Your Skin's Natural Power, 88.
580 Loren Pickart, "Stimulating Hair Growth through Skin Renewal and Skin Remodeling Copper Peptides," accessed July 7, 2010 http://reverseskinaging.com/hairloss7.html.
581 Pickart, "Stimulating Hair Growth through Skin Renewal and Skin Remodeling Copper Peptides."
582 Pickart, Reverse Skin Aging: Using Your Skin's Natural Power, 105.

Unless you have prostate problems, the obvious conclusion would be to consider the copper peptide product, Folligen, first. If you are not sure which type you have, see a physician. For natural remedies to the prostate problem see the nutritional section. In conjunction with copper peptides and/or emu oil use any one of the shampoos listed in Appendix II, one to three times per week. Dr. Peter H. Proctor's hair re-growth products also contain copper peptides (Appendix II).

But not all agree that copper peptides are the answer. In her book, "Don't Go Shopping for Hair Care Products Without Me," Paula Begoun says that "copper peptides are overhyped and unproven for stimulating hair growth in humans."[583] She further dismisses the Boston University study about emu oil cited on Pickart's website, and found that the study was neither published nor substantiated. Begoun may have a point.

On the other hand, scientific research and getting anything published in writing is a very costly and time-consuming business. Thus, Dr. Michael Holick may have the data of the benefits of emu oil, but may lack the funding for an extensive research and writing project. There are always a plethora of research projects to do. One must bear in mind that Dr. Loren Pickart is a renowned scientist in his own right. So it seems doubtful that Pickart would misquote or misrepresent another colleague, then publish this quote for the whole world to see on his website, and to do so over the course of many years.

Hopefully, a detailed study about emu oil will be published in writing some day. But until then, please recall that emu oil is very close in nature to human skin oil. The truth of the matter is that we are stripping too much of our own natural oil away by using harsh detergent-laden shampoos. Once you stop using these harsh shampoos perhaps your scalp will heal itself over time even with its own oil, sebum. However, to speed up the healing process copper peptides or emu oil or both may help heal your scalp at a faster rate initially than doing nothing at all. Although Paula Begoun's review includes an impressive 4,000 products, she did not mention anything about the more natural shampoos recommended in this book, such as Giovanni, Nature's Gate and Real Purity. She also missed what may prove to be two of the best products in the world. These are Super Hair Energizer and clinically proven Thymuskin®. The importance of scalp oil cannot be emphasized enough. Even the primary ingredient in Super Hair Energizer is jojoba oil!

583 Paula Begoun, Don't Go Shopping for Hair Care Products without Me (Seattle, WA: Beginning Press, 2004), 339.

Super Hair Energizer

The first time I found out about Super Hair Energizer was from a report purchased through ebay called "How I Stopped Going Bald & Stopped My Hair Loss." This author named John suggests four main causes of hair loss: (1) DHT, (2) sodium lauryl sulfate, (3) waxy sebum buildup within the follicle, and (4) when the scalp becomes thinner and tighter. These are all excellent conclusions based on his independent research and experience. Obviously, John stopped using shampoos with sodium lauryl sulfate and he came to understand that the negative effects of DHT can be minimized. His research unveiled that the hair growth phase (anagen) is reduced to months rather than the normal two to seven years. Even worse, he found that the hair loss, or shedding phase called telogen, is stretched from the normal three months to an incredible four years by the damaging effects of sodium lauryl sulfate! When the shedding phase is stretched up to four years, baldness occurs. To decrease the negative effects of DHT, John uses the natural herb Saw Palmetto (see nutrition section) in lieu of Propecia®.

Since John began using Super Hair Energizer his hair loss completely stopped. He gradually grew his hair back in receding and balding areas over the course of two years, "with awesome results." Patience is vital. He faithfully used the shampoo, follicle stimulator, and jojoba oil as directed. The products remove the hardened buildup in the follicles. The scalp and hair return to a "normal, healthy, vibrant growing state." He refers to Super Hair Energizer as the "miracle product." He remarked that it takes two years to turn a "peach fuzz" vellus hair follicle into a mature coarser hair (full diameter terminal hair). After a little more than two years his re-growth began to slow down to his satisfaction. He then began to use Thymuskin® (see below) in conjunction with Super Hair Energizer's shampoo. After using Thymuskin® (apparently the "treatment") for five months his hair regrowth rate increased significantly.

After he worked on his scalp over this time period, his picture now shows a man with a full head of hair. Along with Super Hair Energizer, John did several things every day to stimulate his scalp. His scalp was thin and tight especially in balding areas. He said that it is imperative that the connective tissue of the scalp is kept "loose and pliable." So he massaged his scalp, firmly combed his hair and scalp, and used electrical stimulation. John used his fingertips and applied firm pressure while massaging in small circles. The combing of the scalp helped loosen compacted waxy buildup of the follicles. To keep his connective tissue loose, he used a device called a "Magic Comb," which provided electrical stimulation. When I purchased his report, he sent his photograph (with his face blanked out for privacy). His hair was short, probably about one to two inches in length, typical for many modern males. Presumably, he probably wore it short most of his life prior to going bald. All the things John did to stimulate his scalp seem to mimic the effects of longer hair. The weight and movement of longer hair naturally keeps the scalp looser, more pliable and stimulated. An added benefit is that sebum can be combed down a longer hair shaft so that it does not build up on the scalp and within the follicles. Massaging the scalp, like he did, in firm small circles is an excellent way to keep the scalp pliable and healthy.

Super Hair Energizer can be purchased through a few places on the Internet. One particularly helpful company is Hair Growth Solutions. The owner began using the product in 1999 when he was 38 years old. Within three to four days his hair loss stopped. In three weeks he noticed baby fine hair. He still has some receding area that has not filled in, but he and many others are happy with the results. He now sells the product. Contact information for Super Hair Energizer can be found in Appendix II.

Hair Growth Solutions website has several other testimonies about the product.[584] As an example, here are two of them:

I've used Rogaine for years, with practically no results. After a month, I've had what I consider an amazing fill-in to the Vee that was moving my front hairline back towards my ears.

It's growing like magic. Now I have long hair in my old bald spot.

Another major distributor for Super Hair Energizer (Paul Oberdorf – see contact information in Appendix II) claims to have more than 10,000 testimonies. Oberdorf has been selling the product since 1996 and has pages of testimonies he will send you or you can see on his website.[585] Hair loss stops after a short time of use. Testimonies also include the healing of eczema, which can also cause hair loss, psoriasis, and flaky scalp. Hair becomes more manageable and most importantly, there is hair re-growth. Others also call it a miracle product, just like the testimony from John. The product has been manufactured since 1975. Back when I was healing my scalp I used the product and find it to be excellent, and it is reasonably priced.

---

584 http://www.hairgrowthsolutions.com/.
585 Paul Oberdorff, NMS Publishing, 5711 14th Avenue, Brooklyn, NY 11219 Ph: 718-871-1363 accessed July 7, 2010 http://www.superhair.net/.

A primary ingredient in Super Hair Energizer is jojoba oil. The positive effects of jojoba oil for skin and hair have been well known for many years. Hofstein remarks that jojoba oil is very beneficial by being structurally "very similar to the sebum" produced by the follicle.[586] But the effects of hair *re-growth* from pure jojoba oil alone are negligible according to Oberdorf. However, a fermented version of jojoba apparently does cause dormant hair (vellus hairs or peach fuzz) to re-grow into visible terminal hair. Super Hair Energizer is made from a proprietary blending process of 26 botanicals and the pulp of the jojoba bean, involving 23 steps over a three-month aging period! Botanical extraction, fermentation, bacterial cultivation, distillation and an enzymatic sequence all results in an exclusive product ingredient called Ferm-T®.

Ferm-T® (in the Super Hair Energizer products) produces wondrous results with pure herbal ingredients, free of chemicals, pollutants, drugs, and strong detergents. The amount of ammonium lauryl sulfate is very small, like it should be. In fact, the first application of the product foams little. Recall that many typical store bought shampoos may contain 20 percent lauryl sulfate based detergents, which is far too much for the scalp. Both the pH of 7.1 to 7.2 and the small amount (approximately 2.1 percent) of ammonium lauryl sulfate are in the acceptable range. According to the literature, as discussed previously, ammonium lauryl sulfate is milder than sodium lauryl sulfate. The bottom line is that Super Hair Energizer is backed by thousands of testimonials. The product is manufactured by Ferm-T Worldwide, Tempe, Arizona.

Thymuskin®

Thymuskin® is one of the most scientifically backed products on the market. If you believe your hair loss is caused by an autoimmune disorder then this may be the product for you. It was developed in Germany and proven clinically effective in hundreds of patients during nine independent studies over the last 19 years. At least eight universities were, and still are, involved, along with the German Cancer Research Center in Heidelberg and the Ministry of Science and Technology in Bonn-Bad Godesberg. The product was originally developed to stop hair loss during cancer treatments such as chemotherapy, which is cytotoxic to the body. Cancer treatments are extremely hard on the immune system. As we proved earlier, hair loss in males and females causes stress. Stress due to hair loss causes the defenses of the body's immune system to diminish even more. The researchers

586 Hofstein, 68.

found that the healing process during cancer treatments becomes severely hindered due to stress when patients lost their hair. According to Professor Hagedorn, when Thymuskin® "treatment" and "shampoo" are massaged into the scalp right from the beginning of cytotoxic therapy (i.e., cancer treatment), the patient's hair will not fall out. He states there are also "spectacular results for hair regrowth in patients with long-standing total baldness."[587]

Besides all the manmade causes of thinning hair cited in this book, some doctors believe baldness is an autoimmune disease.[588] In this type of baldness the immune system goes "haywire." The body's own immune system turns various sets of hair follicles into autoantigens, a perceived invader. Autoantibodies, white blood cells, are then produced to attack the perceived invaders, the hair follicles! Any part of the immune system can malfunction in this way. Recall earlier that some my have a sensitive skin organ, including sensitive follicles, while others may have a sensitive heart, sensitive kidneys, etc. Thymuskin® was developed to address this autoimmune disease. What if there is another possibility? Could it be that skin irritants like sodium lauryl sulfate and methylisothiazolinone can change the hair follicles into such a damaged thing, that the white blood cells are actually attacking the follicles simply because they are no longer recognizable as follicles? This is just a thought, but it may make a good research project for some young medical student.

The primary organ of the immune system is the thymus, a gland located deep in the chest beneath the breastbone. Professor Hagedorn says the thymus gland acts as a regulator of the immune system. As a person gets older, the thymus gland shrinks and this condition correlates with the augmentation of autoimmune diseases. Under the microscope baldness has been shown to be an autoimmune disease where white blood cells (leukocytes consisting of lymphocytes and macrophages) actually attack hair follicles and cause them to go into dormancy.[589]

Thymuskin® stops this autoimmune attack on hair follicles. Thymuskin® is not a drug, but a stimulative natural substance possessed by every person. The substance is called thymosin, a hormone secreted by the thymus gland, is abundant in youth but diminishes with age. Thymosin the product also includes herbs and other nutrients. Along with hair re-growth, other positive benefits include increased numbers of T-lymphocytes in the

---

587 Morton Walker, Bald No More, 9-10.
588 Morton Walker, How to Stop Baldness and Regrow Hair, 49.
589 Morton Walker, How to Stop Baldness and Regrow Hair, 8, 17.

bloodstream to fight of bacterial infections, and it fights off toxic metals, foreign proteins, viral organisms, cancer cells, and other true antigens that attempt to break down the body's immunity. Thymuskin® makes hair follicles less vulnerable to hormonal changes when body chemistry has gone awry. In men, and some women, it is believed to make hair follicles less sensitive to DHT. In short, it boosts the immune system.

The good news is that dormant follicles (i.e. peach fuzz) can be re-activated. Recall the scientific term for common hair thinning and baldness in men and women is called *alopecia androgenetica (or hereditaria)*. Recall that what you really inherent from your ancestors is a pre-disposition, or sensitive skin, for going bald or having thinning hair problems. The clinical studies in Germany have an extraordinary success rate to reverse so-called common baldness, androgenetic alopecia. These were "conducted by nine scientific investigators in eight medical departments at eight locations in Germany and Austria" with "several hundred patients." The incredible results are that 67 percent of men and 94 percent of women have reversed their hair loss.[590] But again patience is required. After one to three months of use, hair loss is greatly reduced. Hair re-growth occurs anywhere from from nine to 24 months. If hair loss has been heavy and present for more than four years, then do not expect new and stronger hair until up to eighteen months of application. In the U.S. Thymuskin® can be purchased through Biotechne Complex, Inc. where the product has been sold since 1995 (see Appendix II).

Thymuskin® is manufactured in Manheim, Germany. Thymuskin® "Treatment" is the product designed to re-grow hair. It can be applied to the scalp twice per day or at a minimum, once per day. Thymuskin® "Shampoo" must be used in conjunction with the "Treatment." The shampoo is especially designed to clean and penetrate the roots of the follicles. The pH of 5.4 is excellent and perfectly in line with the skin's natural acidity. Although Biotechne's representatives may suggest using the shampoo daily, the scientists involved in the study say to shampoo every other day or perhaps just twice a week. It may depend on how oily your scalp and hair is. Try not to use other products while using Thymuskin® "Treatment" and "Shampoo."

According to representatives at Biotechne, other products can plug up the hair follicles. The possible exception to this is Super Hair Energizer's shampoo, at least according to John's testimony given earlier. Use the "Gel" in lieu of the "Treatment" if you have dry scalp (see Thymuskin's

---

590 Morton Walker, Bald No More, 173-174.

website). Two detailed testimonies in Walker's book indicate that hair re-growth occurred between six to nine months of continuous use.[591] Other good testimonies can be found on Biotechne's website. Use Thymuskin® for 18 months, maybe up to 24 months. Thymuskin® is fairly expensive, but the success rate is very high. After two years of application, you do not have to use it anymore. Chances are good that your hair grew back. After completion of Thymuskin® be sure to grow your hair longer, and use any of the shampoos already mentioned, Super Hair Energizer, Giovanni 50/50, Ginesis, Avalon Organics or the other shampoos listed in Appendix II.

In 2003 and 2004, scientists in the United States discovered that thymosin stimulates hair growth. These fairly recent studies indicate that "a novel small molecule" called thymosin beta4 "increases hair growth by activation of hair follicle stem cells."[592] It appears that the United States is nearly 20 years behind the Germans.

Riquette Hofstein's Method

In her book, "Grow Hair Fast," Hofstein says "when you were born, you had the capacity to live your entire life with a full head of healthy, attractive hair."[593] She understands the damage caused by store-bought hair "care" products, the importance of natural scalp oil (sebum), and the importance of blood flow to the papilla (Figures 2-1; 3-2). Concerning so-called male pattern baldness, the production of keratin is disrupted and sebum begins to build up in the follicle. "The follicle then becomes blocked, inducing further damage to the tiny structure."[594] She believes sebum buildup within the follicle is the literal "root cause of hair loss." Her method addresses this problem (a probable form of seborrheic dermatitis) and takes from three months to about one year.

Hofstein's seven step program has been tested on thousands of clients over the last 30 years. The first two steps of her program are the "magic haircut" and proper brushing.[595] Every tiny dormant vellus hair or peach fuzz is carefully lifted and cut. Second, the hair is to be brushed once or twice a day – a boar's hair brush is recommended. Ironically, these first two

---

591 Morton Walker, Bald No More, 90-92; 127-130. It takes several months to re-grow hair.
592 D. Philp, M. Nguyen, B. Scheremeta, S. St-Surin, A.M. Villa, A. Orgel, H.K. Kleinman and M. Elkin, "Thymosin beta4 increases hair growth by activation of hair follicle stem cells," FASEB J., 2004 Feb;18(2):385-7. Epub 2003 Dec 4. PMID: 14657002 accessed April 16, 2006 http://www.ncbi.nlm.nih.gov/entrez/query.fcgi?CMD=Display&DB=pubmed.
593 Hofstein, 6.
594 Hofstein, 21.
595 Hofstein, 41-46.

steps have more to do with stimulating the hair follicle. The "lifting" of each hair combined with the gentle "pulling" effect during brushing both stimulates blood flow to the scalp. This "lifting and pulling" encourages the proper function of the tiny *erector pili* muscles, whose job is to squeeze the sebaceous glands. Lifting and pulling mimics extra weight. This lubricates the hair with sebum, which promotes a more lustrous, healthy condition. She never quite makes the connection that longer hair is healthier and the weight thereof also causes stimulation of the follicle. The reader should recall that the extra weight of longer hair actually tugs or pulls on the follicle too, the "longer the hair, the stronger the root."[596]

Steps three through seven in her book "Grow Hair Fast" show you in recipe format how to make your own scalp stimulator, sloughing solution, shampoo, and protective sealing solution to restore the acid mantle of the hair and scalp. She gives pages upon pages of recipes with ingredients, including herbs that can be easily purchased just about anywhere. If you do not want to make your own solutions, contact her organization directly. She too has many testimonies and other information on her website. Her contact information is located in Appendix II.

According to her book, one chief ingredient in the shampoo is castile soap. Castile soap can be purchased through several sources – you should inquire of its pH. If you go this route find one that is pH balanced. On the other hand, if you purchase the products from Riquette International directly, follow the directions from them. Even if the pH of their shampoo turns out to be high (on the basic or alkaline side of the pH scale), bear in mind that the follow-up to the shampoo is the "protective sealing lotion," the purpose of which is to restore the skin's natural acid balance.[597]

Laser Hair Comb

Along with the use of non-harmful topical products, hair re-growth success is being achieved with laser hair combs. We already discussed the importance of adequate sunlight. When laser light is applied to the scalp it energizes the bio-chemical cellular function of the follicles. The process is called photo bio-stimulation. The method is clinically proven by many independent researchers and has no side effects. A 90 percent user satisfaction is claimed. Dr. David Kingsley has independently verified good results on his patients with a laser hair comb at his trichology clinic in New

---

596 Pickart, Reverse Skin Aging: Using Your Skin's Natural Power, 117. It is also interesting that Riquette Hofstein's methods mimic the effects of longer hair.
597 Hofstein, 55, 59-61.

York.[598] Manufacturers of laser hair combs can be found in Appendix II. Much more information can be gained through their websites.

Topical Niacin

Along with the laser hair comb, Dr. Kingsley uses topical niacin (i.e., nicotinic acid or vitamin B3) as part of his overall scalp treatment strategy.[599] As Kingsley recognizes, hair loss must be addressed from the outside (topical) and from the inside, meaning good health and healthy food. Dr. Peter H. Proctor's NANO shampoo has also found great success with hair re-growth by using nicotinic acid in his formulations (Appendix II). Topical niacin combined with a good vitamin B dietary supplement discussed earlier could do much good.

598 David H. Kingsley, The Hair-Loss Cure, A Self-Help Guide (Bloomington, IN: iUniverse, 2009), 49-50.
599 Kingsley, 50-51.

Chapter 14: Crown of Life

‖‖

Blessed is the man that endureth temptation: for when he is tried, he shall receive the crown of life, which the Lord hath promised to them that love him (James 1:12).

As you learned, human beings have the potential for a full head of healthy hair for life. The problem is man's interference. In modern times men are often peer-pressured to shear their heads. As the blind lead the blind they all fall in the ditch, having a barren head with dead follicles, or even worse, skin cancer. Only a strong man can stand against the temptation to become addicted to the scissors and razor. The online article *Skin Cancer Primary Prevention and Education Initiative* has an interesting quote by Dr. David Satcher:

> There is good news: skin cancer can be prevented. The challenge, however, lies in changing the attitudes and behaviors that increase a person's risk of developing skin cancer.[600]

So what attitudes really need changed? The negative attitude against male hair must stop. What behavior must change? How about this: stop cutting yourself short! The facts gathered in this book are here to help you solve real manmade problems. The trichotemnomania, or hair-cut madness, of the 20th century military, some religious institutions and churches, some corporations, and marketers have, in my opinion, caused great damage. Sadly, most have no idea that they are, in part, responsible for these diseases. If an organization forces you to close-crop your head, share this knowledge with them. Find out the origin of the rule and talk to that person only, the decision maker. If they repent, they will

---

600 "Skin Cancer Primary Prevention and Education Initiative," accessed November 3, 2005 http://www.cdc.gov/cancer/nscpep/.

256

be like the wise man who believes in the health and well being of their employees.

If not, then they are like a foolish man who obviously cares not about your health and well being, you are nothing to them. Do you want to work for such a person? Do you want to attend church or a so-called "Bible" college in such a place? Ultimately you must take charge for your own health. Try standing up for yourself, but be sure to do it in a respectful way. Thanks to those corporations and religious institutions who allow their men to wear long natural hair without godless manmade rules. Who knows, perhaps modern men will once again gain the same freedom that our long-haired founding fathers had. Females have been freed from the veil and display their long hair. Many of them wish for their men to grow out their hair, so why are men less free now than when the country was founded? Why are men less free than women? True equality is for both sexes to display their long hair as God designed.

The publication of this book will be controversial, not because of the common sense and truth it provides, but more about its implications to certain businesses. Businesses apt to dismiss this book include those who sell artificial hair care products, razors, drugs, and surgical services, since they do little to promote prevention. The health care industry should do more with regards to teaching prevention. But we live in a time when large corporations do not want to be liable for fear of law suits. But the truth is all marketers only care about one thing, which is making money at your expense. They too are especially ignorant about the overuse of scissors and razors, and the awful effects caused by chemical-laden poisonous shampoos, hair dyes, chlorine, artificial foods and so forth. Other than excessive hair cutting and cutting head hair too short, shorter than body hair, here again are the acts of self-flagellation people do to themselves: poor diet, no exercise, no peace, over-washing with harsh detergents, baking the scalp in the sun since the hair is too short to protect it, chemicals placed on the head, shaving head and neck hair, which causes razor burn, cuts, scabs, rash, warts, scars, viral infections, bacterial infections and various other skin eruptions. Why keep your dermatologist busy by fighting these things when all you have to do is grow some hair? These are not the marks of a sane society, but shear nonsense.

And what about the cost of skin cancers of the head, ears and neck? Surgeons are then employed to dissect these cancers with the knife, or burn them off with a torch. Their job is to remove it, not teach you how to prevent it in the first place. Is short hair worth skin cancer? Now that you know the truth, only you can make real changes. By following the guidelines stated in this book, you will be on your way to saving and keeping your hair, and even re-activate your dormant hair follicles for a fuller head of hair. Longer hair means cancer prevention. Less cancer means less surgery. For your sake, use common sense.

The products cited in this book to help re-grow hair are backed by thousands of testimonies. They are superior products worthy of attention. Use them. But do not forget about spinal care, proper nutrition, exercise, stress relief and the host of other things necessary for good health. You are the one ultimately responsible for the health of your own body. You can listen to those who only preach drugs and surgery, who prevent or heal nothing. Or you can listen to reason as outlined in the preceding pages. Many of your male children do not wish to go bald. Young people express this concern all the time. When they see their father go bald, they automatically believe that they will to, that it is inevitable. Hopefully you no longer believe that fable. For such a belief is utter nonsense as long as they are taught the facts. Teach your children how to take care of their crown properly. The crown or scalp is a very delicate area in humans. Prevention of hair loss is better than trying to re-grow hair. Thus, for your own children's sake, you must be willing to share this knowledge with them. Why pass a generational curse along to them when you can pass along great knowledge instead? Please do not be a person who is destroyed by ignorance. Obviously, if you made it to this point in the book, congratulations, you are no longer unaware.

Hair is your natural crown. Its symbolism is quite profound. Remember, in old age white hair is called a "crown of glory" (Proverbs 16:31). Apparently, it was assumed that an old person's hair would turn white like John Wesley's long hair did, and not go bald. With the knowledge you just gained by reading this book your chances of white, long hair in old age, instead of a shiny, sweaty, bald head, have been greatly advanced. In reality, baldness could be called a crown of death. This is true because, as we already learned, baldness is a disease caused by cell damage or cell death in the scalp. And the manmade causes of this damage are striking as already stated throughout this book.

In Scripture, some people originally had a crown of life, a full head of long hair, but later received a crown of death, baldness, either temporarily or permanently. Job (pronounced Jōbe) is a case in point. When Job received word that his entire family was killed, he shaved his head, a picture of death to mourn the loss (Job 1:20). After this, Job was inflicted with boils all over his body including his "crown" or scalp, a punishment attributed to Satan. This infection could have damaged his hair follicles greatly. To make matters worse, Job scratched the sores with a broken piece of pottery (Job 2:7-8). He likely became bald, or very thin, for he was stripped of his "glory" and the "crown" was taken from his "head" (Job 19:9). He must have looked like he had mange. For the record, Job, like many people, did not deserve to go bald, for he was considered a righteous man (Job 1:8). In this case, God was testing his faith. After he passed the test his scalp was probably restored to a degree unknown. A crown of death was also given to certain lewd women who were described as being arrogantly proud and wanton, unduly extravagant, cruel, merciless and inhumane.

Therefore the Lord will smite with a scab the crown of the head of the daughters of Zion, and the Lord will discover their secret parts (Isaiah 3:17).

These proud females were inflicted with sores called "scabs" (scalp cancer?) on "the crown of the head," which led to baldness (Isaiah 3:16-24). Their "secret parts" could be seen. The secret parts are obviously all the nooks, crannies, lumps, bumps, and other scalp blemishes now exposed. For women and men alike, one purpose of head hair is to hide such unsightly features, which obviously become visible on a bald or thinning head. Thus the common epithets of potato head, lump head, or block head were coined especially for crop-headed men. These two stories convey the point that the crown or scalp of your head is a very, very sensitive area. Stress in one form or fashion may have played a significant role in these cases of baldness. Your crown should not be taken for granted. Instead, head hair must be handled with care. If not, problems will arise. Naturally, when the scalp becomes inflamed and irritated with boils, sores and scabs, hair loss is the result. The funny thing in modern times is God does not have to punish our heads. We do it to ourselves.

All the researchers cited in this book agree that you have the capability to have a full head of healthy hair for life. Possible exceptions to this would be those born with rare skin diseases. A healthy head of long hair is a crown of life. This crown symbolizes "eternal life." This is especially true in the case of the long, uncut hair of the Nazarite all around the circumference of the head. In fact, healthy hair is so well constructed that often it is the only thing that remains, besides the skeleton, in the most ancient of burial sites. One could say that this virtually incorruptible hair is nearly immortal or eternal, even in the physical realm. Remarkably, a "crown of life" is promised to all those who love the Lord (James 1:12). The long hair extending in all directions from the head means that eternal life is offered to all peoples of all cultures everywhere on earth, even the utmost corners thereof. This eternal life is granted to all who come to faith in the One resurrected from the dead, the ultimate Nazarite, Jesus Christ, the Son of the Most High.

According to Enoch's vision, the righteous citizens (white sheep) of Heaven have long, uncut, pure, hair:

The sheep were all white, with wool long and pure (Enoch 89:42).

God wants you to have a crown of life. What would you rather have?

Appendix I
Greek Analysis of 1 Corinthians 11:14-15

‖‖

When writing the books of the New Testament, punctuation was rare, and no accents were placed above Greek words, and the Bible verse numbering system did not exist. Here is a quick history of Bible translation:

1. The signs for the accents were not regularly employed in manuscripts until after 600 A.D.[601]
2. In the 4th and 5th centuries Jerome (347 – 420 A.D.) began to add the comma and colon and these were inserted in many more ancient manuscripts.
3. The stroke that we call a comma (,) was invented in the 8th century.
4. The Greek note of interrogation (;) was first used in the 9th century. This has become our question mark (?).
5. In the middle of the 16th century (1551 A.D.) verses in which the New Testament is now divided was introduced by Robert Stephens.[602]

Because of these problems it becomes clear that difficult or controversial passages be translated from the Greek text as original as possible, without the later additions of accents and punctuation. Many scholars have recognized this problem. Thanks to Logos Bible Software, Stephen's Textus Receptus (1550) with Morphology (Stephanus) is an original Greek without accents and punctuation.[603] This is the Greek text utilized in this appendix. With the use of this tool translations can begin afresh without the bias of another person's idea about punctuation and accents being imposed upon the text.

---

601 Herbert Weir Smyth, Greek Grammar (Cambridge, MA: Harvard University Press, 1920. Revised by Gordon M. Messing, 1956. Renewed 1984), 38.

602 Thomas Hartwell Horne, An Introduction to the Critical Study and Knowledge of the Holy Scriptures (New York: Robert Carter and Brothers, 1854) 213-215. Bullet points 2-5 (above) are from this source.

603 Robertus Stephanus and Maurice A. Robinson, Stephen's Textus Receptus (1550) With Morphology (Logos Research Systems, Inc., 2002).

14

2228	3761	846	2228	5449	1321	5209	3754	435	3303	1437	2863	819	846	2076
η	ουδε	αυτη	η	φυσις	διδασκει	υμας	οτι	ανηρ	μεν	εαν	κομα	ατιμια	αυτω	εστιν
ay	oude	aute	ay	phusis	didaskei	humas	hoti	aner	men	ean	koma	atimia	auto	estin
-	neither	itself	-	nature	teach	you	that	man	indeed	if	long hair	dishonor	him	is
or	not even				teaches						adorn hair	disgrace		

15

1135	1161	1437	2863	1391	846	2076	3754	2228	2864	473	4018	1325	846
γυνη	δε	εαν	κομα	δοξα	αυτη	εστιν	οτι	η	κομη	αντι	περιβολαιου	δεδοται	αυτη
gune	de	ean	koma	doxa	aute	estin	hoti	ay	kome	anti	peribolaiou	dedotai	aute
woman	but	if	long hair	glory	her	is	that	the	hair	for	veil	given	[her]
	and		adorn hair						long hair		mantle		

her long hair

tresses or beautified hair

According to Robinson, the early Greek Textus Receptus (TR) editions generally reflect, but not completely, the "Byzantine Textform," otherwise called the "Majority" or "Traditional" text, which predominated throughout the period of manual copying of Greek New Testament manuscripts.

An English transliteration of the Greek alphabet occurs below each Greek term. The numbers, above each Greek word, are those utilized in Green's Interlinear Bible, which is based on Strong's numbering system. The most common English words used by translators occur below the Greek. Various translations are possible depending on what assumptions are made.

Now that we have ridded ourselves of the later additions of punctuation and accented words, there are still a few issues. The issues even with this untainted Greek text are, (1) is the writer posing a question or a statement? (2) what does "nature itself" mean? and (3) what do the Greek words *koma* and *kome* mean in the context of this passage? It is over these primary issues why disagreement exists amongst scholars leading to the various interpretive translations.

Question or Statement?

Thus, the first problem is how verse 14 should begin. Tyndale – 1534 and "The Interlinear Bible" (Green) translate η as *or*, which is certainly legitimate. Other translators do not. Most translators think η marks the beginning of another question with "or" or without "or" at the beginning of the statement.

In this regard η as a "particle" at the beginning of a statement is often not translated, hence the dash (-) placed under the Greek as a word, but is either used to, (1) begin an alternative question that follows a simple direct question, or (2) not introduce an alternative to a previous question, but substitutes another question, which is more specific and intended to anticipate the answer to the first question, or (3) introduce an argument to the contrary, which is used when a person wishes to refute with irony, or (4) introduces questions asking merely for information and imply nothing as to the expected answer.[604] However, others believe η at the

---

604 Herbert Weir Smyth, Greek Grammar (Cambridge, MA: Harvard University Press, 1920. Revised by Gordon M. Messing, 1956. Renewed 1984). Smyth's book defines the particle η with accents for these various meanings, but since the original Greek New Testament had accents the particle must be interpreted. See his #2656 through 2661 (p. 599-600); #2856 through 2861 (p. 648-649).

beginning of verse 14 to be a later insertion, not in the original Greek.[605] This makes it difficult to know whether we are dealing with a question or non-question. This is why some translations are questions while others are simply sentences.

Nature Itself

Some commentators think that Paul's use of "nature itself" has to do with customs or culture rather than what is physically natural. However, φυσις, *phusis* (Strong's number 5449) means nature, natural, natural growth; from 5453 *phuo: grow, sprout, produce*; phusikos, meaning *physical* is from *phusis*; the study of physics descended from these words. The article η can be written either between words or before the words in which a word relationship is shown.[606] Thus, the phrase such as αυτη η φυσις, *aute ay phusis* in verse 14 means *nature itself* (or *nature herself*). This emphasis is very important and indicates that Paul is referring to what is physically natural. It certainly is natural for a man to have long hair. The rendering *nature herself* is very similar to the common American phrase *mother nature*.

Hair, Long Hair, Adorn the Hair, Ornate Hair, Tresses, Beautified Hair?

The following is how the words κομα, *koma and* κομη, *kome* are generally defined:[607 608 609]

2863 κομα, *koma* is from 2864 κομη, *kome (see below)*. κομα, *koma* (or *coma*) – *wear tresses of hair* (Strong); *have long hair* (Strong; Thayer); to *let the hair grow* (Thayer); *hair* generically and figuratively used for other things such as plaited hair or tresses (Tischendorf). The exact meaning over this word in context is problematic.

---

605 Nestle-Aland Novum Testamentum Graece Et Latine. Stuttgart: Deutsche Bibelgesellschaft. Apparently the Alexandrian text that underlies this Greek edition does not have the particle η thus they believe it to be a later insertion.

606 Smyth, 296.

607 James Strong, Greek Dictionary in Strong's Exhaustive Concordance of the Bible (Gordonsville, TN: Dugan Publishers, Inc.).

608 Joseph H. Thayer, Thayer's Greek-English Lexicon of the New Testament (Originally published by T. & T. Clark, Edinburgh, 1896. Peabody, MA: Hendrickson Publishers, first printing – June 1996).

609 Tischendorf, Constantinus Von. Novum Testamentum Graece: To Which Is Added A Greek And English Lexicon With Examples of All The Irregular And More Difficult Inflections (1860). Dublin: W.B. Kelly, p. 46.

2864 κομη, *kome – hair of the head; locks, as ornamental* thus differing from 2359, the usual words for hair: θριξ, *thrix* and τριχες, *trichos*, which denotes merely scalp hair. Thayer says it means "hair, head of hair … by designating the hair as an ornament (the notion of length being only secondary and suggested)." Κομη from the same as 2865 *komizo*, which is from *komeo – to tend* or *to provide for* (Strong; Thayer). The etymology of the English word *coma* is from the Greek κομη (*kome*), hair of the head. In astronomy, the English word *comet* in Greek is κομητης (*kometes*), from κομη, head of hair, tail of comet.[610] Forms of κομη are also found in the ancient Greek Septuagint (LXX) translation of Leviticus 19:27 and Numbers 6:5d. In Leviticus 19:27, the forbidden rounding of the "corners" (Hebrew *payaw*) is translated κομης, *komes*. The plural "corners" occur not just before the ears, but also behind the ears, therefore the hair of men in general was not permitted to be cut off short. Then there is the κομην τριχα, *komen tricha*, or *long hair* (locks, *pera* in Hebrew meaning *to treat delicately*) of Numbers 6:5d: he shall be holy, and shall let the *locks* of the hair of his head grow (AV); he shall be holy, cherishing the *long hair* [Gr. *komen tricha*] of the head (LXX).

As you can see from the above definitions, translators must decide what they think is the true meaning. Do the terms mean long hair or do they mean ornamented hair?

Here are differing translations from the Online Parallel Study Bible:

Is not even nature itself teaching you that if a man, indeed, should have tresses, it is a dishonor to him, yet if a woman should have tresses, it is her glory, seeing that tresses have been given her instead of clothing?[611]

Nor does nature itself teach you that it is a disgrace to a man to have long hair, but it is woman's glory, because her hair has been given her instead of a veil.[612]

As you can see, very different assumptions were made regarding the meaning of words and what is meant by the passage. One translation

---

610 Ernest Weekley, An Etymological Dictionary of Modern English, vol. 1, A – K (New York: Dover Publications, 1967).

611 Concordant Literal Version, accessed July 7, 2010 http://studybible.info/CLV/1%20 Corinthians%2011

612 Accessed July 7, 2010 http://studybible.info/MNT/1%20Corinthians%2011

considers long hair by length only, and indicates that nature itself teaches us that long hair on a man is certainly not a disgrace. The other has to do with "tresses," a word from "tresser" meaning "to weave, plait."[613] This has to do with curling and weaving the hair like women do in long female-type styles and fashion, which differs markedly from unaltered manly long hair. Thirdly, one puts it as a question while the other simply makes it a statement. For these reasons, this is why it has been a difficult passage to translate and several translations are possible (see Chapter 7). In any regard, an honest assessment of the Greek indicates that a man with long natural hair is not disgraceful. If anything, Paul may be saying that a woman's long stylized hair being intentionally beautified is too much of a distraction for men so she should be willing to cover it during prayer in front of others in church.

613 Ernest Weekley, An Etymological Dictionary of Modern English, vol. 2, L – Z (New York: Dover Publications, 1967).

Appendix II
Products to Help Prevent Hair Loss and Restore Your Scalp

||||||||||||||||||||||||||||||||||||||||||||||||||||||||||||||||||||||||||||||||||||||||||||||||||||||||||||||||||||||||||||||||||||||||||||||||||||||||||||||||||||||||||||||||

The following companies sell pH balanced (pH of ~ 5.5-7.0) shampoos without Sodium Lauryl Sulfate. Many of these do not contain any detergent at all. Others contain a milder detergent, such as sodium laureth sulfate, in low amounts. You need to decide, based on your physiology, which shampoo is best for you. Product ingredients can be found on many of their websites. Contact the manufacturer directly with questions.

I. Shampoos to help Prevent Hair Loss

Avalon Organics www.avalonorganics.com pH balanced shampoos with no lauryl or laureth sulfates	**Morrocco Method International** 2743 Rodman Ave. Los Osos, CA 93402 Tel: 805-534-1600 www.morroccomethod.com Five different shampoos to alternate. Testimonials include hair regrowth.
Ginesis www.ginesis.com Tel: 256-767-8256 pH balanced chemical-free shampoo	**Nature's Gate** 9200 Mason Avenue Chatsworth, CA 91311 www.natures-gate.com Tel: 818-882-2951
Giovanni Their shampoos are available at several places on the internet and health food/ vitamin stores	**Real Purity** www.realpurity.com Tel: 800-253-1694 pH balanced shampoo

Healthy Hair Plus	ShiKai Products
www.healthyhairplus.com	www.shikai.com
	Tel: 707-544-0298
Emu Shampoo	Find at several places on the internet and health food/vitamin stores
Hugo Naturals	**Skin Biology, Inc.**
	4122 Factoria Blvd., Suite 200
Chatsworth, CA 91311	Bellevue, WA 98006
www.HugoNaturals.com	www.skinbiology.com
Tel: 818-576-9917 or 866-576-4846	Tel: 425-644-0160
	Folligen therapy spray or lotion for
Several shampoos to choose.	hair retention and regrowth.
	Folligen shampoo.

II. Shampoos and Scalp Treatments to Prevent Hair Loss and Proven to Re-Grow Hair in Many People

The following specialty products are excellent, and are backed by many testimonies of hair re-growth. You may wish to try all these products and see which one is best for you. But remember, you must use these products faithfully for a minimum of 18 - 24 months.

Thymuskin®

Biotechne Complex, Inc.
www.thymuskin.com
Tel: 800-214-8631
Tel: 770-297-9811

Thymuskin can prevent balding during cancer treatments in most cases; and has re-grown hair in about two out of three men, and 95 percent of women with *alopecia androgenetica*, common baldness. Use Thymuskin "Treatment" once or twice a day, and Thymuskin "Shampoo" up to three times per week. Contains sodium laureth sulfate.

Super Hair Energizer

Super Hair Energizer is a fermented jojoba oil based product – it is an herbal treatment backed by more than 10,000 testimonies according to Paul Oberdorf. The product only contains about 2.1 percent ammonium lauryl sulfate. It can be purchased from the following places:

Hair Growth Solutions
www.hairgrowthsolutions.com
Tel: 503-806-3721

NMS Publishing
57`` 14th Avenue, Dpt. JF
Brooklyn, NY 11219-4622
Paul Oberdorff @ Tel: 718-871-1363

Sim, Inc.
554 Green Tree Cv, Suite 201
Collierville, TN 38017
www.hairenergizer.net
Tel: 888-849-8686

Use the "Follicle Stimulator" daily and "Shampoo" up to three times per week. Jojoba Oil is a third product you will need, but you can buy a larger quantity at a better price at a local health food/vitamin store.

Riquette International
269 S. Beverly Drive, Suite 200
Beverly Hills, CA 90212
Tel: 800-747-8388 or 310-551-5253
www.riquette.com info@Riquette.com

Dr. Peter H. Proctor
5555 W. Loop South, Suite 225
Bellaire, Texas 77401
drproctor@drproctor.com
www.drproctor.com
Tel: 713-960-1616

Dr. Proctor has been screening hair loss treatment and hair regrowth-inducing agents for more than 25 years. He has nine U.S. patents for his products. Dr. Proctor offers both prescription and non-prescription formulations for the treatment of balding, alopecia, and hair-loss. Our LONG HAIRitage, being a holistic health book, recommends his non-drug formulations, Proxiphen-N topical treatment and NANO Shampoo and Conditioner. His NANO Shampoo and Conditioner also contains copper peptides, as Dr. Loren Pickart's products at Skin Biology have, and has a minoxidil-like hair growth stimulator NANO (nicotinic acid N-Oxide).

III. Chlorine Shower Filters

Sprite Industries: Chlorine Showerhead Filter

Sprite shower heads with internal replacement cartridges are readily available at hardware stores such as Lowes and Home Depot. Replace filter every six months. You will notice the difference even with the first shower.

IV. Laser Hair Combs

Re-grow hair with clinically proven success with a laser hair comb. Here are two of the primary manufacturers:

HairMax Laser Comb

Lexington International
777 Yamato Rd., Suite 105
Boca Raton, FL 33431
Tel: 561-417-0200 or 866-527-3726
info@lasercomb.net
www.hairmax.com

Leimo Laser Hair Comb

VeryGood.com.sg
(International Sales & Administration)
1028A upper serangoon Road
singapore, 534766
Singapore
Tel: +65-96855151
www.laserhaircomb.com

X-5 Hair Laser

Spencer Forrest
7271 Paramount Blvd.
Pico Rivera, CA 90660
Tel: 800-844-2536
www.spencerforrest.com

The products on these foregoing pages were designed to help you combat hair loss associated with skin and follicle damage caused by seborrheic dermatitis, alopecia follicularis, androgenetic alopecia (common baldness), DHT, and the immune system. Get rid of unnatural harsh chemical-laden hair care products that contribute to these skin disorders, so you can heal your scalp, your crown. Your hair health is in your hands and it would be beneficial for you to determine the true causes of your balding problem. Now, after you heal your scalp, be sure to grow your hair longer as designed. In this way you will avoid future problems.

V. Natural Tanning

MEXITAN™ Dark Tanning Oil
The Secret of Acapulco®

Mexitan is an all natural blend of pure oils, no chemicals, and offers natural sunburn protection. It encourages your skin to produce melanin, nature's own sunburn protection, and allows you to tan darker, faster. Remember to start tanning little by little in the spring. Apply the oil generously. My own personal testimony is that it substantially increases the time you can spend in the sun, similar to a sunscreen but without harsh chemicals. MexitanTM encourages tanning. If you would like added protection or prefer a lotion, try the SPF 8 with Zinc Oxide, a safe mechanical sunscreen. Green Tea's Natural Healing Properties reduce UV damage and helps to prevent skin cancer. It makes a splendid after-bath moisturizer and has been found to repel insects naturally.

Ingredients: Sunflower Oil, Green Tea Extract, Coconut Oil, Cocoa Butter, Almond Oil, Lanolin, Vitamins E and C, and Eucalyptus Oil.

MexitanTM can be purchased from:

Barnacle Kove

PO Box 367126
Bonita Springs, FL 34136
www.barnaclekove.com
Tel: 239-947-1327 (ask for Barnacle Kove)

Mexitan Products, Inc.

www.mexitanproducts.com

For your head, ears, and neck, there is no better sunblock than your hair. It is never a good idea to put a defined parting in your hair. However, if do part your hair so that the skin of the scalp can be seen, then wear a hat or bandana when the sun is directly overhead.

SUN SALVE
SPF 27 Herbal Sunblock

Purchase from:

The Super Salve Company
HC 61 Box 300
Mogollon, NM 88039

www.superslave.com
Tel: 888-956-8466

Glossary

||||||||||||||||||||||||||||||||||||||||||||||||||||||||||||||||||||||||||||||||||||||||||||||||||||||||||||||||||||||||||||||||||||||||||||||||

Acid mantle – a protective layer formed by sebum and sweat as it is extruded onto the skin surface. It creates a pH of 4.0 – 5.5 to ward off unwanted bacteria.

Actinic kerotoses – precancerous growth on the skin.

Alopecia androgenetica or androgenetic alopecia – a word used for common hair thinning or baldness problems in males or females thought to be due to genetic problems or heredity.

Alopecia follicularis – inflammation of the hair follicles of the scalp, resulting in hair loss from the affected area.

Anagen – growth phase of the hair cycle in which each hair has an average lifespan of about four years under normal conditions.

Barbermonger – a man who frequents the barber's shop, or prides himself in being dressed by a barber; a fop. This word occurs in Noah Webster's 1828 dictionary, but is missing in most modern dictionaries probably because most men now have become addicted to the barber.

Basal cell carcinoma – slow-growing non-melanoma skin cancer, and is the most common type of all skin cancers.

Catagen – the resting phase of the hair cycle when anagen ceases in any given follicle. It lasts about three months, then the hair is shed (telogen).

Coarse hair – has the largest circumference and can feel heavy and rough.

Cortex – the middle layer of a hair shaft just beneath the outer cuticle.

Crophead or crop-head - a word for anyone who cuts their hair too short; derived from Crop-Head. Adjective: crop-headed people, corporations,

273

etc. Plural: cropheads or croppies, the later used primarily to describe the youth being trained by cropheads.

Crop-Head - a word used by the Prophet Jeremiah to describe certain Arab groups who cut the corners of their hairline against God's laws. Close-cropping the head is akin to cutting down crops.

Cuticle – the outermost layer of the hair shaft with unique markings characteristic of the individual.

DHT – dihydrotestosterone, an active synthetic male hormone thought to be related to hair loss by a hormonal imbalance.

Dreadlocks or dredlocks – when tightly coiled or spiral hair naturally intertwines and locks with other hairs it forms larger diameter rope-like strands or locks. When white people first observed the hair style on blacks, particularly in Jamaica, they were appalled and considered it dreadful, thus the term dreadlocks was coined.

Fine hair – has the smallest circumference and can feel very soft and silky, like feathers. It generally has a much thinner cortex than other hair textures and generally does not contain the inner medulla.

Hair cycle – the growth (anagen), rest (catagen), and shedding (telogen) phases of hair.

Hair follicle – place where the hair is formed, the root.

Hair shaft – the visible part of the hair seen above the skin surface.

Hippie – word used to describe the youth of the countercultural movement of the late 1960s, which involved anti-war demonstrations and hip clothing as opposed to the crop-headed stiffs in business suits. Originally derived from hipster which replaced the earlier word, beatnik. Although most of the so-called hippies wore long hair, the word has been misapplied by ignorant superficial people to any man who wears long hair.

Keratin – a key structural component in the outer layer of human skin, hair and nails. In hair, this insoluble protein forms rope-like filaments designed to be tougher than the skin surface that it protects.

Keratoacanthoma – a form of squamous cell carcinoma. These rapid-growing skin cancers resemble "volcanoes."

Longhair - an enthusiast of the arts and especially of classical music.

Mechanoreceptors - nerve fibers that surround each hair follicle respond to mechanical deformation or movement stimulating the scalp.

Medium dense hair – neither thick nor thin, yet adequately covers the scalp.

Medium hair – the most common type of texture and typically has lots of body and bounce.

Medulla – innermost layer of a terminal hair shaft generally absent in those with fine hair.

Melanoma – a deadly tumor of malignant cancer of the skin.

Nazarite (or Nazirite) – a vow of holiness taken on a temporary or permanent basis by males and females in which the hair of the head was not to be touched by scissors and razors.

Razorite – those addicted to the razor; opposite of a Nazarite.

Seborrhea – disturbance of sebaceous glands marked by the occurrence of an excessive discharge of sebum from the follicles, forming white or yellowish, greasy scales or cheesy plugs within the follicles and on the scalp.

Seborrheic dermatitis – an inflammatory disease of the skin characterized by yellowish, greasy scaling of the skin of the scalp, usually accompanied by itching.

Sebum – oily substance secreted by the sebaceous gland near each hair follicle. The oil is released through the follicle to protect the hair and skin surface.

Squamous cell carcinoma – non-melanoma skin cancer.

Sweat - the salty, watery solution produced by sweat glands, which have their own separate microscopic openings to the skin surface. Sweat is not released by the hair follicles, but is extruded by the sweat pores, a distinct structure from the hair follicle.

Telogen – part of the hair cycle when a hair is shed.

Terminal Hair – the thick, pigmented hairs found on the scalp, beard, armpits, and pubic area.

Thick Hair – many hairs per unit area such that the scalp cannot be seen (remains adequately concealed) whether the hair is wet or dry.

Thin Hair – sparse coverage so that the scalp can be seen through the hair.

Trichologist – person trained to treat or heal scalp disease by natural holistic methods.

Trichology - the holistic scientific study of the hair and scalp.

Trichophobia – psychological disorder in which a person has a morbid dread of hair.

Trichotemnomania - the obsessive-compulsive habit of cutting or shaving the hair; also called "hair cut madness."

Trichotillomania - the obsessive-compulsive habit of plucking out the hair.

Vellus Hair – the short, very fine, silky, and usually unpigmented hairs found on the seemingly hairless areas of the body such as the forehead, nose, eyelids, and bald scalp.

List of Abbreviations

A.D. – the years corresponding to the common or Christian era (C.E.) since the time of Christ, originally from *anno Domini* (Latin), meaning "in the year of the Lord."

B.C. – before Christ

cm – centimeter

DHT - dihydrotestosterone

DNA - deoxyribonucleic acid

Ed. - editor

FBI - Federal Bureau of Investigation

FDA – U.S. Food and Drug Administration

g – gram(s)

Gr. - Greek

L. – Latin

MIT - methylisothiazoline

mm - millimeter

MPB – Male Pattern Baldness

pH – measure of the acidity or alkalinity of an aqueous solution

SLS – Sodium Lauryl Sulfate

SPF – sun protection (or protectant) factor

Trans. - translator

UV – ultraviolet rays (or radiation)

Bible Versions Referenced in the Text

ESV – English Standard Version

IB – The Interlinear Bible, 2nd edition. Jay P. Green, General Editor and Translator. Peabody, MA: Hendrickson Publishers, 1986.

ISV – International Standard Version

JB – The Jerusalem Bible, a product of the Second Vatican Council (1962-1965) originally published in 1966.

KJV – King James Version. Please note – unless indicated differently this is the version quoted in the book.

LXX – Septuagint, the Greek translation of the Old Testament.

NASB – New American Standard Bible

NEB – New English Bible

NIV – New International Version

NKJV – New King James Version

RSV – Revised Standard Version

About the Author

||

Roger Sigler is a scientific and biblical researcher, author, and lecturer. As an avid enthusiast for natural health, Roger's expertise in long hair and scalp issues began with his observations and studies in environmental science, a field he has worked for more than twenty-five years. Once a person understands how to properly treat the environment of the scalp, hair loss can be overcome. The truth is of utmost importance to him, and his chief desire is to share his knowledge with others for their benefit. Roger is a member of the American Holistic Health Association, Creation Research Society and is an adjunct science instructor at Wharton County Junior College in the Houston, Texas area where he lives with his wife Selene.

Index

223, 229, 232, 236, 250, 251,
252, 256, 257, 258, 259, 268,
271, 273, 274, 275
cell death 38, 39, 42, 45, 86, 175, 258
central medulla 7
central nervous system 36, 37, 42, 43
chlorine 38, 40, 222, 223, 234, 235,
257, 270
Christ 56, 66, 87, 90, 91, 100, 101,
102, 105, 108, 110, 112, 113,
114, 115, 116, 117, 118, 119,
120, 121, 122, 124, 126, 132,
141, 146, 147, 148, 154, 158,
180, 192, 260, 277
copper peptides 32, 33, 38, 40, 240,
242, 245, 246, 247, 269
Corinth 60, 67, 124, 125, 130, 131,
142, 152
Corinthians 6, 61, 63, 70, 79, 125,
126, 127, 128, 129, 132, 134,
135, 136, 137, 138, 141, 142,
161, 176, 261
cortex 7, 10, 273, 274
Crop-head 152, 162, 163, 167, 182,
228, 229, 273, 274
crown (of head) 21, 29, 30, 31, 42, 44,
45, 52, 61, 70, 71, 76, 79, 84,
96, 97, 98, 108, 110, 123, 129,
149, 150, 153, 160, 164, 192,
200, 205, 206, 208, 210, 221,
226, 227, 228, 243, 256, 258,
259, 260, 271
custom 49, 50, 51, 53, 58, 59, 61, 62,
64, 65, 66, 68, 90, 112, 120,
127, 128, 130, 132, 134, 135,
136, 142, 150, 153, 154, 156,
157, 160, 163, 179, 264
Cut Hair
castration 162, 163
circumcision 141, 162, 163
emasculation 65
idolatry 54, 57, 115, 151, 152
war 50, 61, 145, 152, 155, 161, 163,
274
cuticle 7, 8, 219, 220, 222, 273, 274

D

David vii, 2, 25, 26, 27, 33, 34, 50, 51,
68, 70, 81, 82, 83, 84, 85, 87,
88, 90, 93, 129, 131, 133, 135,
152, 156, 169, 208, 216, 254,
255, 256
Deborah 76, 77, 163
Delilah 79, 80, 83, 87, 164
dermis 7, 28, 29
detergent 17, 188, 196, 211, 212, 213,
214, 215, 217, 219, 220, 221,
243, 244, 245, 247, 250, 257,
267
DHT 31, 32, 33, 35, 236, 239, 240,
242, 246, 248, 252, 270, 274,
277
disease 3, 12, 15, 29, 30, 31, 36, 38,
42, 47, 51, 53, 54, 115, 117,
118, 119, 156, 160, 165, 167,
169, 170, 174, 189, 204, 207,
209, 220, 223, 225, 236, 251,
256, 258, 259, 275, 276
DNA 34, 277
Dreadlocks 22, 23, 24, 25, 26, 81, 149,
210, 222, 274

E

Edessa 115, 117, 118, 119, 120, 121
Egypt 25, 49, 56, 57, 72, 73, 75, 102,
149, 152, 162
Egyptian 56, 57, 72, 74, 75
Elijah 90, 91, 100, 101
endocrine system 35, 36
epidermis 28, 38, 173, 218
erector pili muscle 222, 226, 254
Eusebius 115, 119, 120, 121, 148,
149, 160
exercise 6, 31, 37, 40, 42, 43, 45, 48,
92, 93, 216, 221, 228, 235, 257,
258
Ezekiel 50, 57, 96, 97, 185, 233

F

fast food 4, 236, 240

follicle 4, 7, 9, 10, 15, 16, 21, 31, 32,
33, 34, 37, 38, 39, 42, 43, 44,
45, 46, 47, 48, 54, 78, 87, 110,
114, 162, 185, 188, 189, 203,
209, 210, 211, 212, 213, 214,
215, 217, 219, 220, 222, 223,
224, 226, 227, 228, 231, 234,
235, 236, 238, 239, 240, 242,
245, 246, 248, 249, 250, 251,
252, 253, 254, 256, 258, 259,
269, 270, 273, 274, 275

G

Gamaliel 113, 114, 118
gene 19, 32, 33, 34, 35, 38, 39, 167,
220
genetic code 3, 10, 12, 18, 20, 33, 34,
39, 81, 126, 142, 200, 219
Greek 57, 58, 60, 61, 63, 64, 66, 68,
93, 103, 104, 105, 106, 107,
108, 109, 110, 128, 130, 131,
133, 134, 136, 138, 140, 141,
142, 143, 144, 146, 149, 150,
207, 231, 233, 261, 263, 264,
265, 266, 277, 278

H

Habakkuk 96, 97
Hair
care of 157, 258
cycle 15, 19, 46, 217, 219, 273, 274,
275
growth rates 6, 10, 11, 12
re-growth 234, 247, 248, 249, 250,
251, 252, 253, 254, 255, 268
shed 16, 19, 47, 59, 220, 238, 273,
275
shedding 15, 19, 248, 274
strength of 17
symbolism of 67
thick 9, 10, 33, 48, 54, 56, 72, 76,
78, 86, 91, 173, 188, 201, 204,
206, 221, 232, 236, 275, 276
thinning 1, 2, 4, 6, 29, 31, 32, 46,

61, 86, 189, 209, 217, 219, 220,
234, 235, 242, 251, 252, 259,
273
types 9, 18, 19, 21, 24, 26, 31, 38,
43, 44, 55, 67, 72, 82, 87, 108,
112, 116, 132, 133, 134, 141,
174, 202, 207, 210, 215, 218,
227
Hair loss causes 1, 27, 31, 33, 34, 35,
36, 37, 39, 40, 41, 47, 173, 202,
225, 238, 239, 248, 250, 253
chlorine 38, 40, 222, 223, 234, 235,
257, 270
dermatitis 38, 218, 220, 242, 243,
253, 270, 275
DHT 31, 32, 33, 35, 236, 239, 240,
242, 246, 248, 252, 270, 274,
277
dyes 2, 38, 39, 41, 208, 210, 235,
257
excessive cutting 2, 3, 6, 44
hard hats 187, 189
high heat 38, 223
hot oil treatments 224
immune system 35, 170, 228, 242,
250, 251, 252, 270
nerve destruction 215
nutritional deficiencies 35, 236
shampoos 4, 38, 39, 40, 47, 48, 196,
212, 214, 215, 216, 217, 218,
219, 221, 224, 234, 235, 242,
243, 244, 245, 247, 248, 250,
253, 257, 267, 268
short hair 3, 14, 38, 39, 40, 41, 42,
44, 46, 47, 48, 54, 55, 60, 61,
62, 63, 65, 66, 67, 68, 71, 73,
79, 94, 95, 96, 105, 123, 125,
129, 130, 140, 142, 152, 153,
155, 161, 162, 163, 164, 165,
166, 172, 173, 176, 177, 178,
182, 191, 196, 203, 206, 219,
222, 227, 231, 257
smoke 37, 38, 40, 218
spinal lesions 36
stress 4, 6, 35, 36, 39, 40, 43, 44,